A Practical Guide to Child and Adolescent Mental Health Screening, Early Intervention, and Health Promotion, Second Edition

Editor

Bernadette Mazurek Melnyk, PhD, RN, CPNP/NPP, FAAN, FNAP

Assistant Editor

Peter S. Jensen, MD

A Publication of the National Association of Pediatric Nurse Practitioners (NAPNAP)

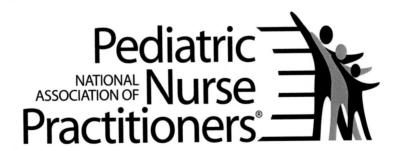

Dedication

This book is dedicated to all children, teens, and college-age youth at risk for and suffering with mental health disorders, especially those children and youth with severe conditions that require hospitalization and those who have little or no access to evidence-based treatment. I have been blessed to care for many of these affected children and adolescents, including those hospitalized at the Elmira Psychiatric Center Children and Youth In-Patient Unit, who enriched my life for almost two decades. These children and youth taught me that "rainbows follow rain" and that, even with the most severe conditions, there is always hope for a brighter tomorrow.

Bernadette Mazurek Melnyk

TABLE OF CONTENTS

Section 1
Assessing Common Mental Health Problems in Children and Adolescents

Introduction 1

Questionnaires and Tools for Screening 2

Performing a Mental Status Exam 3

Example of a Mental Status Assessment Write-up. 4

Rule Out Physical Health Conditions 4

Special Considerations When Interviewing Adolescents About Mental Health Issues. . . . 5

Guidelines for Adolescent Preventive Services (GAPS) 5

KySS Assessment Questions for Parents of Older Infants and Toddlers 6

KySS Assessment Questions for Parents of Preschool Children 8

KySS Assessment Questions For Parents of School-Age Children and Teens 10

Assessment Questions for a Specific Emotional or Behavioral Problem 13

The Pediatric Symptom Checklist (PSC) English. 14

The Pediatric Symptom Checklist (PSC) Spanish 18

The Pediatric Symptom Checklist - Youth Report (Y-PSC) English. 20

The Pediatric Symptom Checklist - Youth Report (PSC-Y) Spanish 22

Pediatric Symptom Checklist (PSC-17) English 24

Pediatric Symptom Checklist (PSC-17) Spanish. 25

The Child Behavior Checklist (CBCL) 26

Guidelines for Adolescent Preventive Services (GAPS) Younger Adolescent
(English) 28

Guidelines for Adolescent Preventive Services (GAPS) Younger Adolescent
(Spanish). 32

Guidelines for Adolescent Preventive Services (GAPS) Middle-Older Adolescent
(English) 36

Guidelines for Adolescent Preventive Services (GAPS) Middle-Older Adolescent
(Spanish). 38

Guidelines for Adolescent Preventive Services (GAPS) Parent/Guardian
(English) 41

Guidelines for Adolescent Preventive Services (GAPS) Parent/Guardian
(Spanish). 43

Important Information about Well-Child Visits for Parents. 45

Internet Resources. 47

References. 49

Section 2
Diagnosing, Managing, and Preventing Mental Health Disorders

Diagnosing Mental Health Disorders 51
General Approach to the Evidence-based Management of Mental Health Disorders in Children and Adolescents 52
Psychopharmacology 54
Prevention of Mental Health/Psychosocial Morbidities in Children and Teens 55
Internet Resources 58
References 59

Section 3
Anxiety Disorders

Information for Healthcare Providers About Anxiety Disorders 61
Common Signs of Anxiety in Children and Teens 62
Medication Guide for Pediatric Anxiety Disorders 65
DSM-5™ Diagnostic Criteria for Separation Anxiety Disorder 66
DSM-5™ Diagnostic Criteria for Generalized Anxiety Disorder 67
DSM-5™ Diagnostic Criteria for Acute Stress Disorder 68
DSM-5™ Diagnostic Criteria for Posttraumatic Stress Disorder 69
DSM-5™ Diagnostic Criteria for Obsessive-Compulsive Disorder 74
The State-Trait Anxiety Inventory for Children 76
The State-Trait Anxiety Inventory for Adults 77
KySS Worries Questionnaire (Ages 10-21 years) 79
KySS Worries Questionnaire for Parents 80
Generalized Anxiety Disorder-7 and Generalized Anxiety Disorder-2 Scales 81
Generalized Anxiety Disorder 7 Item (GAD-7) Scale 82
Screen for Child Anxiety Related Disorders (SCARED) – Child Version 84
Screen for Child Anxiety Related Disorders (SCARED) – Parent Version 86
Information for Parents about Anxiety in Children and Teens 88
Information for Parents on How to Help Your Child/Teen Cope with Stressful Events or Uncertainty 90
Information for Helping Children, Teens, and Their Families Cope with War and/or Terrorism 92
Information for Teens and School-Age Children About Stress and Anxiety 94
Internet Resources 96
References 97

Section 4
Depressive Disorders

Fast Facts 99

Prescribing Information for the Selective Serotonin Reuptake
    Inhibitors Used for the Treatment of Major Depressive Disorder 106

DSM-5™ Diagnostic Criteria for Persistent Depressive Disorder (Dysthymia) 110

DSM-5™ Diagnostic Criteria for Major Depressive Disorder 112

DSM-5™ Diagnostic Criteria for Bipolar I Disorder 114

DSM-5™ Diagnostic Criteria for Bipolar II Disorder. 118

Screening Tools for Child and Adolescent Depression 121

Center for Epidemiological Studies Depression Scale for Children (CES-DC) 123

Patient Health Questionniare-9 (PHQ-9) and PHQ-9 Modified for Teens 124

Edinburgh Postnatal Depression Scale 127

Information on Depression for Parents 130

Information on Depression for Teens. 132

Contract for Self Safety. 134

Contract for Others' Safety 135

Resources for Child and Adolescent Depressive Disorders 136

References. 138

Section 5
Attention-Deficit/Hyperactivity Disorder (ADHD)

Fast Facts 139

DSM-5™ Diagnostic Criteria for Attention-Deficit/Hyperactivity Disorder 141

Changes in ADHD in the DSM-5™ 144

Pharmacotherapy Treatments for Children and Adolescents
    With ADHD: Initial Dose, Kinetics, and Side Effects. 145

Non-Stimulants Used to Treat ADHD 146

The National Initiative for Children's Healthcare Quality (NICHQ)
    Vanderbilt Assessment Scale for ADHD-Parent Informant 147

Swanson, Nolan and Pelham (SNAP-IV-C) 154

Information for Parents About Attention-Deficit/Hyperactivity Disorder (ADHD) 158

Information for Children and Teens About Attention-Deficit/
    Hyperactivity Disorder (ADHD) 160

Internet Resources. 162

References. 163

Section 6
Somatoform Disorders

Fast Facts 165
DSM-5™ Diagnostic Criteria for Somatic Symptom Disorder. 166
DSM-5™ Diagnostic Criteria for Illness Anxiety Disorder. 168
Pharmacological Interventions in Somatic Symptom and Related Disorders. 171
Somatic Symptom Disorders Parent/Caregiver Information 172
Resources for Somatoform Disorders 174
References. 175

Section 7
Disruptive Behaviors in Children and Adolescents

Fast Facts 177
DSM-5™ Diagnostic Criteria for Disruptive Behaviors 181
DSM-5™ Diagnostic Criteria for Adjustment Disorders. 182
DSM-5™ Diagnostic Criteria for Oppositional Defiant Disorder 184
Resources for Providers 190
Resources for Families 190
Information for Parents About Behavior Problems in Children and Teens 191
Handouts for Children to Help Them Cope and Behave in Positive Ways 194
Positive Things About Me 195
Strong Feelings — Anger, Hurt, Fear, Sadness. 196
Taking Control of Your Anger (Strong Feelings) 197
References. 199

Section 8
Eating Disorders

Fast Facts 201
Screening Questions for Eating Disorders. 202
DSM-5™ Diagnostic Criteria for Anorexia Nervosa 203
DSM-5™ Diagnostic Criteria for the Diagnosis of Bulimia Nervosa 205
Management of Anorexia Nervosa. 207
Management of Bulimia Nervosa. 207
Information About Anorexia Nervosa in Children and Teens for Parents. 208
Important Information About Bulimia Nervosa in Children and Teens For Parents. . . . 210
Information About Bulimia Nervosa for Teens 212

Internet Resources. 214
References. 215

Section 9
Autism and Pervasive Development Disorders

Fast Facts 217
Medical History. 220
Medical Conditions With Neurologic Symptoms That Overlap With Those of ASD. . . . 221
DSM-5™ Diagnostic Criteria for Autism Spectrum Disorder 222
Screening Tools for Autism 224
Resources for Parents About ASD in Children. 233
Additional Internet Resources 233
References. 234

Section 10
Helping Children Deal With Death, Loss, and Grief

Fast Facts 235
Age Related Responses to Loss and Grief. 236
The DSM-5™ and the Newly-Emerging Criteria for Persistent
    Complex Bereavement-Related Grief Disorder (CG) 239
Inventory for Complicated Grief-Revised (ICG-RG) for Children 242
How Parents Can Help Children/Teens to Cope with Loss and Grief. 247
How Can I Help My Child Deal with Loss and Grief? 249
Information for Teens about Coping with Loss and Grief 250
What Can I Do to Help Myself Deal with Loss and Grief?. 251
References. 252

Section 11
Marital Separation and Divorce

Fast Facts 255
Typical Responses to Marital Separation. 257
Responses to Marital Separation That Require Immediate
    Assessment and Intervention 257
Critical History-Taking Questions When a Divorce or Separation Has Occurred 258
Early Interventions 258
Screening for Marital Transitions 260
A Dozen Ways to Help your Child Deal with Marital Separation/Divorce 261
Internet Resources. 262
References. 263

Section 12
Child Maltreatment

Fast Facts 265
Screening Tools 268
Information for Parents on Child Maltreatment 271
Information for Adolescents on Child Maltreatment 273
Information on Child Abuse and Neglect for School-Age Children. 275
Internet Resources. 277
References. 278

Section 13
Sexuality

Fast Facts 279
Screening Tools/Questions for Adolescent Sexuality 283
Suggested Reading for Parents About Adolescent Sexuality 284
Internet Resources for Older Teens about Sexuality 285
Internet Resources for Healthcare Providers 286
References. 287

Section 14
Substance Abuse and Addiction Spectrum

Fast Facts 289

Resources on Cultural and Linguistic Competency. 292

Materials that Provide Information on the Signs of a Mental Health for Substance Use
    Problem (SAMHSA, 2011) 293

CRAFT Screening Test 295

The CAGE Questionnaire for Alcohol Use 296

Important Information For Parents on Substance Use Disorders in
    Children and Teens and How to Prevent Them. 297

Important Information For Teens About Alcohol and Other Drugs 299

No Drinking and Driving Contract 301

References. 302

Section 15
Bullying and Violence

Fast Facts 303

DSM-5™ Diagnostic Criteria for Conduct Disorder 309

Resources 312

How to Raise a Nonviolent Child: Information for Parents. 314

References. 317

Section 16
Overweight and Obesity

Fast Facts 319

Evidence-Based Overweight and Obesity Treatment/Management by Stage
    of Overweight/Obesity 324

Psychotropic Medications Associated With Increased Risk of Weight Gain 327

Psychotropic Medications that are Weight Neutral for Most Children
    and Adolescents 327

Resources for Parents and Providers 328

Information About Obesity/Overweight in Children and Teens for Parents 329

References. 331

Section 17
Reimbursement

Fast Facts 333
Time-Based Codes for Counseling 334
Common Diagnoses Used in Primary Care Pediatrics 335

Section 18
Brief Evidence-Based Interventions for Child and Adolescent Mental Health Disorders

Fast Facts 337
Introduction to Cognitive Behavioral Skills Building 344
The Clinical Case 346
COPE: A Cognitive Behavioral Skills-Building Intervention (CBSB) 347
COPE for Children - The Thinking-Feeling-Behaving Triangle 350
COPE for Children - Healthy Coping for Stress and Worry 352
Resources for Healthcare Providers and Parents 354
Internet Resources 354
Tobacco Resources 354
References 355

Section 19
Promoting Mental Health in Schools

Fast Facts 357
The Importance of School Mental Health Promotion 358
Evidence-Based Management, Including Medication Management 360
Federal Policies 365
Screening and Assessment Tools for School Mental Health Promotion 366
Resources Available 369
Appropriate Handouts with Important and Age-Appropriate Information 370
References 371

Index 375

A Practical Guide to Child and Adolescent Mental Health Screening, Early Intervention, and Health Promotion, Second Edition

Editor

Bernadette Mazurek Melnyk*, PhD, RN, CPNP/PMHNP, FAANP, FNAP, FAAN
Associate Vice President for Health Promotion
University Chief Wellness Officer
Dean and Professor, College of Nursing
Professor of Pediatrics & Psychiatry, College of Medicine
The Ohio State University
Columbus, Ohio
Editor, Worldviews on Evidence-based Nursing
Sections: Screening for and Assessing Mental Health Problems in Children & Adolescents,
Diagnosing, Managing and Preventing Mental Health Disorders, Anxiety Disorders,
Mood Disorders, Marital Separation and Divorce & Brief Evidence-based Interventions
for Mental Health Disorders

Assistant Editor

Peter S. Jensen*, MD
President & CEO
The REACH Institute (Resource for Advancing Children's Health)
New York, New York
Co-Director, Division of Child Psychiatry and Psychology, the Mayo Clinic
Sections: Screening for and Assessing Mental Health Problems in Children & Adolescents and
Diagnosing, Managing and Preventing Mental Health Disorders

Contributors

Linda J. Alpert-Gillis, PhD
Associate Professor of Psychiatry, Pediatrics, & Clinical Nursing
Director, Strong Behavioral Health: Child & Adolescent Outpatient Services
Director, Laboratory for Innovation in Child Mental Health Care Delivery
University of Rochester School of Medicine and Dentistry
Rochester, New York
Section: Marital Separation & Divorce

Dawn Anderson-Butcher, PhD, LISW-S
Professor, College of Social Work
The Ohio State University
Columbus, Ohio
Section: Promoting Mental Health in School Settings

Annahita Ball, PhD, LMSW
Assistant Professor
School of Social Work, Louisiana State University
Baton Rouge, Louisiana
Section: Promoting Mental Health in School Settings

Holly E. Brown, DNP, RN, NPP, PMHCS-BC
Assistant Professor of Clinical Nursing
School of Nursing, University of Rochester
Psychiatric Nurse Practitioner
Hillside Children's Center
Rochester, New York
Section: Anxiety Disorders and Autism & Pervasive Developmental Disorders

John V. Campo, MD
Professor and Chair, Department of Psychiatry
The Ohio State University Wexner Medical Center
Columbus, Ohio
Section: Somatic Disorders

Mary Lynn Dell, MD, DMin
Director of Psychosomatic Medicine
Professor of Clinical Psychiatry and Pediatrics
Nationwide Children's Hospital and The Ohio State University
Columbus, Ohio
Section: Somatic Disorders

Ann Guthery, PhD, RN, PMHNP-BC
Family Psychiatric Mental Health Nurse Practitioner
Clinical Associate Professor
Arizona State University
Arizona Family Resource Counseling Center
Phoenix, Arizona
Section: Attention Deficit/Hyperactivity Disorder (ADHD)

Neil E. Herendeen, MD, MMM
Associate Professor of Pediatrics
Golisano Children's Hospital, University of Rochester Medical Center
Rochester, New York
Sections: Child Maltreatment &Reimbursement

Pamela A. Herendeen, DNP, PNP-BC
Professor of Clinical Nursing
Associate Dean for Education & Student Affairs
Director, DNP ProgramUniversity of Rochester School of Nursing
Senior Nurse Practitioner
Golisano Children's Hospital at Strong
Rochester, New York
Section: Child Maltreatment

Aidyn Iachini, PhD, MSW
Assistant Professor
University of South Carolina
Columbia South Carolina
Section: Promoting Mental Health in School Settings

Diana Jacobson, PhD, RN, PNP-BC, PMHS
Assistant Professor
Arizona State University College of Nursing and Health Innovation
Phoenix, Arizona
Section: Assessing & Managing Overweight and Obesity in Children and Teens

Richard E. Kreipe, MD, FAAP, FSAHM, FAED
Elizabeth R. McAnarney Professor in Pediatrics
Golisano Children's Hospital, University of Rochester
Rochester, New York
Section: Eating Disorders

Pamela Lusk, DNP, RN, PMHNP-BC
Clinical Associate Professor
College of Nursing
The Ohio State University
Columbus, Ohio
Psychiatric Nurse Practitioner, Community Health Center of Yavapai County
Prescott, Arizona
Sections: Disruptive Behaviors in Children and Adolescents and Brief Evidence-Based Interventions for Child and Adolescent Mental Health Disorders

Elizabeth A. Mellin, PhD, LPC
Associate Professor
Penn State University
Department of Educational Psychology, Counseling, and Special Education
University Park, Pennsylvania
Section: Promoting Mental Health in School Settings

Mary E. Muscari, PhD, MSCr, CPNP, PMHCNS-BC, AFN-BC
Pediatric Nurse Practitioner, Psychiatric Clinical Specialist, Forensic Clinical Specialist, Criminologist
Associate Professor, Decker School of Nursing
Binghamton University
Binghamton, New York
Affiliate Faculty, Department of Criminology, Regis University
Denver, Colorado
Sections: Bullying and Violence

Deborah A. Napolitano, PhD, BCBA-D
Assistant Professor of Pediatrics
University of Rochester School of Medicine
Rochester, New York
Section: Autism & Pervasive Developmental Disorders=

Patrice Rancour, MS, RN, PMHCNS-BC
Mental Health Clinical Nurse Specialist
Ohio State University Clinic for Integrative Medicine
Columbus, Ohio
Section: Helping Children Deal with Death, Loss and Grief

Leigh Small, PhD, RN, CPNP-PC, FNAP, FAANP
Chair, Department of Family and Community Health Nursing
School of Nursing
Virginia Commonwealth University
Richmond, Virginia
Section: Assessing & Managing Overweight and Obesity in Children and Teens

Victoria von Sadovszky, PhD, RN
Associate Professor
College of Nursing
The Ohio State University
Columbus, Ohio
Section: Sexuality

Barbara Jones Warren, PhD, RN, APRN-BC, FAAN, CNS-BC, PMH
Professor of Clinical Nursing and Director, Psychiatric Nurse Practitioner Program
The Ohio State University College of Nursing
Columbus, Ohio
Section: Substance Abuse

* Individuals with an asterisk have disclosed financial interests/arrangements/affiliations. Unless otherwise indicated the contributors have disclosed no relevant financial relationships or affiliations. The individuals below have disclosed the following:

Bernadette Mazurek Melnyk: President, COPE for HOPE, LLC and Founder COPE2Thrive, LLC.

Peter S. Jensen: Received grant or research support from Shire, Inc.; paid consultant for and has received honoraria from Shire, Inc. and Janssen-Cilag, Inc.; on the Board of The REACH Institute; and shareholder of CATCH Services, Inc.

Foreword

A Practical Guide to Child and Adolescent Mental Health Screening, Early Intervention, and Health Promotion, Second edition

I have both a very personal, as well as a professional, connection to the life challenges that affect mental health. I was homeless for the first time when I was six years old, and throughout my youth continued to struggle with hunger and homelessness, in part because my parents both had problems with substance abuse. In addition, I have been a soldier, serving in times of both peace and war and seeing firsthand the emotional devastation that can occur during combat, and even years after combat. As a registered nurse, I have cared for patients with emotional or mental illnesses that interfered with or complicated their physical health. As a law enforcement officer, I have been on the frontlines of rescuing children and teens from abusive situations that left them fearful and emotionally bereft. And, I have focused as a trauma, burns, and critical care surgeon on saving hearts and minds damaged by attempted suicides and other tragedies. I understand on a very deep level what it means to be mentally unhealthy.

When I became the 17th Surgeon General of the United States in 2002, I had the privilege of bringing my training and experience to bear on the largest practice in the world – the 310 million people across our great nation, as well as serving as an advisor to world leaders beyond our own country who often seek the counsel of the U.S. Surgeon General to benefit their own populations. Mental health is a major public health concern for our nation and the world. Daily mental health challenges exist at a magnitude that can only be described as critical. Through the wider lens available to me as the nation's doctor, I practiced with colleagues addressing the multivariate issues that are involved, including a drastic shortage of child and adolescent mental health professionals; increases in mental health problems among youth; the still unrelenting stigma associated with mental illness; and the lack of a comprehensive, coordinated approach to the early diagnosis and treatment of mental illness.

Among children and teens, the need for help can be particularly challenging for health professionals because of acting-out behaviors or the opposite – their silent suffering. The support and treatment our children need may not be readily available due to lack of access to services, the shortage of trained mental health professionals who focus on children and adolescents, as well as the widespread bias against acknowledging mental illness.

An important strategy for addressing these very real and current challenges is to provide information, education, and resources to the health professionals who stand at the gateway of care. Pediatricians, family practice and primary care physicians, physician's assistants, nurse practitioners, and other members of the medical community can be even more effective members of the mental health network. This book, edited by my friend and colleague Bernadette Melnyk, is a thorough and relevant first step for health professionals to learn about mental illness among children and adolescents, from diagnosis to treatment to resources. Now is the time to get involved and give our youth the help they so desperately need.

Richard H. Carmona, M.D., M.P.H., FACS
17th Surgeon General of the United States

Preface

For the millions of children, teens, and college youth at risk for or affected by mental health problems, time is running out to provide them with the evidence-based treatment they need to become healthy adults capable of functioning to their full capacity. We must act NOW to better screen for, identify, manage, and prevent mental health disorders, which are currently affecting one out of every four to five children and adolescents in the United States.

I was 15 years of age and home alone with my mother when she died suddenly right in front of me from a sneeze that precipitated a stroke. Crippled by guilt that I could do nothing to save her, along with suffering from terrible symptoms of post-traumatic stress disorder, I did not sleep through the night for at least a few years after my mother's death as I continually played the recording of that terrible day over and over again in my head. I also had continual fears of losing my father, having learned that death could come to anyone I loved at any time. After six months with these symptoms, I was taken for help to my family physician, who wrote a prescription for Valium and told me I would be fine if I took one of those pills to help me sleep every night. There was no psychological evaluation and no mental health counseling for me -- just a pill. I took one of those pills that night, which left me feeling groggy in the morning, so I refused to take any more and resigned myself to having to "tough it out" and learn skills on my own to help cope with my tragic loss. In the next four years after my mother's death, I lost a cousin following a motor vehicle accident as well as the only grandparent I ever knew, and my beloved father nearly died from a heart attack - a tremendous amount of stress and loss in a short period of time during those challenging adolescent years. However, I was fortunate to be blessed with both resiliency and a close connection to my much older sister, Chris, which helped me through many dark nights and protected me from ongoing mental health issues as an adult. It is this personal experience, along with caring for so many children and teens affected by mental health problems who were not identified by their primary care providers or treated until they either attempted suicide or became hospitalized with severe mental illness, that fueled my passion to commit much of my career to developing initiatives to promote child and teen mental health, compiling this guide, and testing and implementing programs that could help youth who suffer for years without being identified and treated for mental health problems.

Unfortunately, many children today who are suffering with mental health disorders do not have protective factors to buffer them from developing serious mental illness. Further, fewer than 25% of affected children and teens receive any treatment. It is unfortunate that, even with all of the accumulated knowledge we have today about evidence-based screening and treatment, primary care practices are still not routinely screening for depression and other mental health issues in teens despite the fact that suicide remains the third leading cause of death in adolescents aged 14 years and older. Teens with depression may receive an antidepressant from their primary care provider, but the majority do not receive gold-standard cognitive behavioral therapy or skills building, in large part due to the severe shortage of mental health providers in so many areas across the nation.

Primary care providers are ideally suited to screen for, identify, and manage common mental health disorders in children and teens because of established relationships with their families and a practice setting that lessens stigma, which remains attached to these disorders.

Academic programs that prepare healthcare providers also have been slow to integrate in-depth content on the assessment and management of common mental health disorders in children and teens. Thus, primary care providers often report not having the knowledge and skills believed necessary to appropriately and accurately identify and manage common child and adolescent mental health disorders. Further, although there is finally more emphasis nationally on the importance of integrating physical and mental healthcare, the merging of the two remains slow and problematic issues with reimbursement continue. Horrific mass shootings with unnecessary loss of lives often prompt some national action, but too often, the events pass, the momentum once again slows, and our children and teens along with their families continue to suffer. Therefore, we must stay consistent and persistent in our efforts to improve the lives of so many families impacted by mental health disorders.

The second edition of this guide has been strengthened with new sections, updated diagnostic criteria from the recently published *Diagnostic and Statistical Manual of Mental Disorders*, Fifth Edition (DSM-5™), evidence-based programs, updated educational materials for families, and resources to assist clinicians in being more effective in screening, identifying, managing, and preventing common mental health disorders in children and teens. A major feature of this guide is that it delivers the best "nuts and bolts" evidence-based content in a format that is user-friendly and contains screening tools and interventions that can be readily used in practice.

In conclusion, I challenge everyone who cares for children and teens to ACT NOW and enhance their knowledge and skills in screening for and identifying mental health disorders, using evidence-based treatments, and implementing prevention strategies to reverse the alarming prevalence of mental health disorders among our children and youth. The future of our children and our society depends on it.

Bernadette Mazurek Melnyk, PhD, RN, CPNP/PMHNP, FNAP, FAANP, FAAN
Associate Vice President for Health Promotion
University Chief Wellness Officer
Dean and Professor, College of Nursing
Professor of Pediatrics and Psychiatry, College of Medicine
The Ohio State University

Acknowledgments

The vision and beginnings of this mental health guide began while teaching a pediatric primary care course and recognizing the need for a user-friendly guide on mental health screening, intervention, and health promotion that could be used with nurse practitioner and medical students to enhance their knowledge and skills in caring for the mental health/psychosocial needs of children and their families. With Dr. Leigh Small, a long-time friend and colleague who was teaching the course with me, and six of our students (Marie Dunn, Christine Emmerson, Kelly Fagan, Kristina Moss, Anita O'Brien, and Nancy Swank), we comprised a rudimentary first draft of this guide that future students said was instrumental in assisting them to be more effective in caring for the mental health needs of children and teens. As a result, I would like to acknowledge each of these individuals for their wonderful contributions to a resource that is now widely used by healthcare providers and colleges across the nation. I also would like to thank each of the terrific experts who contributed to the first and now the second edition of this guide, all of whom share a deep passion for promoting the mental health of children/teens and their families. In addition, I would like to acknowledge the following staff at NAPNAP for their assistance, including Dolores Jones, Heather Keesing, and Alison Kahn. Finally, I would like to thank my husband John and my three daughters, Angela, Megan, and Kaylin, for their love, support and understanding during the writing of this second edition.

Bernadette Mazurek Melnyk

SECTION 1
Bernadette Mazurek Melnyk

Introduction to Screening for and Assessing Common Mental Health Problems in Children and Adolescents

Mental health/behavioral disorders affect approximately one out of four to five children and adolescents, creating a major public health problem (Merikangas et al., 2010). Early detection of and evidence-based intervention for mental health/behavioral problems is critical in order to prevent serious ongoing adverse outcomes. However, pediatric primary care settings are underutilized venues for implementation of evidence-based recommendations and guidelines for screening and behavioral counseling (Melnyk et al., 2012).

The incidence of mental health problems is believed to be underestimated due, in large part, to inadequate screening, intervention, and referral by primary care providers as well as denial by families that a problem exists. Findings from research indicate that screening for mental health problems can substantially increase the number of children and adolescents identified as possibly having a mental health problem (Brown & Wissow, 2010). Screening youth for mental health problems is especially important since half of adults with mental health problems have symptoms by 14 years of age, and 75% have symptoms by 24 years of age (Kessler et al., 2005). The three most common mental health problems in children and teens are anxiety disorders, depressive disorders, and attention-deficit/hyperactivity disorder.

Significant health disparities also exist in the receipt of mental health services, with a disproportionate number of Hispanic and African-American children affected (Husky et al., 2012). Mental health problems/psychosocial morbidities are now surpassing physical health problems in children and youth, including asthma and diabetes. There are many reasons for this, including:

- Family instability and malfunctioning

- Stigma associated with mental health problems

- Access to care and reimbursement issues

- Lack of screening

- Inadequate numbers of mental health professionals

- Genetics

Every encounter with a child or adolescent, whether for a well-child or illness visit, is an opportunity to screen for and assess a mental health or psychosocial problem. Each healthcare encounter also is an excellent time to provide preventive counseling and educational information on how to recognize these conditions early, before the problems become more resistant to early interventions.

Because there is much stigma associated with mental health/behavior problems and parents often feel guilty about their children having them, use of screening tools can prompt parents to talk about these issues with their healthcare providers. However, it should be remembered that screening tools cannot replace a developmentally sensitive and comprehensive clinical interview. Screening tools are useful in raising "red flags," which can signal underlying mental health disorders. Since fewer than 25% of children with mental health problems are diagnosed and treated, screening is critical for early recognition and intervention (Foy, 2010).

Risk Factors for Mental Health Disorders in Children and Teens

Risk factors for mental health disorders in children and teens are important to assess and include:

- Parents who have mental health problems, including use of substances
- Poor self-esteem
- Lack of other developmental assets (e.g., good coping skills, optimism)
- Altered parenting
  (e.g., overprotective; controlling; rigid; permissive; lack of supervision and limit setting)
- Parental conflict/separation/divorce
- Chronic illness or handicap of the child or family member
- Hospitalization/life-threatening medical procedures
- Learning disabilities
- Deteriorating grades
- Presence of multiple stressors/recent stressful life events
- Peers who engage in risk-taking behaviors
- Social isolation
- Bullying by peers
- Traumatic event(s)
- Difficult temperament
- Behavior problems
- Stressful home or school environment
- Gay or bisexual orientation
- Substance use

Questionnaires and Tools for Screening

The following questionnaires in this section of the mental health guide can be used for the purpose of collecting information on potential mental health/psychosocial problems from families in primary care or other types of pediatric and adolescent clinical settings. Parents can complete the questionnaires while they are waiting for their child's appointment, or the questionnaires can be mailed to them prior to their scheduled visits. It is a good idea to request that parents arrive 15 minutes early if they have not completed the questionnaires so that they have the chance to finish them during their visit. Included also in this section are screening tools that can be provided to adolescents.

These questionnaires explore issues that parents and teens may be thinking about or reveal areas of concern. The items on the KySS (Keep your children/yourself Safe and Secure) mental health assessment questionnaires were developed by pediatric and mental health experts through a consensus-building process. Once completed, the questionnaires provide healthcare providers with a quick overview of potential or actual mental health/psychosocial issues that need to be more fully assessed during the clinical interview.

An excellent general mental health screening tool for use in primary care that is in the public domain and can be downloaded free of charge is the Pediatric Symptom Checklist (both the 35-item checklist and the 17-item version) (Jellinek, 2002). Information about this screening tool and others is contained in this section.

The United States Preventive Services Task Force (USPSTF) also recommends screening all adolescents (12-18 years of age) for major depressive disorder (MDD) when systems are in place to ensure accurate diagnosis, psychotherapy (cognitive behavioral or interpersonal), and follow-up (see http://www.uspreventiveservicestaskforce.org/uspstf/uspschdepr.htm).

At every well and ill child visit, it is important to pose the following question to parents:

Do you have any concerns or worries about your child's mental/emotional health or his/her behaviors, or has there been a change in how he/she usually behaves at home or at school?

If the response from the parents is affirmative, assessment of the concern should include:

- Degree of impairment
- Distress (by patient and caregiver)
- Severity of symptoms
- Frequency
- Intensity
- Duration
- Actions being taken to deal with the concern, and degree to which they are helpful

If problems are occurring at home and at school, the problem is more serious. Additional questions for assessing mental health/behavior concerns are included in this section.

Performing a Mental Status Exam

If a child is suspected of having a mental health problem after screening and clinical interview, it is important to perform a mental status exam along with a thorough physical exam to rule out potential physical causes of mental health problems. For example, children or teens with depression could have underlying iron deficiency or hypothyroidism.

Components of the mental status exam include the following:

- Appearance (e.g., how is the child dressed and groomed?)
- Attitude and interaction (e.g., is the child cooperative, guarded, or avoidant?)
- Activity level/behavior (e.g., is the child calm, active, or restless; are psychomotor activity, abnormal movements, and/or tics present?)
- Speech (e.g., is the child's speech loud or quiet, flat in tone or full of intonation, slow or rushed? How are words formed? Does the child understand what is being said to him or her? Does the child express himself or herself appropriately?)
- Thought processes (e.g., coherent, disorganized, flight of ideas [rapid skipping from topic to topic], blocking [inability to fill memory gaps], loosening associations [the shifting of topics quickly even though unrelated, echolalia [mocking repetition of another person's words], perseveration [repetition of verbal or motor response])
- Thought content (including delusions [false, irrational beliefs, such as "I am Superman"], obsessions [persistent thoughts or impulses], perceptual disorders [including hallucinations, i.e., altered sensory perceptions, such as hearing voices inside or outside his/her head that others are unaware of], phobias [irrational fears], hypochondriasis [excessive worry about personal health without an actual reason])
- Impulse control (e.g., is the child able to control aggressive, hostile, and sexual impulses?)
- Mood/affect (e.g., depressed, anxious, flat, ambivalent, fearful, irritable, elated, euphoric, inappropriate)

- Suicidal and/or homicidal behavior/ideation
- Cognitive functioning (e.g., orientation to surroundings, attention span/concentration, memory [recent and remote], ability to abstract, insight/judgment)
- Parent-child interaction (e.g., warm, nurturing, conflicted, rejecting, appropriate use of limit setting, in tune with child's feelings/needs, affectionate, eye contact, and other body language)

Example of a Mental Status Assessment Write-up

Shannon is a well-groomed, healthy-appearing, overweight adolescent who is cooperative and pleasant in her conversation. She sits calmly without making abnormal movements and makes good eye contact. Her rate and quality of speech are normal. Her thought processes are generally well organized and free of delusions. Shannon states that she can go quickly from a 0 to 10 in terms of anger. It is evident that she has a pattern of depressive cognitive thinking as she degrades herself frequently.

On a scale of 0 to 10, Shannon rates her depression as 6-7 on average and talks about the fact that she sometimes worries, especially about how other people view her. She denies hallucinations or any sleep problems. Shannon states that she needs help with anger management. She has poor impulse control as evidenced by frequent anger outbursts in her home. Shannon denies suicidal or homicidal ideations. She has some insight into her problems and talks about her desire to be a landscape designer. Short and long-term memories are intact.

Rule Out Physical Health Conditions

When a child has a suspected mental health disorder, it is important to rule out physical conditions as etiological factors, although remember that **many children with mental health problems present with somatic symptoms that often lead to inappropriate medical testing and interventions.**

Obtain a general health history, including:

- A thorough review of all systems (e.g., has your child ever had or does he or she now have problems with his head [headaches, head injuries], with his eyes [difficulty seeing, blurry vision], or with his ears [ear infections, hearing]?)
- Hospitalizations or surgeries
- Chronic illnesses such as diabetes, asthma, or seizures
- Medications, dosages, and side effects your child has experienced from these medications
- Prenatal, natal, and developmental history, including whether the child attained developmental milestones on time

Conduct a thorough physical exam and laboratory testing as indicated by the history.

Rule out

– Vision or hearing problems	– Premenstrual syndrome	– HIV / AIDS
– Anemia	– Diabetes mellitus	– Mitral valve prolapse
– Hypothyroidism	– Head trauma	– Systemic lupus erythematosus
– Mononucleosis	– Central nervous system (CNS) lesions	– Chronic conditions
– Chronic fatigue syndrome		– Developmental delays
– Eating disorders	– Seizures	– Failure to thrive
– Substance abuse	– Cushing syndrome	

Special Considerations When Interviewing Adolescents About Mental Health Issues

It is very important to assure teens about confidentiality before the clinical interview begins. Not informing teens of confidentiality is the main reason that they do not confide in their healthcare providers. However, it also is critical to inform them that you cannot hold their information confidential if they tell you that they want to hurt themselves or that someone else has hurt them.

If time for the interview is limited, the HEADSS (Home, Education, Activities, Drugs, Sexuality, Suicide/Depression) Assessment, developed by J.M. Goldenring and E. Cohen, can be very helpful in identifying potential mental health problems.

- **Home** (e.g., where is the teen living?; who lives in the home?; how is the teen getting along with people in the home?; has the teen ever run away or been incarcerated?)

- **Education** (e.g., how is the teen functioning in school in terms of grades, teacher and peer relations, suspensions, missed school days?)

- **Activities** (e.g., what extracurricular and sports activities is the teen involved in?; what does he or she do with his or her friends?)

- **Drugs** (e.g., which drugs, including intravenous (IV) drugs, alcohol, cigarettes, and caffeine, have been and are used by the teen, his/her family, and friends?)

- **Sexuality** (e.g., when was the first time the teen had sex?; what is the teen's sexual preference?; does the teen use contraceptives – and, specifically, does the teen use condoms?; how many partners has he or she had?; what is the teen's past history of sexually transmitted infections, pregnancy and abortion, sexual or physical abuse?)

- **Suicide** (e.g., has the teen had any suicidal ideations or past history of suicidal attempts?; if there have been suicidal ideations, does the teen have a plan and access to means to commit suicide?)

Guidelines for Adolescent Preventive Services (GAPS)

The American Medical Association (AMA) has a set of Guidelines for Adolescent Preventive Services (GAPS) materials with tools that provide a framework, an assessment system, and resources for preventive health services in adolescents. The GAPS recommendations were created to be delivered as a preventive services package during health visits between the ages of 11 and 21 (see http://www.ama-assn.org/ama/pub/physician-resources/public-health.page). The GAPS questionnaires are available in this section.

Remember, if you do not screen for or ask questions regarding the mental health of the children and adolescents for whom you care, you will not discover and have the opportunity to provide evidence-based preventive information and treatment for potential disorders that can have serious adverse outcomes for the children themselves, their families, and society.

Bottom Line: Screen, Ask, and Assess!

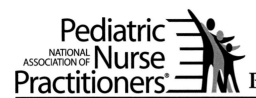
Child's Name_____ DOB_____ Age_____

Parent's/Guardian's Name_____ Relationship to Child _____

Because your child's physical as well as mental/emotional health are very important, please complete each of the following questions. We will have the opportunity to talk about some of these issues during your visit. Please indicate which items are most important to talk about today by placing a check mark in front of those items.

1. What worries or concerns you most about your child's emotions and/or behaviors at this time?

2. Have there been changes in your family in the past year, such as marital separation, remarriage, move, family illness or death)? If yes, what: No Yes

3. Are you afraid of anyone in your home? If yes, who: No Yes

4. Do you ever feel so frustrated that you may hit or hurt your child? No Yes

5. On a scale of 0 (Not at all) to 10 (a lot), how stressed is your child on a day-to-day basis? _____

6. Have you been worried about your child being angry, irritable, sad, fearful, or having a change in behavior in the last month? If yes, what is worrying you: No Yes

7. Do you have any worries about your child being sad? No Yes

8. Are you concerned about your child's weight? If yes, what concerns you: No Yes

9. Who usually watches your child when you are not with him or her?

10. What is the easiest part about being your child's parent?

11. What is the hardest part about being your child's parent?

12. What worries you most about your child?

13. On a scale of 0 (Not at all) to 10 (a lot), how stressed are you on a day-to-day basis? _____

14. On a scale of 0 (Not at all) to 10 (a lot), how depressed are you from day-to-day? _____

15. How do you discipline your child?

16. Do you think that the way that you discipline your child is effective? No Yes

17. Do you think that your child has ever been abused? If Yes, when: No Yes

18. Has your child ever been through a traumatic or very frightening experience (for example, a motor vehicle accident, hospitalization, death of a loved one, watching arguments)?
If Yes, when and what was the trauma?　　　　　　　　　　　　No　　Yes

19. Has your child ever been diagnosed with an emotional, behavioral, or mental health problem? If yes, what and when:　　　　　　　　　　　　No　　Yes

20. Has your child ever been on medication for an emotional, behavioral, or mental health problem? If yes, what medication and when:　　　　　　No　　Yes

21. Do you have guns in your home?　　　　　　　　　　　　　　　No　　Yes

22. Are there stressful things that your family has been dealing with recently? If yes, what?　　No　　Yes

23. On a scale of 0 (Not at all) to 10 (very), how emotionally connected do you feel with your child?　　　　　　　　　　　　　　　　　　_____

24. On a scale of 0 (very easy) to 10 (very difficult), how is your child's temperament?　　_____

25. Does your child have difficulty sleeping? If yes, what specifically (for example, difficulty falling asleep; waking up with nightmares):　　　　　　No　　Yes

26. Does anyone in your home smoke? If yes, who:　　　　　　　　No　　Yes

27. Does anyone in your home use alcohol or drugs to the point that you wish they would stop?　　　　　　　　　　　　　　　　　　　　　　　　No　　Yes

28. On a scale of 0 (None) to 10 (a lot), how much arguing goes on in your home?　　_____

29. On a scale of 0 (Not at all) to 10 (a lot), do you overprotect your child?　　_____

30. On a scale of 0 (Not at all) to 10 (very much so), how satisfied are you with being a parent to your child?　　　　　　　　　　　　　　　　　　_____

31. On a scale of 0 (Not at all) to 10 (very much so), how consistent are you in setting limits with your child?　　　　　　　　　　　　　　　　　　_____

32. Have you or any other of your child's blood relatives ever been diagnosed with a mental health disorder? If yes, who and what:　　　　　　　　No　　Yes

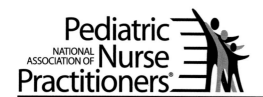

KySS Assessment Questions for Parents of Preschool Children

Child's Name_____ DOB_____ Age_____

Parent's/Guardian's Name_____ Relationship to Child _____

Because your child's physical as well as mental/emotional health are very important, please complete each of the following questions. We will have the opportunity to talk about some of these issues during your visit. Please indicate which items are most important to talk about today by placing a check mark in front of those items.

1. What worries or concerns you most about your child's emotions and/or behaviors at this time? _____

2. Have there been changes in your family in the past year, such as marital separation, remarriage, move, family illness or death)? If yes, what: No   Yes

3. Are you afraid of anyone in your home? If yes, who: No   Yes

4. Do you ever feel so frustrated that you may hit or hurt your child? No   Yes

5. On a scale of 0 (Not at all) to 10 (a lot), how much does your child worry on a day-to-day basis? _____

6. What does your child worry most about?

7. On a scale of 0 (Not at all) to 10 (a lot), how stressed is your child on a day-to-day basis? _____

8. Have you been worried about your child being angry, irritable, sad, fearful, or having a change in behavior in the last month? If yes, what is worrying you? No   Yes

9. How often does your child complain of headaches or stomachaches?
a. Never, b. 1x/month, c. 2x/month, d. 1x/week, c. more that 1x/week _____

10. Do you have any worries about your child being sad or depressed? No   Yes

11. Are you concerned about your child's weight? If yes, what concerns you: No   Yes

12. Who usually watches your child when you are not with him or her?

13. Do you talk about safety with your child? No   Yes

14. What is the easiest part about being your child's parent?

15. What is the hardest part about being your child's parent?

16. What worries you most about your relationship with your child?

17. On a scale of 0 (Not at all) to 10 (a lot), how stressed are you on a day-to-day basis? _____

18. On a scale of 0 (Not at all) to 10 (a lot), how depressed are you on a day-to day basis? _____

19. On a scale of 0 (Not good at all) to 10 (excellent), how does your child cope with stress? _____

20. How do you discipline your child?

21. Do you think that the way that you discipline your child is effective?   No   Yes

22. Do you think that your child has ever been abused? If Yes, when: No   Yes

23. Has your child ever been through a traumatic or very frightening experience (for example, a motor vehicle accident, hospitalization, death of a loved one, watching arguments)? If Yes, when and what was the trauma?   No   Yes

24. Has your child ever been diagnosed with an emotional, behavioral, or mental health problem? If yes, what and when: No   Yes

25. Has your child ever been on medication for an emotional, behavioral, or mental health problem? If yes, what medication and when: No   Yes

26. Do you have guns in your home?   No   Yes

27. Are there stressful things that your family has been dealing with recently? If yes, what?   No   Yes

28. On a scale of 0 (poor) to 10 (excellent), how is your child's self-esteem? _____

29. On a scale of 0 (Not at all) to 10 (very), how emotionally connected do you feel with your child? _____

30. On a scale of 0 (very difficult) to 10 (very easy), how is your child's temperament? _____

31. Does your child have difficulty sleeping? If yes, what specifically (for example, difficulty falling asleep; waking up with nightmares):   No   Yes

32. Does anyone in your home smoke? If yes, who: No   Yes

33. Does anyone in your home use alcohol or drugs to the point that you wish they would stop?   No   Yes

34. On a scale of 0 (None) to 10 (a lot), how much arguing goes on in your home? _____

35. On a scale of 0 (Not good) to 10 (very good), how well does your child get along with his/her peers or friends? _____

36. On a scale of 0 (Not at all) to 10 (a lot), do you overprotect your child _____

37. On a scale of 0 (Not at all) to 10 (very much so), how satisfied are you with being a parent to your child? _____

38. On a scale of 0 (Not at all) to 10 (very much so), are you consistent in setting limits with your child? _____

39. Is your child ever cruel to animals?   No   Yes

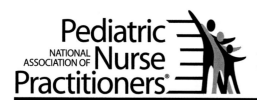

KySS Assessment Questions For Parents of School-Age Children and Teens

Child's Name_____ DOB_____ Age_____

Parent's/Guardian's Name_____ Relationship to Child _____

Because your child's physical as well as mental/emotional health are very important, please complete each of the following questions. We will have the opportunity to talk about some of these issues during your visit. Please indicate which items are most important to talk about today by placing a check mark in front of those items.

1. What worries or concerns you most about your child's emotions and/or behaviors at this time? _____

2. Have there been changes in your family in the past year, such as marital separation, remarriage, move, family illness or death)? If yes, what:　　　　　　　　　　　　　No　　Yes

3. Are you afraid of anyone in your home? If yes, who:　　　　　　　　　　　　　No　　Yes

4. Do you ever feel so frustrated that you may hit or hurt your child?　　　　　　　No　　Yes

5. On a scale of 0 (Not at all) to 10 (a lot), how much does your child worry on a day-to-day basis? _____

6. What does your child worry most about?

7. On a scale of 0 (Not at all) to 10 (a lot), how stressed is your child on a day-to-day basis. _____

8. Have you been worried about your child being angry, irritable, sad, fearful, or having a change in behavior in the last month? If yes, what is worrying you:　　　　　　No　　Yes

9. How often does your child complain of headaches or stomachaches?

10. a. Never, b. 1x/month, c. 2x/month, d. 1x/week, c. more that 1x/week _____

11. Do you have any worries about your child being depressed?　　　　　　　　　　No　　Yes

12. If yes, do you ever think that your child thinks about hurting him- or herself?　　No　　Yes

13. Are you concerned about your child's weight? If yes, what concerns you:　　　　No　　Yes

14. Does your child make negative comments about his or her body or weight?　　　No　　Yes

15. Where does your child spend his/her free time?

16. Who usually watches your child when you are not with him or her?

17. Do you talk about safety with your child?　　　　　　　　　　　　　　　　　No　　Yes

18. What is the easiest part about being your child's parent?

19. What is the hardest part about being your child's parent?

20. What worries you most about your relationship with your child?

21. On a scale of 0 (Not at all) to 10 (a lot), how stressed are you on a day-to-day basis? _____

22. On a scale of 0 (Not at all) to 10 (a lot), how depressed are you on a day-to-day basis? _____

23. On a scale of 0 (Not good at all) to 10 (excellent), how does your child cope with stress? _____

24. How do you discipline your child?

25. Do you think that the way that you discipline your child is effective? No   Yes

26. Has your child ever been through a traumatic or very frightening experience (for example, a motor vehicle accident, hospitalization, death of a loved one, rape)? If Yes, when and what was the trauma? No   Yes

27. On a scale of 0 (Not at all) to 10 (a lot), how comfortable do you feel in talking with your child about sexuality? _____

28. Are you worried about your child becoming sexually active? No   Yes

29. Are you worried about your child and drug or alcohol use? No   Yes

30. Are you worried about your child and cigarette smoking? No   Yes

31. Does your child ever get bullied? No   Yes

32. Has your child ever been diagnosed with an emotional, behavioral, or mental health problem? If yes, what and when: No   Yes

33. Has your child ever been on medication for an emotional, behavioral, or mental health problem? If yes, what medication and when: No   Yes

34. Do you have guns in your home? No   Yes

35. Are there stressful things that your family has been dealing with recently? If yes, what? No   Yes

36. On a scale of 0 (poor) to 10 (excellent), how is your child's self-esteem? _____

37. On a scale of 0 (Not at all) to 10 (very), how emotionally connected do you feel with your child? _____

38. On a scale of 0 (very difficult) to 10 (very easy), how is your child's temperament? _____

39. Has your child had a recent decline in his or her school performance/grades? If yes, when and what: No   Yes

40. Does your child have difficulty sleeping? If yes, what specifically (for example, difficulty falling asleep; waking up with nightmares): No   Yes

41. Does anyone in your home smoke? If yes, who: No   Yes

42. Does anyone in your home use alcohol or drugs to the point that you wish they would stop? No   Yes

43. On a scale of 0 (None) to 10 (a lot), how much arguing goes on in your home? _____

44. On a scale of 0 (Not good) to 10 (very good), how well does your child get along with his/her peers or friends? _____

45. On a scale of 0 (Not at all) to 10 (a lot), do you overprotect your child? _____

46. On a scale of 0 (Not at all) to 10 (very much so), how satisfied are you with being a parent to your child? _____

47. On a scale of 0 (Not at all) to 10 (very much so), are you consistent in setting limits with your child? _____

48. Is your child ever cruel to animals? No Yes

49. Have you or any other of your child's blood relatives ever been diagnosed with a mental health disorder? If yes, who and what: No Yes

Section 1 - Screening for and Assessing Common Mental Health Problems

Assessment Questions for a Specific Emotional or Behavioral Problem

When parents report that they have a specific concern or worry about their child's mental/emotional health or behaviors or that there has been a change in the way the child is functioning at home or school, proceed with the following questions regarding history or background to shed more light on the parent's concern:

1. **What?**

   a.   What specifically occurs?

   b.   What precipitated it?

   c.   What are the associated symptoms (e.g., headaches, stomachaches)?

2. **Where?**

   a.   At home and/or school/day care?

3. **When?**

   a.   Time of day? During a transition?

4. **Who?**

   a.   Who is with the child when it occurs and who is involved?

5. **How?**

   a.   How do the parent and others involved react?

   b.   How long has it been going on?

6. **Why**?

   a.   What makes the parent and child think that this is occurring?

Refer to a mental health specialist if the problem has been persistent, increasing in severity, and/or interfering with functioning at home or in school.

The Pediatric Symptom Checklist (PSC)
(M.S. Jellinek & J.M. Murphy)

Description of the PSC

The PSC is a 1-page questionnaire that lists a range of children's emotional and behavioral concerns as perceived by parents. There is also a youth self-reported version of the scale. The PSC can be easily administered in a pediatric or family practice clinic's waiting room and scored by a receptionist or healthcare provider. A high score indicates likelihood of significant psychosocial dysfunction.

Age Range: 4 - 18 years

Psychometric Properties of the PSC

Instructions for Scoring: The PSC consists of 35 items that are rated as "never," "sometimes," or "often" present and scored as 0, 1, and 2, respectively. Item scores are summed and the total score is recoded into a dichotomous variable indicating psychosocial impairment. For children aged 6 through 16 years, the cut-off score is 28 or higher. For 4- and 5-year-old children, the PSC cut-off is 24 or higher (Little et al., 1994; Pagano et al., 1996). Items that are left blank by parents are simply ignored (score = 0). If 4 or more items are left blank, the questionnaire is considered invalid.

How to Interpret the PSC: A positive score on the PSC suggests the need for further evaluation by a qualified health professional (MD, NP, RN) or mental health professional (PhD, LICSW, Nurse Practitioner of Psychiatry). Both false positives and false negatives occur, and only an experienced clinician should interpret a positive PSC score as anything other than a suggestion that further evaluation may be helpful. Data from past studies using the PSC indicate that 2 out of 3 children who screen positive on the PSC will be correctly identified as having moderate to serious impairment in psychosocial functioning. The one child "incorrectly" identified usually has at least mild impairment, although a small percentage of children turn out to have very little actually wrong with them (e.g., an adequately functioning child of an overly anxious parent). Data on PSC-negative screens indicate 95% accuracy, which still suggest that 1 out of 20 children rated as functioning adequately may actually be impaired. The inevitability of both false-positive and false-negative screens underscores the importance of experienced clinical judgment in interpreting PSC scores. Therefore, it is especially important for parents or other lay persons who administer the form to consult with a licensed professional if their child receives a PSC-positive score.

Validity: Using a receiver operating characteristic curve, Jellinek, Murphy, Robinson, and colleagues (1988) found that a PSC cut-off score of 28 has a specificity of 0.68 and a sensitivity of 0.95 when compared with clinicians' ratings of children's psychosocial dysfunction.

Reliability: Test/retest reliability of the PSC ranges from r = 0.84-0.91. Over time, case/not case classification ranges from 83%-87%. (Jellinek & Murphy, 1988; Murphy et al., 1992).

Inter-item Analysis: Studies (Murphy & Jellinek, 1985; Murphy et al., 1996) also indicate strong internal consistency reliability (Cronbach's alpha = 0.91) of the PSC items and highly significant (p < 0.0001) correlations between individual PSC items and positive PSC screening scores.

Qualifications for Use of the PSC: The training required may differ according to the ways in which the data are to be used. Professional school (e.g., medicine or nursing) or graduate training in psychology of at least the Master's degree level would ordinarily be expected. However, no amount of prior training can substitute for professional maturity, a thorough knowledge of clinical research methodology, and supervised training in working with parents and children. There are no special qualifications for scoring.

Source: Jellinek, M.S., Murphy, J.M., Robinson, J., et al. (1988). Pediatric Symptom Checklist: Screening school age children for psychosocial dysfunction. Journal of Pediatrics, 112:201-209. The PSC is one of only a few public domain measures and can be downloaded in English or Spanish at: http://psc. partners.org/ Free of charge.

From: Pediatric Development and Behavior Online, available at http://www.dbpeds.org

The PSC is in the public domain, available in several languages and can be downloaded for use at http://www.massgeneral.org/psychiatry/services/psc_home.aspx.

Please note: It is suggested that the Child Behavior Checklist (CBCL) be administered if a positive score is found on the PSC (see information on the CBCL that follows the PSC in this guide).

Other Versions of the Pediatric Symptom Checklist

The PSC also is available in a 17-item short form (free and downloadable at http://www.massgeneral.org/psychiatry/services/psc_home.aspx). A total cut-off score of 15 has been recommended (Gardner et al., 2007). Although the shorter version of the PSC-17 has similar properties to the PSC-35, research suggests a greater degree of accuracy with the longer 35-item version. As a result, the PSC-35 remains the recommended instrument unless time limitations call for the 17-item version.

The PSC has recently been adapted for young children, 18 to 60 months of age (Sheldrick et al., 2012a) and for children younger than 18 months (Sheldrick et al., 2012b). It also has been psychometrically evaluated with diverse populations of children (Stoppelbein et al., 2012).

Pediatric Symptom Checklist

Child's Name_____Record Number_____

Today's Date_____ Filled out by_____Date of Birth_____

Please mark under the heading that best fits your child:	Never	Sometimes	Often
1. Complains of aches/pains	o	o	o
2. Spends more time alone	o	o	o
3. Tires easily, has little energy	o	o	o
4. Fidgety, unable to sit still	o	o	o
5. Has trouble with a teacher	o	o	o
6. Less interested in school	o	o	o
7. Acts as if driven by a motor	o	o	o
8. Daydreams too much	o	o	o
9. Distracted easily	o	o	o
10. Is afraid of new situations	o	o	o
11. Feels sad, unhappy	o	o	o
12. Is irritable, angry	o	o	o
13. Feels hopeless	o	o	o
14. Has trouble concentrating	o	o	o
15. Has less interest in friends	o	o	o
16. Fights with others	o	o	o
17. Absent from school	o	o	o
18. School grades dropping	o	o	o
19. Is down on him- or herself	o	o	o
20. Visits doctor with doctor finding nothing wrong	o	o	o
21. Has trouble sleeping	o	o	o
22. Worries a lot	o	o	o

23. Wants to be with you more than before............................	o	o	o
24. Feels he or she is bad	o	o	o
25. Takes unnecessary risks	o	o	o
26. Gets hurt frequently..	o	o	o
27. Seems to be having less fun..	o	o	o
28. Acts younger than children his or her age	o	o	o
29. Does not listen to rules	o	o	o
30. Does not show feelings...	o	o	o
31. Does not understand other people's feelings....................	o	o	o
32. Teases others	o	o	o
33. Blames others for his or her troubles................................	o	o	o
34. Takes things that do not belong to him or her	o	o	o
35. Refuses to share...	o	o	o

Total_____

Other comments

Does your child have any emotional or behavioral problems for which he/she needs help?   ( ) N ( ) Y

Are there any services that you would like your child to receive for these problems?   ( ) N ( ) Y

If yes, what services? _____

Additional copies can be obtained on the Pediatric Development and Behavior home page, available at http://www.dbpeds.org/handouts. © 1986, M. Jellinek and M. Murphy. Reprinted with permission.

Estudio Sobre Adaptacion Social Y Emocional de los Ninos

La salud fisica y emocional son importantes para cada niño. Los padres son los primeros que notan un problema de la conducta emocional o de aprendizaje. Ud puede ayudar a su hijo a obtener el mejor cuidado del doctor por medio de contestar estas preguntas. Favor de indicar cual frase describe a su niño/a.

Indique cual síntoma mejor describe a su niño/a:	NUNCA	ALGUNAS	SEGUIDO
1. Se queja de dolores y malestares	o	o	o
2. Pasa mucho tiempo solo(a)	o	o	o
3. Se cansa fácilmente, tiene poca energiá	o	o	o
4. Nervioso, incapaz de estarse quieto	o	o	o
5. Tiene problemas con un maestro	o	o	o
6. Menos interesado en la escuela	o	o	o
7. Es incansable	o	o	o
8. Esta muy un sonador	o	o	o
9. Se distrae facilmente	o	o	o
10. Temeroso/a a nuevas situaciónes	o	o	o
11. Se siete triste, infelix	o	o	o
12. Es irritable, enojon	o	o	o
13. Se siente sin esperanzas	o	o	o
14. Tiene problemas para concentrarse	o	o	o
15. Menos interesado en amistades	o	o	o
16. Pelea con otros niños	o	o	o
17. Se ausenta de la escuela a menudo	o	o	o
19. Se critica a si mismo/a.	o	o	o
20. Visita al doctor sin que le encuentren nada	o	o	o
21. Tiene problemas para dormir	o	o	o
22. Se preocupa mucho	o	o	o

Section 1 - Screening for and Assessing Common Mental Health Problems

23. Quiere estar con usted mas que antes	o	o	o
24. Cree que el/ella es malo/a	o	o	o
25. Toma riezgos innecesarios	o	o	o
26. Se lastima frecuentemente	o	o	o
27. Parece divertirse menos	o	o	o
28. Actua mas chico que niños de su propia edad	o	o	o
29. No obedece las reglas	o	o	o
30. No demuestra sus sentimientos	o	o	o
31. No comprende los sentimientos de otros	o	o	o
32. Molesta o se burla de otros	o	o	o
33. Culpa a otros por sus problemas	o	o	o
34. Toma cosas que no le pertenecen	o	o	o
35. Se rehusa a compartir	o	o	o

Total_____

Necesita su nino(a) ayuda con problemas en el comportamiento con problemas emocionales? ___Si ___No

Pediatric Symptom Checklist - Youth Report (Y-PSC)

Child's Name_____Record Number_____

Today's Date_____ Filled out by_____Date of Birth_____

Please mark under the heading that best fits your child:	Never	Sometimes	Often
1. Complain of aches or pains	o	o	o
2. Spend more time alone..	o	o	o
3. Tire easily, has little energy	o	o	o
4. Fidgety, unable to sit still	o	o	o
5. Have trouble with teacher	o	o	o
6. Less interested in school	o	o	o
7. Act as if driven by motor...	o	o	o
8. Daydream too much	o	o	o
9. Distract easily..	o	o	o
10. Are afraid of new situations	o	o	o
11. Feel sad, unhappy	o	o	o
12. Are irritable, angry..	o	o	o
13. Feel hopeless	o	o	o
14. Have trouble concentrating	o	o	o
15. Less interested in friends	o	o	o
16. Fight with other children	o	o	o
17. Absent from school	o	o	o
18. School grades dropping	o	o	o
19. Down on yourself...	o	o	o
20. Visit doctor with doctor finding nothing wrong	o	o	o
21. Have trouble sleeping..	o	o	o
22. Worry a lot..	o	o	o

23. Want to be with parent more than before	o	o	o
24. Feel that you are bad	o	o	o
25. Take unnecessary risks	o	o	o
26. Get hurt frequently	o	o	o
27. Seem to be having less fun	o	o	o
28. Act younger than children your age	o	o	o
29. Do not listen to rules	o	o	o
30. Do not show feelings	o	o	o
31. Do not understand other people's feelings	o	o	o
32. Tease others	o	o	o
33. Blame others for your troubles	o	o	o
34. Take things that do not belong to you	o	o	o
35. Refuse to share	o	o	o

Total_____

CUESTIONARIO (PSC-Y)

La salud fisica y emocional van juntas. Usted pueda ayudar al doctor/a a obtener el mejor servicio posible, contestando unas pocas preguntas acerca de usted. La informacion que nos de es parte de la visita de hov.

Indique cual síntoma mejor describe a su niño/a:	NUNCA	ALGUNAS	SEGUIDO
1. Se queja de dolores y malestares	o	o	o
2. Pasa mucho tiempo solo(a)	o	o	o
4. Es inquieto(a)	o	o	o
5. Problemas con un maestro(a)	o	o	o
6. Menos interesado en la escuela	o	o	o
7. Es incansable	o	o	o
8. Es muy sonador	o	o	o
9. Se distrae facilmente	o	o	o
10. Temeroso(a) a nuevas situaciónes	o	o	o
11. Se siete triste, infeliz	o	o	o
12. Es irritable, enojon	o	o	o
13. Se siente sin esperanzas	o	o	o
14. Tiene problemas para concentrandose	o	o	o
15. Menos interesado(a) en amigos(as)	o	o	o
16. Pelea con otros niños(as)	o	o	o
17. Falta a la escuela a menudo	o	o	o
18. Estan bejando sus calificaciones	o	o	o
19. Se critica a si mismo(a)	o	o	o
20. Va al doctor y no encuentren nada	o	o	o
21. Tiene problemas para dormir	o	o	o
22. Se preocupa mucho	o	o	o
24. Cree que eres malo(a)	o	o	o

25. Se pone en peligro sin necesidad	o	o	o
26. Se lastima facilmente	o	o	o
27. Parece divertise menos	o	o	o
28. Actua como un nino a su edad	o	o	o
29. No obedece reglas	o	o	o
30. No demuestra sus sentimientos	o	o	o
31. No comprende el sentir de otros	o	o	o
32. Molesta a otros	o	o	o
33. Culpa a otros de sus problemas	o	o	o
34. Toma cosas que no le pertenecen	o	o	o
35. Se rehusa a compartir.	o	o	o

Total_____

Necesita usted ayuda con problemas de comportamiento, emocionales o aprendizaje? _____Si _____No

Pediatric Symptom Checklist (PSC-17)

Please mark under the heading that best describes your child:

	(0) NEVER	(1) SOMETIMES	(2) OFTEN
1. Feels sad, unhappy	–	–	–
2. Feels hopeless	–	–	–
3. Is down on self	–	–	–
4. Worries a lot	–	–	–
5. Seems to be having less fun	–	–	–
6. Fidgety, unable to sit still	–	–	–
7. Daydreams too much	–	–	–
8. Distracted easily	–	–	–
9. Has trouble concentrating	–	–	–
10. Acts as if driven by a motor	–	–	–
11. Fights with other children	–	–	–
12. Does not listen to rules	–	–	–
13. Does not understand other people's feelings	–	–	–
14. Teases others	–	–	–
15. Blames others for his/her troubles	–	–	–
16. Refuses to share	–	–	–
17. Takes things that do not belong to him/her	–	–	–

Does your child have any emotional or behavioral problems for which she/he needs help? __No __Yes

Lista de Síntomas Pediátricos (Pediatric Symptom Checklist –PSC)

La salud física y emocional son importantes para cada niño. Los padres son los primeros que notan un problema de la conducta emocional o del aprendizaje de su hijo(a). Ud. puede ayudar a su hijo(a) a obtener el mejor cuidado de su doctor por medio de contestar estas preguntas. Favor de indicar cual frase describe a su hijo(a)

Indique cual síntoma mejor describe a su hijo/a:

	NUNCA (0)	ALGUNAS VECES (1)	FRECUENTEMENTE (2)
1. Se siente triste, infeliz	1._____	_____	_____
2. Se siente sin esperanzas	2._____	_____	_____
3. Se siente mal de sí mismo(a)	3._____	_____	_____
4. Se preocupa mucho	4._____	_____	_____
5. Parece divertirse menos	5._____	_____	_____
6. Es inquieto(a), incapaz de sentarse tranquilo(a)	6._____	_____	_____
7. Sueña despierto demasiado	7._____	_____	_____
8. Se distrae fácilmente	8._____	_____	_____
9. Tiene problemas para concentrarse	9._____	_____	_____
10. Es muy activo(a), tiene mucha energía	10._____	_____	_____
11. Pelea con otros niños	11._____	_____	_____
12. No obedece las reglas	12._____	_____	_____
13. No comprende los sentimientos de otros	13._____	_____	_____
14. Molesta o se burla de otros	14._____	_____	_____
15. Culpa a otros por sus problemas	15._____	_____	_____
16. Se niega a compartir	16_____	_____	_____
17. Toma cosas que no le pertenecen	17._____	_____	_____

Total_____

¿Tiene su hijo(a) algún problema emocional o del comportamiento para el cual necesita ayuda? __Si __No

M.S. Jellinek and J. M. Murphy, Massachusetts General Hospital. Reprinted with permission.
Spanish PSC Gouverneur Revision 2-7-03

The Child Behavior Checklist (CBCL)
(T. Achenbach & C.S. Edelbrock)

Description

The Child Behavior Checklist (CBCL) is a tool used by parents or other individuals to rate a child's problem behaviors and competencies. This Likert-Scale tool can either be self-administered or administered through an interview and now includes DSM-oriented scales. The CBCL also can be used to measure a child's change in behavior over time or following a treatment. The first section of the CBCL consists of 20 competence items and the second section consists of 120 items on behavior or emotional problems during the past 6 months (e.g., aggression, hyperactivity, bullying, conduct problems, defiance, and violence). Parents rate their child for how true each item is now or was within the past 6 months using the following scale: 0 = not true (as far as you know); 1 = somewhat or sometimes true; and 2 = very true or often true. Teacher Report Forms (TRF), Youth Report Forms (YRF), and Direct Observation Forms are also available. It is suggested that the CBCL be used for further evaluation if a positive score is found on the PSC.

Age Range: Two versions of the tool exist: one for children 1½ to 5 years of age and another for **ages 6 to 18.** The Youth Self-Report tool is targeted for teens 11 to 18 years of age.

Psychometric Properties of the CBCL

The CBCL has been extensively studied and supported by multiple studies to be a valid and highly reliable tool for use with African-American, Caucasian, and Hispanic/Latino children across all socioeconomic levels. The range of internal consistency reliability is reported as 0.78 to 0.97.

Manual and computer scoring is available.

Examiner Qualifications: Master's degree

Permission Required to Use Instrument: Yes

Contact Information for Ordering the CBCL:

Achenbach System of Empirically Based Assessment
1 South Prospect Street, Room 6436
Burlington, Vermont 05401-3456
Phone: 802-656-8313
Fax: 802-656-2608
Email: mail@aseba.org
Website: www.ASEBA.org

Sources:

Achenbach, T. (1991). Integrative guide to the 1991 CBCL/4-18, YSR, and TRF Profiles.
Burlington, VT: University of Vermont, Department of Psychology.
Achenbach, T. & Edelbrock, C.S. (1983). *Manual for the Child Behavior Checklist and Revised Child Behavior Profile.*
Burlington, VT: University of Vermont.

Guidelines for Adolescent Preventive Services

Several tools have been designed to support implementing the American Medical Association's (AMA) Guidelines for Adolescent Preventive Services (GAPS) program in your clinical setting. The 6 forms that follow include the Younger Adolescent Questionnaire in English and Spanish, Middle-Older Adolescent Questionnaire in English and Spanish, and the Parent/Guardian Questionnaire in English and Spanish. The questionnaires are considered master copies that you can reproduce but not alter, modify, or revise without the expressed written consent of the Child and Adolescent Health Program at the American Medical Association.

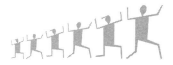

Chart# _____

Name_____ Today's Date_____
　　　　　　Last　　　　　　　　First　　　　　　　Middle Initial　　　　　　　　　　　　month　　day　　year

Birthdate _____ Grade in School _____ **Boy** or **Girl** (*circle one*)   Age _____
　　　　month　　day　　year

Address_____ City_____State_____Zip_____

Phone Number_____ Pager/Beeper Number_____
　　　　　area code

What languages are spoken where you live? _____

Are you:　　　☐ White　　　　　　　　　☐ African-American　　　　　　☐ Asian/Pacific Islander
　　　　　　　☐ Latino/Hispanic　　　　　☐ Native American　　　　　　☐ Other _____

Medical History

1. Why did you come to the clinic/office today?_____

_____

2. Are you allergic to any medicines?
　☐ No　☐ Yes, name of medicine(s): _____　☐ Not Sure

3. Do you have any health problems?
　☐ No　☐ Yes, problem(s): _____　☐ Not Sure

4. Are you taking any medicine now?
　☐ No　☐ Yes, name of medicine(s): _____　☐ Not Sure

5. Have you been to the dentist in the last year? ....☐ No　☐ Yes　☐ Not Sure

6. Have you stayed overnight in a hospital in the last year? ....☐ No　☐ Yes　☐ Not Sure

7. Have you ever had any of the problems below?

	Yes	No	Not Sure		Yes	No	Not Sure
Allergies or hay fever	☐	☐	☐	Seizures	☐	☐	☐
Asthma	☐	☐	☐	Cancer	☐	☐	☐
Tuberculosis (TB)	☐	☐	☐	Diabetes	☐	☐	☐

For Girls Only

8. Have you started having periods? .... ☐ No ☐ Yes

    a. *If yes*, are your periods regular (once a month) ? .... ☐ No ☐ Yes

    b. *If yes*, what was the 1st day of your last period? Month _____ Day _____

9. Have you ever been pregnant? .... ☐ Yes ☐ No

Family Information

10. Who do you live with? (Check all that apply).
    ☐ Mother   ☐ Stepmother   ☐ Brother(s)/ages_____
    ☐ Father   ☐ Stepfather   ☐ Sister(s)/ages_____
    ☐ Guardian   ☐ Other adult relative   ☐ Other/(explain)_____

11. Do you have older brothers or sisters who live away from home? .... ☐ Yes ☐ No ☐ Not Sure

12. During the past year, have there been any changes in your family such as: (Check all that apply)
    ☐ Marriage   ☐ Loss of job   ☐ Births   ☐ Other changes_____
    ☐ Separation   ☐ Moved to a new neighborhood ☐ Serious Illness/Injury   _____
    ☐ Divorce   ☐ A new school   ☐ Deaths   _____

Specific Health Issues

13. Please check whether you have questions or are worried about any of the following:

☐ Height	☐ Neck or back	☐ Muscle or pain in arms/legs	☐ Anger or temper
☐ Weight	☐ Breasts	☐ Menstruation or periods	☐ Feeling tired
☐ Eyes or vision	☐ Heart	☐ Wetting the bed	☐ Trouble sleeping
☐ Hearing or earaches	☐ Coughing or wheezing	☐ Trouble urinating or peeing	☐ Fitting in/belonging
☐ Colds/runny or stuffy nose	☐ Chest pain or trouble breathing	☐ Drip from penis or vagina	☐ Cancer
☐ Mouth or teeth or breath	☐ Stomach ache	☐ Wet dreams	☐ HIV/AIDS
☐ Headaches	☐ Vomiting or throwing up	☐ Skin (rash/acne)	☐ Dying
☐ Other_____			

These questions will help us get to know you better. Choose the answer that best describes what you feel or do. Your answers will be seen only by your health care provider and his/her assistant.

Health Profile

Eating/Weight/Body

14. Do you eat fruits and vegetables every day? .... ☐ No ☐ Yes

15. Do you drink milk and/or eat milk products every day? .... ☐ No ☐ Yes

16. Do you spend a lot of time thinking about ways to be skinny? .... ☐ Yes ☐ No

17. Do you do things to lose weight (skip meals, take pills, starve yourself, vomit, etc) .... ☐ Yes ☐ No

18. Do you work, play, or exercise enough to make you sweat or breathe hard at least 3
    times a week? .... ☐ No ☐ Yes

19. Have you pierced your body (not including ears) or gotten a tattoo? .... ☐ Yes ☐ No

School

20. Is doing well in school important to you? .... ☐ No ☐ Yes
21. Is doing well in school important to your family and friends? .... ☐ No ☐ Yes
22. Are your grades this year worse than last year? .... ☐ Yes ☐ No ☐ Not Sure
23. Are you getting failing grades in any subjects this year? .... ☐ Yes ☐ No ☐ Not Sure
24. Have you been told that you have a learning problem? .... ☐ Yes ☐ No
25. Have you been suspended from school this year? .... ☐ Yes ☐ No

Friends and Family

26. Do you know at least one person who you can talk to about problems? .... ☐ No ☐ Yes
27. Do you think that your parent(s) or guardian(s) usually listen to you and take your
    feelings seriously? .... ☐ No ☐ Yes
28. Have your parents talked with you about things like alcohol, drugs, and sex? .... ☐ No ☐ Yes ☐ Not Sure
29. Are you worried about problems at home or in your family? .... ☐ Yes ☐ No ☐ Not Sure
30. Have you ever thought seriously about running away from home? .... ☐ Yes ☐ No

Weapons/Violence/Safety

31. Is there a gun, rifle, or other firearm where you live? .... ☐ Yes ☐ No ☐ Not Sure
32. Have you ever carried a gun, knife, club, or other weapon to protect yourself? ...... ☐ Yes ☐ No
33. Have you ever been in a physical fight where you or someone else got hurt? .... ☐ Yes ☐ No
34. Have you ever been in trouble with the police? .... ☐ Yes ☐ No
35. Have you ever seen a violent act take place at home, school, or in your neighborhood? ..... ☐ Yes ☐ No
36. Are you worried about violence or your safety? .... ☐ Yes ☐ No ☐ Not Sure
37. Do you usually wear a helmet and/or protective gear when you rollerblade,
    skateboard, or ride a bike? .... ☐ No ☐ Yes
38. Do you always wear a seat belt when you ride in a car, truck, or van? .... ☐ No ☐ Yes

Tobacco

39. Have you ever tried cigarettes or chewing tobacco? .... ☐ Yes ☐ No
40. Have any of your close friends ever tried cigarettes or chewing tobacco? .... ☐ Yes ☐ No
41. Does anyone you live with smoke cigarettes/cigars or chew tobacco? .... ☐ Yes ☐ No

Alcohol

42. Have you ever tried beer, wine, or other liquor (except for religious purposes)? ..... ☐ Yes ☐ No
43. Have any of your close friends ever tried beer, wine, or other liquor
    (except for religious purposes)? .... ☐ Yes ☐ No
44. Have you ever been in a car when the driver has been using drugs or drinking
    beer, wine or other liquor? .... ☐ Yes ☐ No
45. Does anyone in your family drink so much that it worries you? .... ☐ Yes ☐ No ☐ Not Sure

Drugs

46. Have you ever taken things to get high, stay awake, calm down or go to sleep? ..... ☐ Yes ☐ No ☐ Not Sure
47. Have you ever used marijuana (pot, grass, weed, reefer, or blunt)? .... ☐ Yes ☐ No ☐ Not Sure
48. Have you ever used other drugs such as cocaine, speed, LSD, mushrooms, etc.? ..... ☐ Yes ☐ No ☐ Not Sure
49. Have you ever sniffed or huffed things like paint, 'white-out', glue, gasoline, etc.? ..... ☐ Yes ☐ No ☐ Not Sure

50. Have any of your close friends ever used marijuana, other drugs, or done other things to get high? .... ☐ Yes ☐ No ☐ Not Sure

51. Does anyone in your family use drugs so much that it worries you? .... ☐ Yes ☐ No ☐ Not Sure

Development/Relationships

52. Are you dating someone or going steady? .... ☐ Yes ☐ No ☐ Not Sure

53. Are you thinking about having sex ("going all the way "or "doing it")? .... ☐ Yes ☐ No ☐ Not Sure

54. Have you ever had sex? .... ☐ Yes ☐ No ☐ Not Sure

55. Have any of your friends ever had sex? .... ☐ Yes ☐ No ☐ Not Sure

56. Have you ever felt pressured by anyone to have sex or had sex when you did not want to? .... ☐ Yes ☐ No ☐ Not Sure

57. Have you ever been told by a doctor or a nurse that you had a sexually transmitted disease like herpes, gonorrhea, or chlamydia? .... ☐ Yes ☐ No ☐ Not Sure

58. Would you like to receive information on abstinence ("how to say no to sex")? .... ☐ Yes ☐ No ☐ Not Sure

59. Would you like to know how to avoid getting pregnant, getting HIV/AIDS, or getting sexually transmitted diseases? .... ☐ Yes ☐ No ☐ Not Sure

Emotions

60. Have you done something fun during the past two weeks? .... ☐ No ☐ Yes

61. When you get angry, do you do violent things? .... ☐ Yes ☐ No

62. During the past few weeks, have you felt very sad or down as though you have nothing to look forward to? .... ☐ Yes ☐ No

63. Have you ever seriously thought about killing yourself, made a plan, or tried to kill yourself? .... ☐ Yes ☐ No

64. Is there something you often worry about or fear? .... ☐ Yes ☐ No

65. Have you ever been physically, emotionally, or sexually abused? .... ☐ Yes ☐ No ☐ Not Sure

66. Would you like to get counseling about something that is bothering you? .... ☐ Yes ☐ No ☐ Not Sure

Special Circumstances

67. In the past year have you been around someone with tuberculosis (TB)? .... ☐ Yes ☐ No ☐ Not Sure

68. In the past year, have you stayed overnight in a homeless shelter, jail, or detention center? .... ☐ Yes ☐ No

69. Have you ever lived in foster care or a group home? .... ☐ Yes ☐ No

Self

70. What two words best describe you?

1)_____ 2)_____

71. What would you like to be when you grow up?

_____

72. If you could have three wishes come true, what would they be?

1)_____

2)_____

3)_____

AA61:98-301:3/98

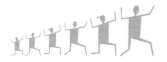

Archivo #_____

Nombre_____ Fecha de Hoy _____
    (Apellido)   (Nombre)   (Inicial)   mes/día/año

Fecha de Nacimiento_____ Año/Curso Escolar_____ Niño o Niña *(marque con círculo)* Edad_____
         mes/día/año

Dirección_____ Ciudad_____ Código Postal/Zip_____

Teléfono (   )_____ Anunciador/Pager/Beeper (   )_____
   Código

¿ Cuales idiomas se hablan donde vive Ud.? _____

¿Es Ud.?:   ☐ Blanco   ☐ Afro-Americano   ☐ Asiático/Isleño del Pacífico
                ☐ Latino/Hispano   ☐ Indígena Norteamericano   ☐ Otro

Historia Médica

1. ¿Porqué vino al consultorio hoy?_____

_____

2. ¿Tiene alergias a cualquier medicina?
   ☐ No   ☐ Sí, (nombre(s) de la(s) medicina(s):_____) ☐ No estoy seguro

3. ¿Tiene cualquier problema con la salud?
   ☐ No   ☐ Sí, (problema(s): _____) ☐ No estoy seguro

4. ¿Esta tomando medicinas actualmente?
   ☐ No   ☐ Sí, (nombre de la medicina(s):_____) ☐ No estoy seguro

5. ¿En el último año ha consultado al dentista?... ☐ No ☐ Sí ☐ No estoy seguro

6. En el último año Ha pasado la noche en el hospital?........................... ☐ No ☐ Sí ☐ No estoy seguro

7. ¿Alguna vez padeció cualquiera de los siguientes problemas de salud?

	Sí	No	No estoy seguro		Sí	No	No estoy seguro
Alergias o "hay fever"	☐	☐	☐	Convulsiones/Ataques	☐	☐	☐
Asma	☐	☐	☐	Cáncer	☐	☐	☐
Tuberculosis (TB)	☐	☐	☐	Diabetes	☐	☐	☐

Unicamente para Niñas

8. Ha comenzado a tener su período/ la regla? ....☐ No ☐ Sí
   a. Si ya comenzó Le viene regularmente (una vez al mes)?........................☐ No ☐ Sí
   b. Si es el caso, ¿Cual fue el primer día de la última regla?....................Mes _____ Día_____

9. ¿Alguna vez ha estado embarazada? ....☐ No ☐ Sí

Información Familiar

10. ¿Con quién vive? (Marque todas que sean ciertas).

☐ Madre   ☐ Madrastra   ☐ Hermanos/edades

☐ Padre   ☐ Padrastro   ☐ Hermanas/edades

☐ Guardián Legal   ☐ Otro pariente adulto   ☐ Otra/(explique)

11. ¿Tiene hermanos mayores que no viven en casa?.................................. ☐ Sí ☐ No ☐ No estoy seguro

12. En el último año Han habido cambios importantes en su familia? (Marque todas que sean ciertas),

☐ Matrimonios   ☐ Alguien perdi su empleo   ☐ Nacimientos   ☐ Otros cambios

☐ Separaciones   ☐ Mudanzas a otros vecindarios   ☐ Enfermedades graves

☐ Divorcios   ☐ Cambio de escuela   ☐ Muertes

Problemas Específicos de la Salud

13. Por favor, marque a continuación si tiene preguntas o alguna preocupación sobre:

☐ Estatura/desarrollo físico   ☐ Cuello o espalda   ☐ Músculos o dolor en los brazos/piernas   ☐ Enojo o mal genio

☐ Peso   ☐ Pechos/senos   ☐ Menstruación o la regla   ☐ Cansancio

☐ Ojos/la vista   ☐ Corazón   ☐ Mojarse la cama   ☐ Dificultad al dormir

☐ Dificultad para oir o dolor del oído   ☐ Tos o le chilla el pecho   ☐ Dificultad para orinar o hacer pipí   ☐ Su relación con los compañeros

☐ Catarro/moquillo o las narices tapadas   ☐ Dolor del pecho o dificultad en respirar   ☐ Gota del pene o la vagina   ☐ Cáncer

☐ Boca o dientes o aliento   ☐ Dolor del estómago   ☐ Sueño mojado   ☐ VIH/SIDA

☐ Dolores de cabeza   ☐ Vómito o náuseas   ☐ Piel (salpullido/espinillas)   ☐ La muerte

☐ Otro _____

Estas preguntas nos ayudarán a conocerle mejor. Escoja la respuesta que mejor indica lo que siente o hace.
Sus respuestas ser n vistas nicamente por su médico/enfermera y su asistente.

Su Salud

Comer/Peso/Cuerpo

14. ¿Come Ud. frutas y vegetales cada día? ....☐ No ☐ Sí

15. ¿Toma Ud. leche y/o come productos lácteos cada día? ....☐ No ☐ Sí

16. ¿Gasta mucho tiempo pensando en como adelgazar? ....☐ Sí ☐ No

17. ¿Trata de bajar de peso (evita comidas, toma pastillas, ayuna, vomita, eta) .....☐ Sí ☐ No

18. ¿Trabaja Ud, juega, o hace suficiente ejercicio como para sudar o respirar fuerte por lo menos 3 veces por semana? ....☐ No ☐ Sí

19. Ha perforado su cuerpo (sin incluir las orejas) o ha puesto un tatuaje? ....☐ Sí ☐ No

La Escuela

20. ¿Salir bien en sus estudios es importante para Ud.? ....☐ No ☐ Sí

21. ¿Salir bien en sus estudios es importante para su familia y sus amigos?..........☐ No ☐ Sí

22. ¿Sus notas (calificaciones) son peores este año ? ....☐ Sí ☐ No ☐ No estoy seguro

23. ¿Está saliendo mal en alguna materia ? ....☐ Sí ☐ No ☐ No estoy seguro

24. ¿Le han dicho que tiene dificultad en aprender? ....☐ Sí ☐ No

25. ¿Le han suspendido de clases este año?..☐ Sí ☐ No

Los Amigos y la Familia

26. ¿Conoce al menos una persona con quien puede hablar si tiene un problema? ☐ No ☐ Sí
27. ¿ Cree Ud. que sus padres o su guardián le
escuchan y toman en serio sus sentimientos?..☐ No ☐ Sí
28. ¿Sus padres han hablado con Ud. sobre alcohol, drogas, y sexo ? ....☐ No ☐ Sí   ☐ No estoy seguro
29. ¿Está preocupado por problemas en su casa o en su familia ? ....☐ Sí ☐ No   ☐ No estoy seguro
30. ¿Alguna vez ha contemplado seriamente fugarse de la casa? ....☐ Sí ☐ No

Las Armas/la Violencia/la Seguridad

31. ¿Hay una pistola, rifle u otra arma de fuego en la casa donde vive ? ....☐ Sí ☐ No   ☐ No estoy seguro
32. ¿Alguna vez ha portado una pistola, cuchillo,
palo u otra arma para protegerse?..☐ Sí ☐ No
33. ¿Alguna vez ha estado en una pelea donde Ud. u otra persona fue lesionado?..☐ Sí ☐ No
34. ¿Alguna vez ha tenido problemas con la policía? ....☐ Sí ☐ No
35. ¿Alguna vez ha visto un acto de violencia en la casa, la escuela,
o en el vecindario?..☐ Sí ☐ No
36. ¿Está Ud. preocupado por la violencia o por su seguridad? ....☐ Sí ☐ No   ☐ No estoy seguro
37. ¿Normalmente usa Ud. un casco y/o equipo protectivo cuando patina
("roller blade," "skateboard", o monta a bicicleta? ....☐ No ☐ Sí
38. ¿Siempre usa Ud. el cinturón de seguridad cuando monta
en un auto, vehículo de carga, o camioneta? ....☐ No ☐ Sí

El Tabaco

39. Ha probado Ud. cigarrillos o tabaco de mascar (rapé)?..........................☐ Sí ☐ No
40. ¿Alguno de sus mejores amigos ha probado cigarrillos o tabaco de mascar?......☐ Sí ☐ No
41. ¿Alguien con quien vive Ud. fuma cigarrillos/puros o usa tabaco de mascar?....☐ Sí ☐ No

El Alcohol

42. ¿Alguna vez ha probado Ud. cerveza, vino, u otro licor
(fuera de propósitos religiosos)? ....☐ Sí ☐ No
43. ¿Alguno de sus mejores amigos ha probado cerveza, vino, u otro licor
(fuera de propósitos religiosos)? ....☐ Sí ☐ No
44. ¿Alguna vez ha estado en un veh culo cuando el motorista ha estado
tomando drogas, cerveza, vino, u otro licor? ....☐ Sí ☐ No
45. ¿Hay alguien en su familia que toma tanto que le preocupa?..................☐ Sí ☐ No   ☐ No estoy seguro

Las Drogas

46. ¿Alguna vez ha tomado sustancias para elevarse, para
mantenerse despierto, calmarse, o para dormir?..................................☐ Sí ☐ No   ☐ No estoy seguro
47. ¿Alguna vez ha usado marijuana
(hierba, pasto, maría, mota, "refer, o pot")?..☐ Sí ☐ No   ☐ No estoy seguro
48. ¿Alguna vez ha usado otras drogas como la coca na,
la metanfetamina "speed", LSD, hongos.?..☐ Sí ☐ No   ☐ No estoy seguro
49. ¿Alguna vez ha inhalado sustancias: pintura, "white-out",
gases de los pegantes o gomas, gasolina? ....☐ Sí ☐ No   ☐ No estoy seguro
50. ¿Alguno de sus mejores amigos ha usado la marijuana, otras drogas o
hecho otras cosas para elevarse o sentirse "bien"? ....☐ Sí ☐ No   ☐ No estoy seguro
51. ¿Hay alguien en su familia que usa tanta droga que le preocupa? ....☐ Sí ☐ No   ☐ No estoy seguro

El Desarrollo/Relaciones Personales

52. ¿Tiene novio(a) o esta saliendo con alguien?......................................☐ Sí ☐ No ☐ No estoy seguro
53. ¿Está pensando en tener relaciones sexuales (en hacerlo, tener sexo)?............☐ Sí ☐ No ☐ No estoy seguro
54. ¿Quisiera recibir información sobre como abstenerse
(como decir que "no" a tener sexo)?..☐ Sí ☐ No ☐ No estoy seguro
55. ¿Alguna vez ha tenido relaciones sexuales?....................................☐ Sí ☐ No ☐ No estoy seguro
56. ¿Alguno de sus amigos ha tenido relaciones sexuales ya?......................☐ Sí ☐ No ☐ No estoy seguro
57. ¿Alguna vez ha sido presionado por alguien a tener
relaciones o ha tenido relaciones cuando no quería? ....☐ Sí ☐ No ☐ No estoy seguro
58. ¿Alguna vez un médico le ha dicho que tuvo una enfermedad
transmitida sexualmente como el herpes, la gonorrea, o la sífilis?.............☐ Sí ☐ No ☐ No estoy seguro
59. ¿Quisiera saber como evitar el embarazo, el VIH/SIDA,
o una enfermedad "venérea"?...☐ Sí ☐ No ☐ No estoy seguro

Las Emociones

60. ¿ Ha hecho algo divertido en las últimas dos semanas? ....☐ No ☐ Sí
61. ¿Cuando se pone enojado, se hace cosas violentas?...........................☐ No ☐ Sí
62. ¿Durante las últimas semanas ha sentido muy triste,
desanimado, desalentado? ....☐ No ☐ Sí
63. ¿Alguna vez ha pensado seriamente en matarse,
ha hecho un plan, o ha intentado matarse? ....☐ No ☐ Sí
64. ¿Hay algo que le preocupa o teme con frecuencia?..........................☐ No ☐ Sí
65. ¿Alguna vez ha sido abusado físicamente, emocionalmente, o sexualmente?....☐ No ☐ Sí ☐ No estoy seguro
66. ¿Quisiera hablar con un(a) consejero(a) de algo que le preocupa? ....☐ No ☐ Sí ☐ No estoy seguro

Circunstancias Especiales

67. En este año pasado, ¿Ha pasado tiempo con alguien
que tiene la tuberculosis?..☐ Sí ☐ No ☐ No estoy seguro
68. En este año pasado, ¿Ha pasado la noche en un albergue,
la cárcel, o un centro detención juvenil? ....☐ Sí ☐ No
69. ¿Alguna vez ha vivido con padres de crianza, o en una casa juvenil?.................☐ Sí ☐ No

Sí Mismo

70. ¿Cuales dos palabras describen mejor a Ud.? 1)_____ 2)_____

71. ¿Que quiere hacer cuando sea adulto?_____

72. Si podrían concederle tres deseos, cuales serían?

1)_____

2)_____

3)_____

Febrero, 1998

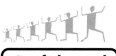

Confidential (Your answers will not be given out.) Chart # _____

Name _____ Date _____
        Last   First   Middle Initial

Date of Birth _____ Grade in School_____ Year in college_____ Sex: Male Female Age _____

Address _____ City _____ Zip _____

Phone number where you can be reached _____ Pager/beeper number_____

What languages are spoken where you live? _____Race _____

Medical History

1. Why did you come to the clinic/office today? _____

2. Do you have any health problems? ☐ Yes ☐ No Problem(s) _____

3. Did you have any health problems in the past 12 months? ☐ Yes ☐ No Problem(s) _____

4. Are you taking any medicine now? ☐ Yes ☐ No Name of medicine _____

For Girls

5. Date when last period started_____ Are your periods regular (monthly)? .... ☐ No ☐ Yes
                           Month   Date
6. Have you had a miscarriage, an abortion, or live birth in the past 12 months? .... ☐ Yes ☐ No

Specific Health Issues

7. Please check whether you have questions or are worried about any of the following:

☐ Height/weight	☐ Mouth/teeth/breath	☐ Frequent or painful urination	☐ Trouble sleeping
☐ Blood pressure	☐ Neck/back		☐ Feeling tired a lot
☐ Diet/food/appetite	☐ Chest pain/trouble breathing	☐ Discharge from penis or vagina	☐ Cancer
☐ Future plans/job		☐ Wetting the bed	☐ Dying
☐ Skin (rash, acne)	☐ Coughing/wheezing	☐ Sexual organs/genitals	☐ Sad or crying a lot
☐ Headaches/migraines	☐ Breasts	☐ Menstruation/periods	☐ Stress
☐ Dizziness/fainting	☐ Heart	☐ Wet dreams	☐ Anger/temper
☐ Eyes/vision	☐ Stomach ache	☐ Physical or sexual abuse	☐ Violence/personal safety
☐ Ears/hearing/ear aches	☐ Nausea/vomiting	☐ Masturbation	☐ Other (explain)
☐ Nose	☐ Diarrhea/constipation	☐ HIV/AIDS	_____
☐ Lots of colds	☐ Muscle or joint pain in arms/legs		_____

Health Profile

These questions will help us get to know you better. Choose the answer that best describes what you feel or do. Your answers will be seen only by your health care provider and his/her assistant.

Eating/Weight

8. Are you satisfied with your eating habits?.. ☐ No ☐ Yes

9. Do you ever eat in secret? .... ☐ Yes ☐ No

10. Do you spend a lot of time thinking about ways to be thin? .... ☐ Yes ☐ No

11. In the past year, have you tried to lose weight or control your weight by vomiting, taking diet pills or laxatives, or starving yourself?.. ☐ Yes ☐ No

12. Do you exercise or participate in sport activities that make you sweat and breathe hard for 20 minutes or more at a time at least three or more times during the week?........................... ☐ No ☐ Yes

School

13. Are your grades this year worse than last year?.. ☐ Yes ☐ No ☐ Not in school

14. Have you either been told you have a learning problem or do you think you have a learning problem?............ ☐ Yes ☐ No

15. Have you been suspended from school this year?... ☐ Yes ☐ No ☐ Not in school

Friends & Family

16. Do you have at least one friend who you really like and feel you can talk to?............................ ☐ No ☐ Yes

17. Do you think that your parent(s) or guardian(s) *usually* listen to you and take your feelings seriously? ...... ☐ No ☐ Yes

18. Have you ever thought seriously about running away from home?.................................... ☐ Yes ☐ No ☐ Not sure

Weapons/Violence/Safety

19. Do you or anyone you live with have a gun, rifle, or other firearm? . . . . ☐ Yes ☐ No ☐ Not sure

20. In the past year, have you carried a gun, knife, club, or other weapon for protection? . . . . ☐ Yes ☐ No

21. Have you been in a physical fight during the *past 3 months*? . . . . ☐ Yes ☐ No

22. Have you ever been in trouble with the law? . . . . ☐ Yes ☐ No

23. Are you worried about violence or your safety? . . . . ☐ Yes ☐ No ☐ Not sure

24. Do you usually wear a helmet when you rollerblade, skateboard, ride a bicycle , motorcycle, minibike, or ride in an all-terrain vehicle (ATV)? . . . . ☐ No ☐ Yes

25. Do you usually wear a seat belt when you ride in or drive a car, truck, or van? . . . . ☐ No ☐ Yes

Tobacco

26. Do you ever smoke cigarettes/cigars, use snuff or chew tobacco? . . . . ☐ Yes ☐ No

26. Do any of your close friends ever smoke cigarettes/cigars, use snuff or chew tobacco? . . . . ☐ Yes ☐ No

28. Does anyone you live with smoke cigarettes/cigars, use snuff or chew tobacco? . . . . ☐ Yes ☐ No

Alcohol

29. In the past month, did you get drunk or very high on beer, wine, or other alcohol? . . . . ☐ Yes ☐ No

30. In the past month, did any of your close friends get drunk or very high on beer, wine, or other alcohol? . . . . ☐ Yes ☐ No

31. Have you ever been criticized or gotten into trouble because of drinking? . . . . ☐ Yes ☐ No ☐ Not sure

32. In the past year have you used alcohol and then driven a car/truck/van/motorcycle? . . . . ☐ Yes ☐ No ☐ Does not apply

33. In the past year, have you been in a car or other motor vehicle when the driver has been drinking alcohol or using drugs? . . . . ☐ Yes ☐ No

34. Does anyone in your family drink or take drugs so much that it worries you? . . . . ☐ Yes ☐ No

Drugs

35. Do you ever use marijuana or other drugs, or sniff inhalants? . . . . ☐ Yes ☐ No ☐ Not sure

36. Do any of your close friends ever use marijuana or other drugs, or sniff inhalants? . . . . ☐ Yes ☐ No ☐ Not sure

37. Do you ever use non-prescription drugs to get to sleep, stay awake, calm down, or get high? (These drugs can be bought at a store without a doctor's prescription.) . . . . ☐ Yes ☐ No

38. Have you ever used steroid pills or shots without a doctor telling you to? . . . . ☐ Yes ☐ No ☐ Not sure

Development

39. Do you have any concerns or questions about the size or shape of your body, or your physical appearance? . . . . ☐ Yes ☐ No ☐ Not sure

40. Do you think you may be gay, lesbian, or bisexual? . . . . ☐ Yes ☐ No ☐ Not sure

41. Have you ever had sexual intercourse? (How old were you the first time?_____) . . . . ☐ Yes ☐ No ☐ Not sure

42. Are you using a method to prevent pregnancy? (Which:_____) . . . . ☐ No ☐ Yes ☐ Not active

43. Do you and your partner(s) *always* use condoms when you have sex? . . . . ☐ No ☐ Yes ☐ Not active

44. Have any of your close friends ever had sexual intercourse? . . . . ☐ Yes ☐ No ☐ Not sure

45. Have you ever been told by a doctor or nurse that you had a sexually transmitted infection or disease? . . . . . . ☐ Yes ☐ No ☐ Not sure

46. Have you ever been pregnant or gotten someone pregnant? . . . . ☐ Yes ☐ No ☐ Not sure

47. Would you like to receive information or supplies to prevent pregnancy or sexually transmitted infections? . . . ☐ Yes ☐ No ☐ Not sure

48. Would you like to know how to avoid getting HIV/AIDS? . . . . ☐ Yes ☐ No ☐ Not sure

49. Have you pierced your body (not including ears) or gotten a tattoo? . . . . ☐ Yes ☐ No ☐ Thinking about it

Emotions

50. Have you had fun during the past two weeks? . . . . ☐ No ☐ Yes

51. During the past few weeks, have you *often* felt sad or down or as though you have nothing to look forward to? . . . . ☐ Yes ☐ No

52. Have you ever *seriously* thought about killing yourself, made a plan or actually tried to kill yourself? . . . . ☐ Yes ☐ No

53. Have you ever been physically, sexually, or emotionally abused? . . . . ☐ Yes ☐ No ☐ Not sure

54. When you get angry, do you do violent things? . . . . ☐ Yes ☐ No

55. Would you like to get counseling about something you have on your mind? . . . . ☐ Yes ☐ No ☐ Not sure

Special Circumstances

56. In the past year, have you been around someone with tuberculosis (TB)? . . . . ☐ Yes ☐ No ☐ Not sure

57. In the past year, have you stayed overnight in a homeless shelter, jail, or detention center? . . . . ☐ Yes ☐ No

58. Have you ever lived in foster care or a group home? . . . . ☐ Yes ☐ No

Self

59. What four words best describe you? _____

60. If you could change one thing about your life or yourself, what would it be? _____
_____

61. What do you want to talk about today? _____

97-892:1.2M:11/97

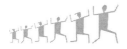

Confidencial (No le diremos a nadie lo que tú nos digas)   Expediente # _____

Nombre_____ Fecha_____
          (apellido)   (nombre)   (inicial del segundo nombre)

Fecha de nacimiento _____Año Escolar _____Año Universitario _____Sexo: ❑ Hombre ❑ Mujer   Edad_____

Dirección_____Ciudad_____Area Postal_____

Teléfono donde te podemos llamar_____Beeper_____

¿Qué idiomas se hablan en tu hogar?_____Raza_____

Historial Médico

1. ¿Por qué viniste hoy a la clínica/oficina? _____

2. ¿Tienes algún problema de salud? ❑ Sí ❑ No Problema(s) _____

3. ¿Has tenido algún problema de salud en el año pasado?   ❑ Sí ❑ No

4. ¿Estás tomando alguna medicina ahora? ❑ Sí ❑ No Nombre de la medicina_____

Para Mujeres Jóvenes

5. ¿Cuál fue el primer día de tu última regla? _____ ¿Te viene la regla regularmente cada mes? .... ❑ No   ❑ Sí

6. ¿Has tenido un aborto (natural o provocado) o has tenido un hijo en los ultimos 12 meses? .... ❑ Sí   ❑ No

Sobre La Salud

7. Si tienes alguna pregunta o preocupación sobre alguno de los siguientes temas, márcalos.

❑ Estatura/peso
❑ Alta o baja presión
❑ Dieta/comida/apetito
❑ Planes para el futuro/trabajo
❑ Piel (sarpullido, acné)
❑ Dolores de cabeza/migrañas
❑ Mareos/desmayos
❑ Ojos/visión
❑ Oídos/dolor de oídos
❑ Nariz
❑ Muchos catarros
❑ Boca/dientes/aliento
❑ Cuello/espalda
❑ Dolor de pecho/dificultad al respirar

❑ Tos/te silba el pecho
❑ Senos (el busto)
❑ Corazón
❑ Dolores de estómago
❑ Náusea/vómitos
❑ Diarrea/estreñimiento
❑ Dolor muscular o en las articulaciones
❑ Orinas frecuentamente o tienes dolor al orinar
❑ Secreción del pene o de la vagina
❑ Te orinas en la cama
❑ Organos sexuales/genitales
❑ Menstruación/regla

❑ Eyaculas cuando sueñas (el despertar mojado)
❑ Abuso físico o sexual
❑ Masturbación
❑ VIH/SIDA
❑ No duermes bien
❑ Cansancio todo el tiempo
❑ Cáncer
❑ La muerte
❑ Triste o lloras mucho
❑ Estrés
❑ Enojo/mal humor
❑ Violencia/seguridad personal

❑ Otros (explica) _____

Tu Salud

Estas preguntas nos ayudarán a conocerte mejor. Escoge la respuesta que mejor describe lo que sientes o haces. Tus respuestas sólo las repasan el doctor y su asistente.

Dieta/Peso

8. ¿Estás satisfecho con tus hábitos alimenticios?..❑ No ❑ Sí

9. ¿Comes a escondidas o en secreto de vez en cuando?..❑ Sí ❑ No

10. ¿Te pasas horas pensando en cómo bajar de peso? ....❑ Sí ❑ No

11. En el año pasado, ¿trataste de bajar o controlar tu peso haciéndote vomitar, usando pastillas, laxantes o purgantes, o dejando de comer? ....❑ Sí ❑ No

12. ¿Haces ejercicios o participas en actividades deportivas tres veces o más durante la semana que te hacen sudar y respirar fuerte y que duran 20 minutos? ....❑ No ❑ Sí

Voltee la página

Escuela

13. ¿Tus notas de este año son peores que las del año pasado? .... ❑ Sí ❑ No ❑ No estoy en la escuela

14. ¿Te han dicho o piensas que tienes problemas para aprender? .... ❑ Sí ❑ No

15. ¿Te han suspendido de clases en la escuela este año? .... ❑ Sí ❑ No ❑ No estoy en la escuela

Amistades y Familia

16. ¿Tienes un amigo a quien estimas mucho y con quien puedes hablar de todo? .... ❑ No ❑ Sí

17. ¿Piensas que tus padres o tus guardianes te escuchan usualmente y te toman tus sentamientos en serio? .... ❑ No ❑ Sí

18. ¿Alguna vez has pensado seriamente en escaparte de tu casa? .... ❑ Sí ❑ No ❑ No estoy seguro(a)

Armas/Violencia/Seguridad

19. ¿Alguna de las personas con quien vives tú mismo tiene una pistola, rifle, o alguna otra arma de fuego? .... ❑ Sí ❑ No ❑ No estoy seguro(a)

20. ¿Has portado una pistola, navaja, garrote o alguna otra arma para protegerte en los últimos 12 meses? .... ❑ Sí ❑ No

21. ¿Has tenido alguna pelea física en los últimos 3 meses? .... ❑ Sí ❑ No

22. ¿Has tenido problemas con la ley? .... ❑ Sí ❑ No

23. ¿Te preocupa la violencia o tu seguridad? .... ❑ Sí ❑ No ❑ No estoy seguro(a)

24. ¿Usas un casco cuando montas en patines, patineta, bicicleta, motocicleta, miniciclo, trimoto o arenero? .... ❑ No ❑ Sí

25. ¿Usas el cinturón de seguridad cuando viajas en carro, camión, o camioneta? .... ❑ No ❑ Sí

Tabaco

26. ¿Fumas cigarrillos/puros, masticas tabaco, o usas "snuff?" .... ❑ Sí ❑ No

27. ¿Alguno de tus amigos fuma cigarrillos/puros, mastica tabaco, o usa "snuff?" .... ❑ Sí ❑ No

28. ¿Alguna de las personas con quien vives fuma cigarrillos/puros, mastica tabaco, o usa "snuff?" .... ❑ Sí ❑ No

Alcohol

29. El mes pasado, ¿tuviste una borrachera con cerveza, vino, o alguna otra bebida alcohólica? .... ❑ Sí ❑ No

30. El mes pasado, ¿alguno de tus mejores amigos tuvo una borrachera con cerveza, vino, o alguna otra bebida alcohólica? .... ❑ Sí ❑ No

31. ¿Alguna vez te han criticado o has tenido problemas porque tomas? .... ❑ Sí ❑ No ❑ No estoy seguro(a)

32. ¿Bebiste alcohol este año pasado, y después manejaste un carro, camión, camioneta o motocicleta? .... ❑ Sí ❑ No ❑ No aplica

33. ¿Estuviste en un carro o algún otro vehículo este año pasado, en el cual el chofer estaba bebido o había usado drogas? .... ❑ Sí ❑ No

34. ¿Te preocupas por alguno de tu familia que toma mucho o usa drogas? .... ❑ Sí ❑ No

Drogas

35. ¿A veces usas marihuana u otras drogas, o inhalas goma o cosas parecidas? .... ❑ Sí ❑ No ❑ No estoy seguro(a)

36. ¿Alguno de tus mejores amigos usa marihuana u otras drogas, o inhala goma o cosas parecidas? .... ❑ Sí ❑ No ❑ No estoy seguro(a)

37. ¿Alguna vez has usado medicinas sin receta médica para poder dormir, estar despierto, calmarte, o ponerte en onda? .... ❑ Sí ❑ No
    (Medicinas que se pueden comprar en cualquier farmacia, sin receta médica)

38. ¿Has usado esteroides en pastilla o como inyección sin receta medica? .... ❑ Sí ❑ No ❑ No estoy seguro(a)

Desarrollo

39. ¿Te preocupa o quieres más información sobre la forma o tamaño de tu cuerpo, o tu apariencia física? .... ❑ Sí ❑ No ❑ No estoy seguro(a)

40. ¿Crees ser homosexual, lesbiana, o bisexual? .... ❑ Sí ❑ No ❑ No estoy seguro(a)

41. ¿Has tenido relaciones sexuales? .... ❏ Sí   ❏ No ❏ No estoy seguro(a)
    ¿Cuántos años tenías la primera vez?_____

42. ¿Estás usando algún método para prevenir el embarazo? .... ❏ No ❏ Sí   ❏ No tengo relaciones
    ¿Cuál? _____

43. ¿Usas condones cuando siempre tienes relaciones sexuales con tus pareja(s)? .... ❏ No ❏ Sí   ❏ No tengo relaciones

44. ¿Alguno de tus mejores amigos ha tenido relaciones sexuales? .... ❏ Sí   ❏ No ❏ No estoy seguro(a)

45. ¿Te ha dicho alguna vez algún doctor o enfermera que tienes una enfermedad o
    infección que se transmite sexualmente? .... ❏ Sí   ❏ No ❏ No estoy seguro(a)

46. ¿Has estado embarazada alguna vez, o has sido tú el que embarazó a alguna joven? .. ❏ Sí   ❏ No ❏ No estoy seguro(a)

47. ¿Quieres información o cosas que te ayuden a evitar embarazos, o infecciones
    transmitidas sexualmente? .... ❏ Sí   ❏ No ❏ No estoy seguro(a)

48. ¿Quieres saber cómo evitar contraer el virus del VIH/SIDA? .... ❏ Sí   ❏ No ❏ No estoy seguro(a)

49. ¿Te has perforaste (excluyendo las orejas) o recibiste algún tatuaje en el cuerpo? .... ❏ Sí   ❏ No ❏ Lo estoy pensando

Emociones

50. ¿Te has divertido en las últimas dos semanas? .... ❏ No ❏ Sí

51. Durante las últimas dos semanas, ¿te has sentido triste con frecuencia,
    o desganado, o como si no tuvieras nada que buscar en la mañana? .... ❏ Sí   ❏ No

52. ¿Alguna vez has seriamente pensado en el suicidio, hecho planes para hacerlo, o
    tratado de matarte? .... ❏ Sí   ❏ No

53. ¿Alguna vez te han abusado físicamente, sexualmente, o emocionalmente? .... ❏ Sí   ❏ No ❏ No estoy seguro(a)

54. ¿Haces cosas violentas cuando te enojas? .... ❏ Sí   ❏ No

55. ¿Deseas tener una consulta profesional sobre algo que te está molestando? .... ❏ Sí   ❏ No ❏ No estoy seguro(a)

Circunstancias Especiales

56. En los últimos 12 meses, ¿estuviste con alguien que tiene tuberculosis? .... ❏ Sí   ❏ No ❏ No estoy seguro(a)

57. ¿Te has quedado alguna noche en un refugio para desamparados, cárcel,
    o prisión juvenil? .... ❏ Sí   ❏ No

58. ¿Has vivido en un hogar adoptivo o una casa para grupos de jóvenes? .... ❏ Sí   ❏ No

Sobre Tu Persona

59. ¿Cuáles son las cuatro palabras que mejor describen cómo eres? _____

60. Si pudieras cambiar algo en tu vida, o en tu persona, ¿qué cosa cambiarías? _____
    _____

61. ¿De qué cosas quieres hablar hoy? _____

97-896:1.2M:11/97

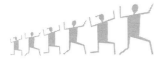

Guidelines for Adolescent Preventive Services
Parent/Guardian Questionnaire

Confidential (Your answers will not be given out.)

Date _____

Adolescent's name _____ Adolescent's birthday _____ Age _____

Parent/Guardian name _____ Relationship to adolescent _____

Your phone number: Home _____ Work _____

Adolescent Health History

1. Is your adolescent allergic to any medicines?
   ☐ Yes ☐ No   If yes, what medicines? _____

2. Please provide the following information about medicines your adolescent is taking.

Name of medicine	Reason taken	How long taken
_____	_____	_____
_____	_____	_____
_____	_____	_____

3. Has your adolescent ever been hospitalized overnight?
   ☐ Yes ☐ No   If yes, give the age at time of hospitalization and describe the problem.

Age	Problem
_____	_____
_____	_____

4. Has your adolescent ever had any serious injuries?
   ☐ Yes ☐ No   If yes, please explain. _____

5. Have there been any changes in your adolescent's health during the past 12 months?
   ☐ Yes ☐ No   If yes, please explain. _____

6. Please check (✔) whether your adolescent ever had any of the following health problems:
   If yes, at what age did the problem start:

	Yes	No	Age		Yes	No	Age
ADHD/learning disability	☐	☐	____	Headaches/migraines	☐	☐	____
Allergies/hayfever	☐	☐	____	Low iron in blood (anemia)	☐	☐	____
Asthma	☐	☐	____	Pneumonia	☐	☐	____
Bladder or kidney infections	☐	☐	____	Rheumatic fever or heart disease	☐	☐	____
Blood disorders/sickle cell anemia	☐	☐	____	Scoliosis (curved spine)	☐	☐	____
Cancer	☐	☐	____	Seizures/epilepsy	☐	☐	____
Chicken pox	☐	☐	____	Severe acne	☐	☐	____
Depression	☐	☐	____	Stomach problems	☐	☐	____
Diabetes	☐	☐	____	Tuberculosis (TB)/lung disease	☐	☐	____
Eating disorder	☐	☐	____	Mononucleosis (mono)	☐	☐	____
Emotional disorder	☐	☐	____	Other: _____	☐	☐	____
Hepatitis (liver disease)	☐	☐	____				

7. Does this office or clinic have an up-to-date record of your adolescent's immunizations (record of "shots")?
   ☐ Yes ☐ No ☐ Not sure

Family History

8. Some health problems are passed from one generation to the next. Have you or any of your adolescent's *blood* relatives (parents, grandparents, aunts, uncles, brothers or sisters), living or deceased, had any of the following problems? If the answer is "Yes," please state the age of the person when the problem occurred and his or her relationship to your adolescent.

	Yes	No	Unsure	Age at Onset	Relationship
Allergies/asthma	☐	☐	☐	_____	_____
Arthritis	☐	☐	☐	_____	_____
Birth defects	☐	☐	☐	_____	_____
Blood disorders/sickle cell anemia	☐	☐	☐	_____	_____

AA59:97-894:11/97

	Yes	No	Unsure	Age at Onset	Relationship
Cancer (type_____)	☐	☐	☐	_____	_____
Depression	☐	☐	☐	_____	_____
Diabetes	☐	☐	☐	_____	_____
Drinking problem/alcoholism	☐	☐	☐	_____	_____
Drug addiction	☐	☐	☐	_____	_____
Endocrine/gland disease	☐	☐	☐	_____	_____
Heart attack or stroke *before* age 55	☐	☐	☐	_____	_____
Heart attack or stroke *after* age 55	☐	☐	☐	_____	_____
High blood pressure	☐	☐	☐	_____	_____
High cholesterol	☐	☐	☐	_____	_____
Kidney disease	☐	☐	☐	_____	_____
Learning disability	☐	☐	☐	_____	_____
Liver disease	☐	☐	☐	_____	_____
Mental health	☐	☐	☐	_____	_____
Mental retardation	☐	☐	☐	_____	_____
Migraine headaches	☐	☐	☐	_____	_____
Obesity	☐	☐	☐	_____	_____
Seiures/epilepsy	☐	☐	☐	_____	_____
Smoking	☐	☐	☐	_____	_____
Tuberculosis/lung disease	☐	☐	☐	_____	_____

9. With whom does the adolescent live most of the time? *(Check all that apply.)*

☐ Both parents in same household   ☐ Stepmother   ☐ Sister(s)/ages _____
☐ Mother   ☐ Stepfather   ☐ Other _____
☐ Father   ☐ Guardian   ☐ Alone
☐ Other adult relative   ☐ Brother(s)/ages _____

10. In the past year, have there been any changes in your family? *(Check all that apply.)*

☐ Marriage   ☐ Loss of job   ☐ Births   ☐ Other _____
☐ Separation   ☐ Move to a new neighborhood   ☐ Serious illness
☐ Divorce   ☐ A new school or college   ☐ Deaths

Parental/Guardian Concerns

11. Please review the topics listed below. Check(✔) if you have a concern about your adolescent.

	Concern About My Adolescent		Concern About My Adolescent
Physical problems	☐	Guns/weapons	☐
Physical development	☐	School grades/absences/dropout	☐
Weight	☐	Smoking cigarettes/chewing tobacco	☐
Change of appetite	☐	Drug use	☐
Sleep patterns	☐	Alcohol use	☐
Diet/nutrition	☐	Dating/parties	☐
Amount of physical activity	☐	Sexual behavior	☐
Emotional development	☐	Unprotected sex	☐
Relationships with parents and family	☐	HIV/AIDS	☐
Choice of friends	☐	Sexual transmitted diseases (STDs)	☐
Self image or self worth	☐	Pregnancy	☐
Excessive moodiness or rebellion	☐	Sexual identity	
Depression	☐	(heterosexual/homosexual/bisexual)	☐
Lying, stealing, or vandalism	☐	Work or job	☐
Violence/gangs	☐	Other: _____	☐

12. What seems to be the greatest challenge for your teen? _____

13. What is it about your teen that makes you proud of him or her? _____

14. Is there something on your mind that you would like to talk about today?

   What is it? _____

15. Can we share your answers to Question 13 with your teen?   ☐ Yes   ☐ No

AA59:97-894:11/97

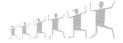

Confidencial (No le diremos a nadie lo que nos diga)

Fecha _____

Nombre del adolescente _____ Fecha de nacimiento _____ Edad _____

Nombre del Padre o Guardián _____ Su relación con el adolescente _____

Su número de teléfono: de casa (_____) _____ del trabajo (_____) _____

Historial Médico del Adolescente

1. ¿Es su adolescente alérgico a alguna medicina?
   ❏ Sí   ❏ No   Si la respuesta es *Sí*, ¿a cuál medicina? _____

2. Por favor, díganos qué medicinas está tomando su adolescente.
Nombre de la medicina	Razón para tomarla	Cuánto tiempo tiene tomándola

3. ¿Alguna vez ha estado hospitalizado su adolescente?
   ❏ Sí   ❏ No   Si la respuesta es *Sí*, escriba la edad que tenía y explique cuál era el problema.
   Edad   Problema

4. ¿Su adolescente alguna vez se ha lastimado seriamente?
   ❏ Sí   ❏ No   Si su respuesta es *Sí*, por favor explique. _____

5. ¿Ha notado cambios en la salud de su adolescente en los últimos 12 meses?
   ❏ Sí   ❏ No   Si su respuesta es *Sí*, por favor explique. _____

6. Por favor, marque (✓) si su adolescente alguna vez padeció de alguno de los siguientes problemas de salud. Si su respuesta es *Sí*, marque cuántos años tenía cuando comenzó el problema.

	Sí	No	Edad		Sí	No	Edad
Problemas de aprendizaje/ADHD	❏	❏	____	Dolores de Cabeza/Migrañas	❏	❏	____
Alergias	❏	❏	____	Falta de Hierro en la Sangre (anemia)	❏	❏	____
Asma	❏	❏	____	Pulmonía	❏	❏	____
Infección de la vejiga o de los riñones	❏	❏	____	Fiebre reumática o enfermed del corazón	❏	❏	____
Enfermedad de la Sangre	❏	❏	____	Escoliosis (columna vertebral curva)	❏	❏	____
Cáncer	❏	❏	____	Convulsiones/Epilepsia	❏	❏	____
Varicela	❏	❏	____	Acné	❏	❏	____
Depresión	❏	❏	____	Problemas Estomacales	❏	❏	____
Diabetes	❏	❏	____	Tuberculosis/enfermedad del pulmón	❏	❏	____
Problemas Alimenticios	❏	❏	____	Mononucleosis	❏	❏	____
Problemas Emocionales	❏	❏	____	Otra(s): _____	❏	❏	____
Hepatitis (enfermedad del hígado)	❏	❏					

7. ¿Tiene esta clínica toda la información sobre las vacunas de su adolescente?
   ❏ Sí   ❏ No   ❏ No estoy seguro

Historial Familiar

8. Algunos problemas de salud se pasan de generación a generación. ¿Hay alún pariente biológico, de su adolescente (padres, abuelos, tíos, o hermanos), que haya tenido alguna de las siguientes enfermedades? Incluya parientes vivos y difuntos. Si la respuesta es *Sí*, marque cuántos años tenía la persona cuando empezó el problema y su relación con su adolescente.

	Sí	No	No estoy seguro	Edad cuando empezó	Relación con el adolescente
Alergias/Asma	❏	❏	❏	_____	_____
Artritis	❏	❏	❏	_____	_____
Defectos de Nacimiento	❏	❏	❏	_____	_____
Enfermedad de sangre	❏	❏	❏	_____	_____
Cáncer (de qué tipo _____)	❏	❏	❏	_____	_____

Voltee la página

	Sí	No	No estoy seguro	Edad cuando empezó	Relación con el adolescente
Depresión	❑	❑	❑	_____	_____
Diabetes	❑	❑	❑	_____	_____
Problema con la bebida/Alcoholismo	❑	❑	❑	_____	_____
Adicción a drogas	❑	❑	❑	_____	_____
Enfermedad del sistema endocrino	❑	❑	❑	_____	_____
Ataques al Corazón o Embolias <u>antes</u> de los 55 años	❑	❑	❑	_____	_____
Ataques al Corazón o Embolias <u>después</u> de los 55 años	❑	❑	❑	_____	_____
Presión Alta	❑	❑	❑	_____	_____
Alto Nivel de Colesterol	❑	❑	❑	_____	_____
Enfermedad de los Riñones	❑	❑	❑	_____	_____
Problemas de Aprendizaje	❑	❑	❑	_____	_____
Enfermedad del Hígado	❑	❑	❑	_____	_____
Salud Mental	❑	❑	❑	_____	_____
Retardo Mental	❑	❑	❑	_____	_____
Migrañas	❑	❑	❑	_____	_____
Obesidad	❑	❑	❑	_____	_____
Convulsiones/Epilepsia	❑	❑	❑	_____	_____
Fumar	❑	❑	❑	_____	_____
Tuberculosis/enfermedad del pulmón	❑	❑	❑	_____	_____

9. ¿Con quién vive el adolescente la mayor parte del año? (Marque todas las que sean ciertas)
   - ❑ Ambos padres en la misma casa
   - ❑ Madre
   - ❑ Padre
   - ❑ Otro pariente adulto
   - ❑ Madrastra
   - ❑ Padrastro
   - ❑ Guardián Legal
   - ❑ Hermanos/edades _____
   - ❑ Hermanas/edades _____
   - ❑ Otra persona _____
   - ❑ Solo

10. En estos últimos 12 meses, ¿han habido cambios importantes en su familia? (Marque todos los que sean ciertos.)
    - ❑ Matrimonios
    - ❑ Separaciones
    - ❑ Divorcios
    - ❑ Alguien perdió el trabajo
    - ❑ Mudanzas a otros vecindarios
    - ❑ Cambio de escuela o universidad
    - ❑ Nacimientos
    - ❑ Enfermedades graves
    - ❑ Muertes
    - ❑ Otros_____
    - _____
    - _____

Preocupaciones de los padres o guardián

11. Por favor, fíjese en los temas que le damos a continuación. Marque (✓) si tiene <u>usted</u> alguna preocupación sobre algún tema con respecto a su adolescente.

	Me preocupa		Me preocupa
Problemas físicos	❑	Pistolas/armas	❑
Desarrollo físico	❑	Malas notas escolares/ausencias/abandono de estudios	❑
Peso	❑	Fumar cigarrillos/mascar tabaco	❑
Cambios en su apetito	❑	Uso de drogas	❑
Hábitos de dormir	❑	Uso de bebidas alcohólicas	❑
Hábitos de comer/nutrición	❑	Noviazgos/Fiestas	❑
La cantidad de actividad física	❑	Conducta sexual	❑
Desarrollo emocional	❑	Relaciones sexuales sin protección	❑
Su relación con sus padres y familia	❑	VIH/SIDA	❑
Tipo de amigos que tiene	❑	Enfermedades Transmitidas Sexualmente	❑
Auto-proyección o auto-estima	❑	El embarazo	❑
Cambios exagerados de carácter o rebelión	❑	Identidad Sexual (heterosexual, homosexual, bisexual)	❑
Depresión	❑	El trabajo u ocupación	❑
Mentir, robar, o vandalismo	❑	Otra_____	
Violencia/pandillas	❑		

12. ¿Cuáles son los retos personales más difíciles para su adolescente? _____

13. ¿Qué lo enorgullece de su adolescente? _____

14. Hoy, ¿Quisiera hablarnos sobre algo en especial? ¿Que? _____

15. ¿Nos permite mostrarle a su adolescente su respuesta a la Pregunta #13?   ❑ Sí   ❑ No

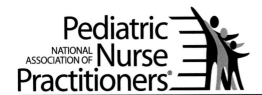

Important Information about Well-Child Visits for Parents

Understanding the Well-Child Visit

Every day, "healthy" children are brought to doctors and nurse practitioners for well-child visits. Leading pediatric authorities recommend routine visits, ideally beginning with a prenatal visit and continuing throughout infancy, childhood, and adolescence. The purpose of these visits is to help families keep children healthy as well as to pick up early signs of potential problems. These visits are so important to a child's health that both private and public insurance companies pay for them. This is because childhood is a unique period of time to lay the foundation for a person's health throughout life.

Yet a funny thing sometimes happens during these visits. The most important part of the visit gets overlooked. Many parents don't even realize that both they and their healthcare provider are forgetting to talk about the biggest threats to their child's well-being.

Many things happen during these visits. Many of the activities are very visible, like weighing a child and providing him or her with necessary immunizations. But sometimes, the most important part of the visit, the part that is not so easy to see, gets forgotten. That is the part of the visit that should be spent talking to your doctor or nurse practitioner about how your child is growing emotionally and mentally and the important role that behavior plays in keeping your child healthy.

Unlike 100 years ago, the greatest threats faced by children in this country today are not infection and physical illnesses. The Surgeon General and others have often called attention to the real risks to children's health today. **Children's health today is threatened most by behaviors**—their own behaviors, the behaviors of their families and friends, or sometimes the behavior of strangers. Many children and adolescents die from accidents and injuries, from homicide, and suicide. One in four has a mental health disorder and many more have behavior problems that interfere with their family relationships, their friendships, and their performance in school. Mental health problems appear in families of all social classes and backgrounds. Child mental health problems often continue into adulthood and worsen if untreated. Yet, more is known today than ever before about how to recognize early mental health problems in children and how to help them during the critical childhood years. It is most important that you talk to your healthcare provider about your child's emotions and behaviors on a regular basis and share your concerns.

There is nothing to be ashamed of if your child has an emotional or behavior problem. The sooner you share your concerns with your child's doctor or nurse practitioner, the faster your child can be helped.

**Please turn the page over to view
a list of steps you can take to keep your child healthy.**

Parents: Did you remember to talk to your doctor/nurse practitioner today about your child's behavior and emotions?

Remember:

Both parents and healthcare providers have a role to play in keeping children mentally and physically healthy.

How Can Parents Assure This Happens

1. Expect your pediatric healthcare provider to talk to you routinely about your child's behavior and emotions. Many doctors and nurse practitioners will use screening tools at every visit to help recognize when children are having more difficulties than usual.

2. Call or make an appointment to talk to your healthcare provider when you have concerns or worries about your child's behavior or emotions.

3. Some concerns can be dealt with in a single visit, but most will require follow-up calls or appointments. Following up is most important.

4. Some pediatric healthcare providers have more experience in behavior/mental health management than others. After taking a careful history, some providers may suggest that you be referred to a mental health clinician. Yet others will talk to you about some short-term interventions they may be able to provide, such as:

    a. Formal screening for mental health problems and strengths

    b. Discussions to help you and your child better understand the problem

    c. Brief solution-focused counseling sessions that help you and your child manage the problem

    d. Participation in group sessions with other parents or children

5. If the problem is not getting better or seems to be getting worse, do not hesitate to ask your healthcare provider for a referral to someone with expertise in the mental healthcare of children.

6. When your healthcare provider suggests certain treatments to deal with the problem, ask him or her for the evidence behind what is being recommended.

7. Keep your pediatric provider informed about your child's progress even after referral to a specialist. Your pediatric primary care provider has an important role to play in helping you to advocate for your child's continued mental and physical health.

Internet Resources and Professional Development Programs in Child and Adolescent Mental Health

American Academy of Child and Adolescent Psychiatry
www.aacap.org

This Website provides excellent information on the assessment and treatment of child and adolescent mental health disorders. Handouts addressing a multitude of problems (i.e., Facts for Families) are available.

American Academy of Pediatrics (AAP): Development and Behavior
http://www2.aap.org/sections/dbpeds/

This Website, sponsored by the AAP Section on Developmental and Behavioral Pediatrics (SODBP), is targeted to professionals interested in child development and behavior, especially in the clinical setting. It houses a variety of screening tools as well as educational handouts on developmental and behavioral problems that are downloadable for use in practice. There is a learning section that features "the toolbox," which is a link to special articles, features, keywords, and evidence. There also is a practice section that emphasizes practical information and tools to support primary care and specialty practice.

KidsHealth
www.kidshealth.org

This is an outstanding Website that contains health information for healthcare providers, parents, teens, and children. Many of the topics relate to emotions and behaviors (e.g., anxiety, fears, depression) and are developmentally sensitive to specific age groups. Physicians and other healthcare providers review all material before it is posted on this Website.

National Association of Pediatric Nurse Practitioners (NAPNAP)
www.napnap.org

This site can be accessed to keep abreast of all ongoing and new initiatives of NAPNAP. Mental health resources for providers are housed at the site in addition to fact sheets on a variety of mental health issues, which can be downloaded and printed for distribution.

National Institute of Mental Health
www.nimh.nih.gov

This Website contains outstanding evidence-based educational resources and publications on a variety of mental health disorders. Health information is arranged by age/gender and treatment across the life span. Fact sheets on a variety of disorders are available for downloading and distribution.

The Ohio State University's KySS℠ Child and Adolescent Mental Health Online Fellowship Program

The KySS program prepares pediatric and family nurse practitioners, family physicians, pediatricians, social workers, and other health professionals who care for children to accurately screen for, identify, and deliver early evidence-based interventions for affected children and teens. It is a collaborative among the Ohio State Colleges of Nursing, Medicine, and Social Work. Uniqueness of the KySS℠ program includes: 12 on-line modules that are self-paced to fit busy schedules, complemented by clinical learning activities, and guided by a faculty mentor with expertise in child and adolescent health. For more information, see **www.nursing.osu.edu**. Upon satisfactory completion of the entire fellowship program, the participants receive a KySS Fellowship Certificate from The Ohio State University and are well prepared to take the Pediatric Nursing Certification Board's pediatric primary care mental health specialist certification exam.

The REACH (REsource for Advancing Children's Health) Institute
http://www.thereachinstitute.org/about-REACH.html

The REACH Institute is dedicated to improving the mental health of American children and adolescents with emotional and behavioral challenges. It provides workshops for healthcare providers that teach the best evidence-based therapies, from psychotherapy to pharmacology, to improve the mental health of children and teens. Excellent resources at the Website are available for healthcare providers, agencies, and families.

United States Preventive Services Task Force (USPSTF)
http://www.ahrq.gov/clinic/uspstfix.htm

The USPSTF is an independent group of national experts in prevention and evidence-based practice that works to improve the health of all Americans by making evidence-based recommendations about clinical preventive services such as screenings, counseling services, or preventive medications. The USPSTF is made up of 16 volunteer members from the fields of preventive medicine and primary care, including internal medicine, family medicine, pediatrics, behavioral health, obstetrics/gynecology, and nursing. Every year, the USPSTF updates the Guide to Clinical Preventive Services, which contains evidence-based recommendations for a variety of topics, including screening for depression and obesity in children and adolescents.

REFERENCES

American Medical Association (1994). Guidelines for Adolescent Preventive Services. Available at **http://www.ama-assn.org/ama/pub/physician-resources/public-health/promoting-healthy-lifestyles/adolescent-health/guidelines-adolescent-preventive-services.page.**

Brown, J.D., & Wissow, L.S. (2010). Screening to identify mental health problems in primary care: Considerations for practice. *International Journal of Psychiatry in Medicine*, 40(1), 1-19.

Foy, J.M. (2010). Enhancing pediatric mental health care: Report from the American Academy of Pediatrics Task Force on Mental Health. *Pediatrics*, 125 Supplement 3, S69-S75.

Gardner, W., Lucas A., Kolko, D.J., & Campo, J.V. (2007). Comparison of the PSC-17 and alternative mental health screens in an at-risk primary care sample. *Journal of the American Academy of Child & Adolescent Psychiatry*, 46(5), 611-618.

Husky, M.M., Kanter, D.A., McGuire, L., & Olfson, M. (2012). Mental health screening of African American adolescents and facilitated access to care. *Community Mental Health Journal*, 48(1), 71-78.

Jellinek, M.S., & Murphy, J.M. (1998). Screening for psychosocial disorders in pediatric practice. *American Journal of Diseases of Children*, 145(11), 1153-1157.

Jellinek, M., Patel, B.P., & Froehle, M. (2002). *Bright Futures in Practice: Mental Health- Vol I. Practice Guide.* Arlington, VA: National Center for Education in Maternal and Child Health.

Jellinek, M., Patel, B.P., & Froehle, M. (2002). *Bright Futures in Practice: Mental Health- Vol II. Tool Kit.* Arlington, VA: National Center for Education in Maternal and Child Health.

Kessler, R.C., Berglund, P., Demier, O., Jin, R., Merikangas, I.K., & Walters, E.E. (2005). Lifetime prevalence and age of onset distributions of DSM-IV disorders in the National Co-morbidity Survey Replication. *Archives of General Psychiatry*, 62(6), 593-602.

Little, M., Murphy, J.M., Jellinek, M.S., Bishop, S.J., & Arnett, H.L. (1994). Screening four- and five-year-old children for psychosocial dysfunction: a preliminary study with the Pediatric Symptom Checklist. *Journal of Developmental and Behavioral Pediatrics*, 15(3), 191-197.

Melnyk, B.M., Grossman, D.C., Chou, R., Mabry-Hernandez, I., Nicholson, W., Dewitt, T.G., Cantu, A.G., & Flores, G.; US Preventive Services Task Force (2012). USPSTF perspective on evidence-based preventive recommendations for children. *Pediatrics*, 130(2), 399-407.

Merikangas, K. R., He, J., Burstein, M., Swanson, S., Avenevoli, S., Cui, L., Benjet, C., Georgiades, K., & Swendesen, J. (2010). Lifetime prevalence of mental disorders in U.S. adolescents: results from the National Co-morbidity Survey Replication – Adolescent supplement (NCS-A). *Journal of the American Academy of Child and Adolescent Psychiatry*, 49(10), 980-989.

Murphy, J.M., Arnett, H.L., Bishop, S.J., Jellinek, M.S., & Reede, J.Y. (1992). Screening for psychosocial dysfunction in pediatric practice. A naturalistic study of the Pediatric Symptom Checklist. *Clinical Pediatrics*, 31(11), 660-667.

Murphy, J.M., Ichinose, C., Hicks, R.C., Kingdon, D., Crist-Whitzel, J., Jordan, P., Feldman, G., & Jellinek, M.S. (1996). Screening for psychosocial dysfunction in pediatric practice. A naturalistic study of the Pediatric Symptom Checklist. *Journal of Pediatrics*, 129 (6), 864-869.

Murphy, J., & Jellinek, M.S. (1985). Development of a brief psychosocial screening instrument for pediatric practice: final report. NIMH Contract No. 84M0213612. Rockville, Md: National Institute of Mental Health.

Pagano, M., Murphy, J.M., Pederson, M., Mosbacher, D., Crist-Whitzel, J., Jordan, P., Rodas, C., & Jellinek, M.S. (1996). Screening for psychosocial problems in four- and five-year-olds during routine EPSDT examinations; validity and reliability in a Mexican-American sample. *Clinical Pediatrics*, 35, 139-146.

Sheldrick, R.C., Henson, B.S., Merchant, S., Neger, E.N., Murphy, J.M., & Perrin, E.C. (2012a). The preschool pediatric symptom checklist (PPSC): development and initial validation of a new social/emotional screening instrument. *Academic Pediatrics*, 12 (5), 456-467.

Sheldrick, R.C., Henson, B.S., Neger, E.N., Merchant, S., Murphy, J.M., & Perrin, E.C. (2012). The baby pediatric symptom checklist: development and initial validation of a new social/emotional screening instrument for very young children. *Academic Pediatrics*, Oct 20. pii: S1876-2859(12)00202-1 doi: 10.1016/j.acap.2012.08.003. [Epub ahead of print].

Stoppelbein, L., Greening, L., Moll, G., Jordan, S., & Suozzi, A. (2012). Factor analysis of the Pediatric Symptom Checklist-17 with African-American and Caucasian pediatric populations. *Journal of Pediatric Psychology*, 37(3), 348-357.

SECTION 2
Bernadette Mazurek Melnyk

Diagnosing, Managing, and Preventing Mental Health Disorders

Diagnosing Mental Health Disorders

The reliable diagnoses of mental health disorders are essential for guiding evidence-based treatment along with identifying prevalence rates for the planning of mental health services and accurately documenting important public health information, such as morbidity and mortality rates. Mental health disorders are diagnosed according to criteria in the Diagnostic and Statistical Manual of Mental Disorders, Fifth Edition (DSM-5™) by the American Psychiatric Association (APA). Diagnostic criteria include symptoms, behaviors, cognitive functions, personality traits, physical signs, syndrome combinations, and durations requiring clinical expertise to differentiate from normal life variation and treatment responses to stress (DSM-5™).

In the former edition, DSM-IV™, mental health disorders were classified according to the following multiaxial classification system that included the following categories:

- Axis I: Psychological disorders (e.g., major depressive disorder, generalized anxiety disorder)

- Axis II: Psychological disorders (e.g., borderline personality)/mental retardation)

- Axis III: General medical conditions (e.g., asthma, diabetes)

- Axis IV: Psychosocial and environmental problems (e.g., problems with primary support group, social environment; educational problems; occupational problems; housing problems; economic problems; problems with access to healthcare services; problems related to interaction with the legal system)

- Axis V: Global assessment of functioning (GAF) (e.g., psychological, social, and work functioning); a score is given on a scale of 100 (superior functioning) to 0 (inadequate information). For example, a score of 21-50 would indicate symptoms of serious impairment in social, occupational, or school functioning.

The DSM-5™ moved to a nonaxial documentation of diagnosis (formerly Axes I, II, and III) in which Axis III is combined with Axes I and II. Therefore, clinicians should continue to list medical conditions that are important to understanding and managing mental health disorders in their documentation. Further, even though the prior Axis IV contained information about psychosocial and environmental issues that could affect mental health disorders, the DSM-5™ recommends using the International Classification of Diseases (ICD-9 CM) codes and the new Z codes contained in ICD-10-CM for these issues. Axis V was dropped from the DSM-IV™ due to its lack of conceptual clarity and questionable psychometric properties (DSM-5™, 2013). Instead, it is recommended that clinicians use the World Health Organization Disability Assessment Schedule (WHODAS 2.0) to assess functioning. This assessment tool, along with several others, which were developed to be administered at the initial patient interview and to monitor treatment progress, are available from the APA at **http://www.psychiatry.org/practice/dsm/dsm5/online-assessment-measures**. A modification of this scale also is available for children/adolescents and their parents (WHODAS-child) and for youths aged 6 to 17 years.

It is important to exercise much caution when conferring DSM-5™ diagnoses on children and adolescents, as stigma and labeling can place additional burdens upon an already stressed family system, especially if the diagnosis is not accurate. However, correctly identifying a diagnosis and beginning early intervention as well as providing comprehensive psycho-education can be of enormous relief and can assist the child and family in obtaining positive outcomes. Before a diagnosis is made, it is necessary to gain collateral information from multiple sources (e.g., the child's parents, day care, school teachers) and to conduct a comprehensive interview with the child and family. If the diagnosis is in doubt and/or the disorder is complex or not responsive to early intervention strategies, it is critical to have the child seen and concurrently managed by a mental healthcare provider (e.g., psychiatrist, psychiatric mental health nurse practitioner, or psychologist).

General Approach to the Evidence-based Management of Mental Health Disorders in Children and Adolescents

Based upon the mental health assessment, a decision must be made to:

- Triage immediately

- Intervene

- Consult with a mental health professional

- Refer to a mental health professional (it is important to know the mental health specialists in your area and preferably to send the family to someone in close proximity; follow-up is critical to assure that the family has adhered to the referral)

— A good referral form template can be accessed at
   www.brightfutures.org/mentalhealth/pdf/index.html.

— Good referral rule of thumb:
   Always refer when a child is exhibiting behaviors that are dangerous to himself or others, including vandalism, fire setting, cruelty to animals, and self-harm.

— Possible referrals include:
   Psychiatrists, psychiatric mental health nurse practitioners, psychologists
   Outpatient services, Partial hospital services, Inpatient services, Emergency and urgent care services, Youth emergency services, lifeline, preventive services of the department of social services

— Barriers to referral include:
   Lack of mental healthcare providers/services
   Family reluctance to accept a mental health diagnosis
   Reluctance to "label" the child

In making a decision about management, **consider severity, persistence, and resistance to change**

Once a mental health problem is identified, support of and therapeutic communications with the family are critical.

Treating a child/teen for a mental health problem typically requires more than one person or system.

Many early interventions, especially with young children, are parent-focused.

School-age and teen interventions need to be skill oriented, and it is best to teach the skills to both children and parents.

Conduct therapeutic communication with the child and family (active listening and acknowledgment of the challenge).

Promote optimism about the process and outcomes:
> *Emphasize that mental health problems are treatable!*

Engage parents and child in an active role.

Focus on one achievable goal – what can be changed?

Children and parents need to learn where to turn for help and information, so it is important to know your community resources.

Encourage families to use multiple resources (reliable Internet resources, books, TV, school staff, healthcare, professionals, clergy, friends, extended family, mental healthcare professionals)

4-Goal Model for the Brief Mental Health Visit

Begin treatment while the diagnostic process is under way:

- Understand the concern (active listening)
- Rule out an emergency
- Make a diagnosis and start treatment
- Agree on a plan (engage the patient/parents and do something!)

From the 15-minute Mental Health Visit Webcast, which can be accessed at **http://www2.aap.org/sections/adolescenthealth/15minutewebcast.cfm.**

Psycho-education

Counseling parents and children/teens about what to expect in dealing with a particular condition is critical, as it will assist them in coping with the condition and adhering to treatment.

Psychosocial Interventions

More evidence exists for psychosocial interventions (e.g., cognitive behavioral therapy/cognitive behavior skills building) than for any other type of intervention in support of their efficacy for treating mood, anxiety, and behavior disorders.

— Lewinsohn and Clark's "Adolescent Coping with Stress and Coping with Depression" courses are evidence-based and downloadable for use without permission at www.kpchr.org/public/acwd/acwd.html.

— The COPE (Creating Opportunities for Personal Empowerment) Program, a 7-session manualized cognitive-behavioral skills building program for teens, is available from Dr. Bernadette Melnyk at cope.melnyk@gmail.com. A child and college age/young adult version of COPE also is available. Evidence to support the positive effects of COPE on depression, anxiety, and self-esteem is accumulating (Lusk & Melnyk, 2011; Melnyk et al., 2009; Melnyk, Kelly & Lusk, in press). A 15-session COPE Healthy Life-styles TEEN (Thinking, Emotions, Exercise, and Nutrition) program that contains the 7-session cognitive-behavioral skills building program with additional sessions on nutrition and physical activity also is available and has been shown to improve healthy lifestyle behaviors, physical and mental health, and social skills in adolescents as well as prevent overweight and obesity (Melnyk et al., 2009; Melnyk et al., in press).

Psychopharmacology

Medications supported as the most effective, on the basis of clinical trials with children and teens, include stimulant medications for attention-deficit/hyperactivity disorder (ADHD) and selective serotonin reuptake inhibitors (SSRIs) for obsessive-compulsive disorder and moderate to severe major depressive disorder (MDD). However, **medication alone is usually not fully effective in treating a mental health disorder.** A combination of medication with therapy/counseling typically leads to the best outcomes. Risperidone also has been empirically supported as an effective treatment for autism.

General rule of thumb when starting medication in children and teens:
Start Low, Go Slow!

Providers without in-depth psychopharmacology education and skills training should be extremely cautious about prescribing medications for mental health disorders in children and teens without consultation from a child psychiatrist or psychiatric mental health nurse practitioner.

Evidence-based management guidelines for some mental health disorders in children and adolescents can be found at **www.guideline.gov**; this is the National Guideline Clearinghouse for evidence-based clinical practice guidelines, sponsored by the Agency for Health Care Research and Quality and the American Medical Association (AMA). For information about how to critically appraise evidence-based guidelines, see Melnyk & Fineout-Overholt (2011).

Excellent Mental Health Resources for Healthcare Providers

The American Academy of Pediatrics' Task Force on Mental Health has created resources and an action tool kit to assist pediatric primary care providers in dealing with child and adolescent mental health problems, which can be downloaded at **www.aap.org/mentalhealth.**

Bright Futures in Practice: Mental Health-Volume I (Practice Guide) and Volume II (Tool kit) (2002) can be downloaded with no charge at: **www.brightfutures.org/mentalhealth/.** Bright Futures is a national health promotion initiative dedicated to the principle that every child deserves to be healthy; it is now housed at the Bright Futures Educational Center at the American Academy of Pediatrics. Although now over a decade since publication, it still contains relevant resources and tools.

Foy, J.M. (2010). Enhancing pediatric mental health care: Report from the American Academy of Pediatrics Task Force on Mental Health (2010). Pediatrics, 125 (Supplement 3). Download at **http://pediatrics.aappublications.org/content/125/Supplement_3.toc**. The supplement contains the following articles:

— Enhancing pediatric mental healthcare: Strategies for preparing a community

— Enhancing pediatric mental healthcare: Strategies for preparing a primary care practice

— Enhancing pediatric mental healthcare: Algorithms for primary care
  The National Institute of Mental Health has a Website that contains outstanding evidence-based educational resources and publications on a variety of mental health disorders for healthcare providers (see www.nimh.nih.gov).

The REACH (REsource for Advancing Children's Health) Institute is committed to accelerating the acceptance and use of evidence-based interventions that foster children's emotional and behavioral health. REACH's web site contains helpful resources for health professionals and families at **http://www.thereachinstitute.org/**

Stahl, S.M. (2011). The Prescriber's Guide. Stahl's Essential Psychopharmacology. New York, NY: Cambridge University Press. This publication is an excellent psychopharmacology handbook.

Knowing is not enough; we must apply. Willing is not enough; we must do.

—GOETHE

Prevention of Mental Health / Psychosocial Morbidities in Children and Teens

Prevention of mental health disorders should occur at the primary, secondary, and tertiary levels. Interventions should target the family, school, and community.

Primary prevention must start during pregnancy or at birth with parenting education and support (e.g., anticipatory guidance about normal developmental milestones and characteristics, temperament, discipline, and positive parenting strategies to facilitate self-esteem and close relationships).

Remember that it is much easier to prevent behaviors that have never started than to curtail negative patterns. It is never too early to begin parent effectiveness training.

Parent Effectiveness Training as a Preventive and Early Intervention Strategy

Important tips to provide to parents:

- Provide positive reinforcement/praise: "Catch children being good!"
- Provide specific praise (e.g., "I like the way you brushed your teeth without me telling you to today" instead of "You are a good girl").
- Promote independence and age-appropriate control.
- Set age-appropriate limits.
- Reward cooperative behavior (e.g., special time together, stickers).
- Provide age-appropriate independence and competencies.
- Give gradual increases in work responsibilities with increasing age.
- Allow children to make choices.
- Allow children to struggle some with challenges to build their coping strategies.
- Do not rush to answer questions for children.
- Help children learn to problem-solve and find resources to address their challenges.
- Define position on at-risk behaviors (e.g., zero tolerance for drug or alcohol use).
- Avoid double standards (e.g., "Do as I say, not as I do"), as modeling is a powerful learning mechanism.
- Don't make excuses for children/teens. (If they think there is a problem, there usually is.)
- Frequently communicate expectations to children regarding behaviors and school performance.
- Become acquainted with their friends and the parents of their friends (hold meetings to determine group rules).

Additional strategies:

- Provide parents with excellent resources for parenting (see section Websites and other resources).
- Caution parents to prevent their children/teens – especially those under 13 years of age – from watching R-rated movies.
- Help parents to assist their children in dealing with the current stressful events in their lives and in our society.
- Encourage parents to take time for themselves to rest or relax, and to seek counseling if highly stressed, anxious, or depressed; emphasize to them that their mood state will affect their children.
- Emphasize the importance of daily physical activity and exercise in releasing stress and anxiety for all family members.
- Encourage family activities and outings.

Important Information about Limit-Setting for Parents

- All feelings are okay; all behaviors are not.

- Work on only 1 or 2 limits at a time.

- Make sure that consequences are age appropriate.

- Follow through on limits set.

- Teach parents structured choices.

- Give children at least 2 choices about something that needs to happen. This increases decision-making ability, cooperation, independence, and self-esteem. For example: "Do you want to do your homework before or after dinner today? You decide -- it's up to you."

Teach Parents How to Help Their School-Age Children and Teens
- Problem-solve

  — Identify the problem.

  — Identify the cause of the problem.

  — Generate solutions.

  — Discuss the consequence of each solution.

  — Choose a solution and put it into action.

- Develop positive patterns of thinking

  — Teach the thinking, behaving, and emotion triangle (i.e., how you think affects how you behave and how you feel. If you think you are stupid, you will feel depressed and not attempt to do better in school). It is necessary to stop the negative thought and turn it into a positive one (e.g., "Okay, I may not have done as well on my math test as I should have, but I'm good at English." The consequence is feeling emotionally better).

- Control anger

  — Help the child identify anger triggers and cues as well as implement cool down strategies, such as:

    - Counting to 10 or saying the alphabet
    - Diaphragmatic breathing
    - Walking away
    - Positive self-talk (e.g., "I am calming down")
    - Writing it down
    - Talking it out
    - Listening to music
    - Communicating his/her anger to the person in appropriate ways
    - Telling the other person he or she is angry, using "I" instead of "You" statements
    - Channeling the anger in appropriate ways (e.g., use physical activity)
    - Learning to accept no for an answer or unchangeable situations (e.g., you cannot change other people, only how to respond to them)

Parents and Children/Teens Need to Know How to Access Resources

- Children/teens and parents need to learn where to turn for help and information.
- It is critical to know your community resources.
- Reinforce to children/teens and parents that you deal with their mental and emotional health just as you deal with their physical health.
- Encourage families to use multiple resources (e.g., the Internet, books, school staff, healthcare professionals, extended family, and mental healthcare professionals).

Other Preventive Strategies

- Screen for mental health/psychosocial morbidities at every healthcare encounter.
- Assess parenting competence, style, stressors, and presence of mental health problems.
- Raise awareness of these problems (e.g., use posters in practice settings, distribute handouts, teach parenting classes).
- Build developmental assets in children/teen and parents as well communities (e.g., teach effective communication strategies, problem-solving skills, refusal skills, and coping strategies; provide children and teens with opportunities for involvement in community education).
- Implement preventive strategies for children and teens at highest risk for psychopathology and for those who have experienced traumatic events, including motor vehicle accidents, hospitalization, and rape, as well as family and neighborhood violence.
- Encourage parents to be actively involved in their children's lives, and to monitor their activities (e.g., who, what, when, and where) as well as the things that they are reading, watching, and listening to.
- Emphasize to parents the importance of mentoring and modeling healthy behaviors.
- Advise parents to require 48-hour advance notice for sleeping over at a friend's house, as most drug and alcohol parties come together at the last minute.
- Encourage parents to spend special time with their children/teens and to listen to them.
- Facilitate mentors for children/teens, as those who have mentors are less likely to use illegal drugs and alcohol and are less likely to skip school.
- Encourage service to others, such as belonging to sport/club/hobby/religious groups.
- Provide opportunities for children to be successful; encourage mastery of skill development; teach coping and problem-solving strategies as well as refusal skills; build relationships with youth.
- Teach children coping and problem-solving skills (e.g., encourage journaling and creative expression with school-age children and teens).
- Detect abuse and neglect early, address poverty, build strong families with supports/resources.
- Use quality resources to promote mental health in your state.

Internet Resources

ACT for Youth (Assets Coming Together)
http://www.actforyouth.net/)
The ACT for Youth Center of Excellence is an excellent resource that links research to practice in areas of positive youth development and adolescent sexual health. The Center provides publications and presentations as well as technical assistance and training and education.

Bright Futures Handouts for Families
www.brightfutures.org/
Encounter forms for each well-child visit throughout childhood and adolescence can be accessed at this site.

The Children's Mental Health Resource Kit: Promoting Children's Mental Health Screens and Assessments
http://www.childrensdefense.org/child-research-data-publications/data/childrens-mental-health-resource-kit.pdf
This Resource Kit can be accessed on the Website or by calling 202-662-3575.

Creating Opportunities for Parent Empowerment (COPE)
http://copeforhope.com/
This Website provides a series of evidence-based intervention materials that can be easily administered in clinical practice settings, aimed at parents with children experiencing marital separation or divorce, hospitalization, critical illness, and those experiencing the birth of a premature infant.

The REACH (REsource for Advancing Children's Health) Institute
http://www.thereachinstitute.org/about-REACH.html
The REACH Institute is dedicated to improving the mental health of American children and adolescents with emotional and behavioral challenges. It provides workshops for healthcare providers that teach the best evidence-based therapies, from psychotherapy to pharmacology, to improve the mental health of children and teens. Excellent resources at the Website are available for healthcare providers, agencies, and families.

REFERENCES

Foye, J.M. (2010). Enhancing pediatric mental health care: Report from the American Academy of Pediatrics Task Force on Mental Health. *Pediatrics*, 125(Suppl 3), S69-S195.

Jellinek, M., Patel, B.P., & Froehle, M. (2002). *Bright Futures in Practice: Mental Health-Vol I. Practice Guide.* Arlington, VA: National Center for Education in Maternal and Child Health.

Jellinek, M. Patel, B.P., & Froehle, M. (2002). *Bright Futures in Practice: Mental Health-Vol II. Tool Kit.* Arlington, VA: National Center for Education in Maternal and Child Health.

Lusk, P., & Melnyk, B.M. (2011). The brief cognitive-behavioral COPE intervention for depressed adolescents: outcomes and feasibility of delivery in 30-minute outpatient visits. *Journal of the American Psychiatric Nurses Association*, 17(3), 226-236.

Melnyk, B.M., & Fineout-Overholt, E. (2011). Evidence-Based Practice in Nursing & Healthcare. *A Guide to Best Practice (2nd edition).* Philadelphia, Pa: Wolters Kluwer/Lippincott Williams & Wilkins.

Melnyk, B.M., Kelly, S., & Lusk, P. (in press). Outcomes and feasibility of a manualized cognitive-behavioral skills building intervention: group COPE for depressed and anxious adolescents in school settings. *Journal of the American Psychiatric Nurses Association.*

Melnyk, B.M., Jacobson, D., Kelly, S., et al. (in press). Promoting healthy lifestyles in high school adolescents. A randomized controlled trial. *American Journal of Preventive Medicine.*

Melnyk, B.M., Jacobson, D., Kelly, S., O'Haver, J., Small, L., & Mays, M.Z. (2009). Improving the mental health, healthy lifestyle choices and physical health of Hispanic adolescents: a randomized controlled pilot study. *Journal of School Health*, 79(12), 575-584.

SECTION 3
Holly Brown & Bernadette Mazurek Melnyk

Anxiety Disorders

Information for Healthcare Providers About Anxiety Disorders

Fast Facts

- Fear and anxiety are a normal part of a child's development, but they should not be excessive, interfere with functioning, or persist beyond developmentally appropriate periods. Routine screening is recommended.

- Fear is the emotional response to a real or perceived impending threat whereas anxiety is anticipation of a future threat.

- Anxiety disorders are among the most common mental health problems in children and teens.

- Children and teens with anxiety disorders experience severe and persistent distress that interferes with their daily functioning; often these disorders are significantly under-reported, undetected, and under-diagnosed.

- Parents describe these children as "worriers."

- Comorbidities are the rule and not the exception, such as depression, oppositional defiant disorder, learning disorders, eating disorders, attention-deficit/hyperactivity disorder (ADHD), and substance abuse.

- Children with anxiety disorders are often misdiagnosed with ADHD.

- Depressive symptoms are often present with anxiety disorders.

- Somatic complaints such as stomach pain, headaches, chest pain, and fatigue are common (see Table 3.1 for common signs of anxiety).

- Panic disorder is characterized by recurrent unexpected panic attacks, which are abrupt surges of intense fear or discomfort that reaches a peak within minutes.

Table 3.1 Common Signs of Anxiety in Children and Teens

Physical	Behavioral	Cognitive
Restlessness and irritability (very common in younger children)	Escape/avoidant behaviors	"What if...?" (cognitive distortions, negativistic thinking)
Agitation	Crying	
	Clinging to/fear of separation from parents	Catastrophic thoughts (threat bias, low perceived control)
Fidgeting	Soft voice	
Headaches	Variations in speech	Worry about things before they happen
Abdominal complaints (e.g., stomachaches, nausea, vomiting, diarrhea)	Nail-biting	
Sleep difficulties	Thumb-sucking	Constant worries or concerns about family, school, friends, or activities
	Vigilance and scanning	
Fatigue	Freezing	
Palpitations, increased heart rate, increased blood pressure	Regression (bedwetting, temper tantrums)	
Hyperventilation or shortness of breath	Insomnia	
Muscle tension	Poor concentration	
	Social withdrawal	
Dizziness, tingling, weakness	Social skills deficits	
Tremors	Anger (especially in adolescents)	

Anxiety Spectrum Diagnoses

- Separation anxiety disorder
- Selective mutism (consistent failure to speak in specific social situations in which one is expected to speak (e.g., at school)
- Specific phobia (marked fear or anxiety about a specific object or situation (e.g., heights, animals, flying)
- Social anxiety disorder (social phobia): marked fear or anxiety about one or more social situations
- Panic disorder (recurrent unexpected panic attacks during which time four of the following symptoms occur: palpitations, pounding heart, or fast heart rate; sweating; trembling or shaking; sensations of shortness of breath; feelings of choking; chest pain or discomfort; nausea or abdominal distress; feeling dizzy, light-headed or faint; chills or heat sensations; paresthesias; derealization (feelings of unreality) or depersonalization (being detached from oneself); fear of losing control or "going crazy"; and fear of dying (DSM-5™).
- Panic attack specifier (when it accompanies another disorder, such as posttraumatic stress disorder)
- Agoraphobia (fear or anxiety about certain situations, such as using public transportation or being outside of the home alone)
- Generalized anxiety disorder
- Substance/medication-induced anxiety disorder
- Anxiety disorder due to another medical condition
- Other specified anxiety disorder
- Unspecified anxiety disorder (from the DSM-5™, 2013)

Other Related Disorders

- Trauma- and stressor-related disorders, which include:

— Posttraumatic stress disorder

— Acute stress disorder

- Posttraumatic stress disorder
- Obsessive compulsive disorder

Critical History-Taking Questions

- Is the anxiety appropriate for the age of the child or teen?
- Does the child have symptoms in response to a specific stimulus (e.g., social situations); is it spontaneous (free-floating or present all the time for no particular reason); or is it anticipatory?
- What are the situations or factors that bring the anxiety symptoms on? What are the reinforcers for anxiety symptoms (e.g., school refusal and parent staying home from work)?
- Has this child/teen experienced a traumatic event (e.g., has the child been a witness to domestic violence, experienced physical/sexual abuse)?
- Is there a history of recent stressful life events, marital transition, or family members with mental health disorders?
- Does the anxiety interfere with or impair the child's daily functioning, such as school attendance and grades, social relationships or activities, or family relationships, routines, and family accommodation for anxiety symptoms?
- What impact do the anxiety symptoms have on the child's sleep, energy, appetite, and concentration?
- Is there a family history of anxiety disorders in biological relatives?
- Are there accompanying signs of depression?

Medical Conditions to be Ruled Out

- Hypoglycemia
- Hyperthyroidism
- Pheochromocytoma
- Seizure disorder
- Cardiac arrhythmia
- Migraine headaches
- Brain tumor
- Hypoxia
- Asthma
- Lead intoxication

Medications/Drugs That May Cause Anxiety

Caffeine (assess intake of: carbonated beverages, energy drinks, coffee)

- Nicotine
- Diet pills
- Antihistamines
- Antiasthmatics (e.g., theophylline)
- Marijuana
- Sympathomimetics (e.g., nasal decongestants such as pseudoephedrine)
- Stimulants (including cocaine)
- Steroids
- Antipsychotics (e.g., side effects such as akathisia)
- SSRIs (e.g., Celexa, Prozac, Luvox, Paxil, Zoloft)

Treatment

Careful screening and assessment; goal is to diagnose and determine severity

- Educate parents and children about common signs and symptoms
- Environmental changes: promote optimal sleep habits, decrease stressors, establish and/or reinforce predictable schedules and/or routines
- Individual therapy (cognitive behavioral therapy [CBT] or cognitive behavioral skills building with the COPE [Creating Opportunities for Personal Empowerment] Program [see depressive disorders section], interpersonal therapy, play therapy); combination CBT and psychopharmacological intervention is safe and more effective than CBT alone to reduce severe anxiety in children diagnosed with these disorders (Walkup et al., 2008).
- Enhance coping skills, both as a preventive intervention and management
- Behavioral intervention: contingency management (e.g. positive reinforcement, shaping of behaviors, extinction)
- Family interventions
  - Parent anxiety management
  - Teaching parents to function as co-therapists in the home environment (i.e., the CBT therapist transfers skills to the parents, who then transfer skills to the anxious child in the home environment)
- Pharmacological intervention
  - First-line: antidepressants (SSRIs)/anti-anxiety agents and buspirone (Buspar)
  - Second-line: venlafaxine (Effexor) and benzodiazepines
  - Alternatives: alpha-adrenergic agents, beta blockers, or antihistamines
  - See Table 3.2 for medications used to treat pediatric anxiety disorders

Table 3.2 Medication Guide for Pediatric Anxiety Disorders

Medication	Indications	Side Effects	Dosing		
			Initial (mg)	Range (mg/day)	Schedule
Selective Serotonin Reuptake Inhibitors (SSRIs)	First-line treatment Nonaddictive Well tolerated	Gastrointestinal (GI) side effects Weight gain or loss Dry mouth Insomnia Somnolence Headaches Irritability Restlessness Sexual side effects Sweating Tremor **Carefully consider Black Box Warning		Use the lowest dose to treat symptoms	
Citalopram (Celexa)			5-20	10-60	QD; QAM
Escitalopram (Lexapro)			5-10	10-20	QD; QAM
Fluoxetine (Prozac)			5-20	10-80	QD; QAM
Fluvoxamine (Luvox)			12.5-50	50-300	BID to TID
Paroxetine (Paxil)			5-10	0-60	QD; QAM or PM
Sertraline (Zoloft)			12.5-25	50-200	QD-BID; QAM
Buspirone (Buspar)	First-line Treatment for generalized anxiety Nonaddictive Well Tolerated	Headache Nausea Dizziness Lightheadedness Somnolence	5 BID	5-60	BID-TID
Benzodiazepines	Second-line treatment	Sedation Cognitive blunting		BID-TID	
Diazepam (Valium)		Dizziness	1-2 HS	0.25-4	HS-BID
Clonazepam (Klonopin)	Addiction potentia and cognitive blunting	Ataxia Memory disturbance Constipation Diplopia	0.125-0.5	0.125-3	HS-BID
Lorazepam (Ativan)	Time-limited circumstances	Hypotension	0.125-0.5 BID	0.125-4	HS-TID

Adapted from: Ghalib, K.D., Vidair, H.B., Woodcome, H.A., Walkup, J.T. & Rynn, M.A. (2011). Assessment and treatment of child and adolescent anxiety disorders. In: Martin, A., Scahill, L., & Kratochvil, C.J. (Eds.), Pediatric Psychopharmacology Principles and Practice, 2nd ed. New York: Oxford University Press, pp. 480-495.

**Note: Caution must be exercised when prescribing SSRIs to children and adolescents with psychiatric disorders, as studies have shown an increased risk for suicidal thinking (suicidality) in the first few months after starting treatment. Patients started on SSRIs should be monitored weekly for the first 4 weeks of treatment for increased anxiety symptoms, presence of or increase in suicidality, or unusual changes in behavior. Families should be advised to monitor for these signs/symptoms and alert their provider if present.

DSM-5™ Diagnostic Criteria for Separation Anxiety Disorder

A. Developmentally inappropriate and excessive fear or anxiety concerning separation from those to whom the individual is attached, as evidenced by at least three of the following:

1. Recurrent excessive distress when anticipating or experiencing separation from home or from major attachment figures.

2. Persistent and excessive worry about losing major attachment figures or about possible harm to them, such as illness, injury, disasters, or death.

3. Persistent and excessive worry about experiencing an untoward event (e.g., getting lost, being kidnapped, having an accident, becoming ill) that causes separation from a major attachment figure.

4. Persistent reluctance or refusal to go out, away from home, to school, to work, or elsewhere because of fear of separation.

5. Persistent and excessive fear of or reluctance about being alone or without major attachment figures at home or in other settings.

6. Persistent reluctance or refusal to sleep away from home or to go to sleep without being near a major attachment figure.

7. Repeated nightmares involving the theme of separation.

8. Repeated complaints of physical symptoms (e.g., headaches, stomachaches, nausea, vomiting) when separation from major attachment figures occurs or is anticipated.

B. The fear, anxiety, or avoidance is persistent, lasting at least 4 weeks in children and adolescents and typically 6 months or more in adults.

C. The disturbance causes clinically significant distress or impairment in social, academic, occupational, or other important areas of functioning.

D. The disturbance is not better explained by another mental disorder, such as refusing to leave home because of excessive resistance to change in autism spectrum disorder; delusions or hallucinations concerning separation in psychotic disorders; refusal to go outside without a trusted companion in agoraphobia; worries about ill health or other harm befalling significant others in generalized anxiety disorders; or concerns about having an illness in illness anxiety disorder.

DSM-5™ Diagnostic Criteria for Generalized Anxiety Disorder

A. Excessive anxiety and worry (apprehensive expectation), occurring more days than not for at least 6 months, about a number of events or activities (such as work or school performance).

B. The individual finds it difficult to control the worry.

The anxiety and worry are associated with three (or more) of the following six symptoms (with at least some symptoms having been present for more days than not for the past 6 months):

Note: Only one item is required in children.

Restlessness or feeling keyed up or on edge.

Being easily fatigued.

Difficulty concentrating or mind going blank.

Irritability.

Muscle tension.

Sleep disturbance (difficulty falling or staying asleep, or restless, unsatisfying sleep).

C. The anxiety, worry, or physical symptoms cause clinically significant distress or impairment in social, occupational, or other important areas of functioning.

D. The disturbance is not attributable to the physiological effects of a substance (e.g., a drug of abuse, a medication) or another medical condition (e.g., hyperthyroidism).

E. The disturbance is not better explained by another mental disorder (e.g., anxiety or worry about having panic attacks in panic disorder, negative evaluation in social anxiety disorder [social phobia], contamination or other obsessions in obsessive-compulsive disorder, separation from attachment figures in separation anxiety disorder, reminders of traumatic events in posttraumatic stress disorder, gaining weight in anorexia nervosa, physical complaints in symptom disorder, perceived appearance flaws in body dysmorphic disorder, having a serious illness anxiety disorder, or the content of delusional beliefs in schizophrenia or delusional disorder).

Reprinted with permission from the Diagnostic and Statistical Manual of Mental Disorders, Fifth Edition,
(Copyright ©2013). American Psychiatric Association. All Rights Reserved.

DSM-5™ Diagnostic Criteria for Acute Stress Disorder

A. Exposure to actual or threatened death, serious injury, or sexual violation in one (or more) of the following ways:

   1. Directly experiencing the traumatic event(s).

   2. Witnessing, in person, the event(s) as it occurred to others.

   3. Learning that the event(s) occurred to a close family member or close friend.

      Note: In cases of actual or threatened death of a family member or friend, the event(s) must have been violent or accidental.

   4. Experiencing repeated or extreme exposure to aversive details of the traumatic event(s) (e.g., first responders collecting human remains, police officers repeatedly exposed to details of child abuse).

      Note: This does not apply to exposure through electronic media, television, movies, or pictures, unless this exposure is work related.

A. Presence of nine (or more) of the following symptoms from any of the five categories of intrusion, negative mood, dissociation, avoidance, and arousal, beginning or worsening after the traumatic event(s) occurred:

Intrusion Symptoms

   1. Recurrent, involuntary, and intrusive distressing memories of the traumatic event(s).

      Note: In children, repetitive play may occur in which themes or aspects of the traumatic event(s) are expressed.

   2. Recurrent distressing dreams in which the content and/or affect of the dream are related to the event(s).

      Note: In children, there may be frightening dreams without recognizable content.

   3. Dissociative reactions (e.g., flashbacks) in which the individual feels or acts as if the traumatic event(s) were recurring. (Such reactions may occur on a continuum, with the most extreme expression being a complete loss of awareness of present surroundings.)

      Note: In children, trauma-specific reenactment may occur in play.

   4. Intense or prolonged psychological distress or marked physiological reactions in response to internal or external cues that symbolize or resemble an aspect of the traumatic event(s).

DSM-5™ Diagnostic Criteria for Posttraumatic Stress Disorder

Posttraumatic Stress Disorder

Note: The following criteria apply to adults, adolescents, and children older than 6 years. For children 6 years and younger, see corresponding criteria below.

A. Exposure to actual or threatened death, serious injury, or sexual violence in one (or more) of the following ways:

   1. Directly experiencing the traumatic event(s).

   2. Witnessing, in person, the event(s) as it occurred to others.

   3. Learning that the traumatic event(s) occurred to a close family member or close friend. In cases of actual or threatened death of a family member or friend, the event(s) must have been violent or accidental.

   4. Experiencing repeated or extreme exposure to aversive details of the traumatic event(s) (e.g., first responders collecting human remains; police officers repeatedly exposed to details of child abuse).

      Note: Criterion A4 does not apply to exposure through electronic media, television, movies, or pictures, unless this exposure is work related.

B. Presence of one (or more) of the following intrusion symptoms associated with the traumatic event(s), beginning after the traumatic event(s) occurred:

   1. Recurrent, involuntary, and intrusive distressing memories of the traumatic event(s).

      Note: In children older than 6 years, repetitive play may occur in which themes or aspects of the traumatic event(s) are expressed.

   2. Recurrent distressing dreams in which the content and/or affect of the dream are related to the traumatic event(s).

      Note: In children, there may be frightening dreams without recognizable content.

   3. Dissociative reactions (e.g., flashbacks) in which the individual feels or acts as if the traumatic event(s) were recurring. (Such reactions may occur on a continuum, with the most extreme expression being a complete loss of awareness of present surroundings.)

      Note: In children, trauma-specific reenactment may occur in play.

   4. Intense or prolonged psychological distress at exposure to internal or external cues that symbolize or resemble an aspect of the traumatic event(s).

   5. Marked physiological reactions to internal or external cues that symbolize or resemble an aspect of the traumatic event(s).

C. Persistent avoidance of stimuli associated with the traumatic event(s), beginning after the traumatic event(s) occurred, as evidenced by one or both of the following:

   1. Avoidance of or efforts to avoid distressing memories, thoughts, or feelings about or closely associated with the traumatic event(s).

1. Avoidance of or efforts to avoid external reminders (people, places, conversations, activities, objects, situations) that arouse distressing memories, thoughts, or feelings about or closely associated with the traumatic event(s).

A. Negative alterations in cognitions and mood associated with the traumatic event(s), beginning or worsening after the traumatic event(s) occurred, as evidenced by two (or more) of the following:

   1. Inability to remember an important aspect of the traumatic event(s) (typically due to dissociative amnesia and not to other factors such as head injury, alcohol, or drugs).

   2. Persistent and exaggerated negative beliefs or expectations about oneself, others, or the world (e.g., "I am bad," "No one can be trusted," "The world is completely dangerous," "My whole nervous system is permanently ruined").

   3. Persistent, distorted cognitions about the cause or consequences of the traumatic event(s) that lead the individual to blame himself/herself or others.

   4. Persistent negative emotional state (e.g., fear, horror, anger, guilt, or shame).

   5. Markedly diminished interest or participation in significant activities.

   6. Feelings of detachment or estrangement from others.

   7. Persistent inability to experience positive emotions (e.g., inability to experience happiness, satisfaction, or loving feelings).

B. Marked alterations in arousal and reactivity associated with the traumatic event(s), beginning or worsening after the traumatic event(s) occurred, as evidenced by two (or more) of the following:

   1. Irritable behavior and angry outbursts (with little or no provocation) typically expressed as verbal or physical aggression toward people or objects.

   2. Reckless or self-destructive behavior.

   3. Hypervigilance.

   4. Exaggerated startle response.

   5. Problems with concentration.

   6. Sleep disturbance (e.g., difficulty falling or staying asleep or restless sleep).

C. Duration of the disturbance (Criteria B, C, D, and E) is more than 1 month.

D. The disturbance causes clinically significant distress or impairment in social, occupational, or other important areas of functioning.

E. The disturbance is not attributable to the physiological effects of a substance (e.g., medication, alcohol) or another medical condition.

Specify whether:

   With dissociative symptoms: The individual's symptoms meet the criteria for posttraumatic stress disorder, and in addition, in response to the stressor, the individual experiences persistent or recurrent symptoms of either of the following:

1. **Depersonalization:** Persistent or recurrent experiences of feeling detached from, and as if one were an outside observer of, one's mental processes or body (e.g., feeling as though one were in a dream; feeling a sense of unreality of self or body or of time moving slowly).

2. **Derealization:** Persistent or recurrent experiences of unreality of surroundings (e.g., the world around the individual is experienced as unreal, dreamlike, distant, or distorted).

Note: To uses this subtype, the dissociative symptoms must not be attributable to the physiological effects of a substance (e.g., blackouts, behavior during alcohol intoxication) or another medical condition (e.g., complex partial seizures).

Specify if:

With delayed expression: If the full diagnostic criteria are not met until at least 6 months after the event (although the onset and expression of some symptoms may be immediate).

Posttraumatic Stress Disorder for Children 6 Years and Younger

A. In children 6 years and younger, exposure to actual or threatened death, serious injury, or sexual violence in one (or more) of the following ways:

1. Directly experiencing the traumatic event(s).

2. Witnessing, in person, the event(s) as it occurred to others, especially primary caregivers.

   Note: Witnessing does not include events that are witnessed only in electronic media, television, movies, or pictures.

3. Learning that the traumatic event(s) occurred to a parent or caregiving figure.

B. Presence of one (or more) of the following intrusion symptoms associated with the traumatic event(s), beginning after the traumatic event(s) occurred:

1. Recurrent, involuntary, and intrusive distressing memories of the traumatic event(s).

   Note: Spontaneous and intrusive memories may not necessarily appear distressing and may be expressed as play reenactment.

2. Recurrent distressing dreams in which the content and/or affect of the dream are related to the traumatic event(s).

   Note: It may not be possible to ascertain that the frightening content is related to the traumatic event.

3. Dissociative reactions (e.g., flashbacks) in which the child feels or acts as if the traumatic event(s) were recurring. (Such reactions may occur on a continuum, with the most extreme expression being a complete loss of awareness of present surroundings.) Such trauma-specific reenactment may occur in play.

4. Intense or prolonged psychological distress at exposure to internal or external cues that symbolize or resemble an aspect of the traumatic event(s).

5. Marked physiological reactions to reminders of the traumatic event(s).

A. One (or more) of the following symptoms, representing either persistent avoidance of stimuli associated with the traumatic event(s) or negative alterations in cognitions and mood associated with the traumatic event(s), must be present, beginning after the event(s) or worsening after the event(s):

Persistent Avoidance of Stimuli

1. Avoidance of or efforts to avoid activities, places, or physical reminders that arouse recollections of the traumatic event(s).

2. Avoidance of or efforts to avoid people, conversations, or interpersonal situations that arouse recollections of the traumatic event(s).

Negative Alterations in Cognition

3. Substantially increased frequency of negative emotional states (e.g., fear, guilt, sadness, shame, confusion).

4. Markedly diminished interest or participation in significant activities, including constriction of play.

5. Socially withdrawn behavior.

6. Persistent reduction in expression of positive emotions.

B. Alterations in arousal and reactivity associated with the traumatic event(s), beginning or worsening after the traumatic event(s) occurred, as evidenced by two (or more) of the following:

1. Irritable behavior and angry outbursts (with little or no provocation) typically expressed as verbal or physical aggression toward people or objects (including extreme temper tantrums).

2. Hypervigilance.

3. Exaggerated startle response.

4. Problems with concentration.

5. Sleep disturbance (e.g., difficulty falling or staying asleep or restless sleep).

C. The duration of the disturbance is more than 1 month.

D. The disturbance causes clinically significant distress or impairment in relationships with parents, siblings, peers, or other caregivers or with school behavior.

E. The disturbance is not attributable to the physiological effects of a substance (e.g., medication or alcohol) or another medical condition.

Specify whether:

With dissociative symptoms: The individual's symptoms meet the criteria for posttraumatic stress disorder, and the individual experiences persistent or recurrent symptoms of either of the following:

1. **Depersonalization:** Persistent or recurrent experiences of feeling detached from, and as if one were an outside observer of, one's mental processes or body (e.g., feeling as though one were in a dream; feeling a sense of unreality of self or body or of time moving slowly).

2. **Derealization:** Persistent or **recurrent experiences of unreality of surroundings (e.g., the world around the individual is experienced as unreal, dreamlike, distant, or distorted).**

Note: To use this subtype, the dissociative symptoms must not be attributable to the physiological effects of a substance (e.g., blackouts, behavior during alcohol intoxication) or another medical condition (e.g., complex partial seizures).

Specify if:

With delayed expression: If the full diagnostic criteria are not met until at least 6 months after the event (although the onset and expression of some symptoms may be immediate).

DSM-5™ Diagnostic Criteria for Obsessive-Compulsive Disorder

A. Presence of obsessions, compulsions, or both:

Obsessions are defined by (1) and (2):

1. Recurrent and persistent thoughts, urges, or images that are experienced, at some time during the disturbance, as intrusive and unwanted, and that in most individuals cause marked anxiety or distress.

2. The individual attempts to ignore or suppress such thoughts, urges, or images, or to neutralize them with some other thought or action (i.e., by performing a compulsion).

Compulsions are defined by (1) and (2):

1. Repetitive behaviors (e.g., hand washing, ordering, checking) or mental acts (e.g., praying, counting, repeating words silently) that the individual feels driven to perform in response to an obsession or according to rules that must be applied rigidly.

3. The behaviors or mental acts are aimed at preventing or reducing anxiety or distress, or preventing some dreaded event or situation; however, these behaviors or mental acts are not connected in a realistic way with what they are designed to neutralize or prevent, or are clearly excessive.
    Note: Young children may not be able to articulate the aims of these behaviors or mental acts.

A. The obsessions or compulsions are time-consuming (e.g., take more than 1 hour per day) or cause clinically significant distress or impairment in social, occupational, or other important areas of functioning.

A. `The obsessive-compulsive symptoms are not attributable to the physiological effects of a substance (e.g., a drug of abuse, a medication) or another medical condition.

A. The disturbance is not better explained by the symptoms of another mental disorder (e.g., excessive worries, as in generalized anxiety disorder; preoccupation with appearance, as in body dysmorphic disorder; difficulty discarding or parting with possessions, as in hoarding disorder; hair pulling, as in trichotillomania [hair-pulling disorder]; skin picking, as in excoriation [skin-picking] disorder; stereotypies, as in stereotypic movement disorder; ritualized eating behavior, as in eating disorders; preoccupation with substances or gambling, as in substance-related and addictive disorders; preoccupation with having an illness, as in illness anxiety disorder; sexual urges or fantasies, as in paraphilic disorders; impulses, as in disruptive, impulse-control, and conduct disorders; guilty ruminations, as in major depressive disorder; thought insertion or delusional preoccupations, as in schizophrenia spectrum and other psychotic disorders; or repetitive patterns of behavior, as in autism spectrum disorder).

Specify if:

With good or fair insight: The individual recognizes that obsessive-compulsive disorder beliefs are definitely or probably not true or that they may or may not be true.

With poor insight: The individual thinks obsessive-compulsive disorder beliefs are probably true.

With absent insight/delusional beliefs: The individual is completely convinced that obsessive-compulsive disorder beliefs are true.

Specify if:

Tic-related: The individual has a current or past history of a tic disorder.

The State-Trait Anxiety Inventory for Children
(C. D. Spielberger, et al.)

Description of the STAIC

The STAIC differentiates between anxiety proneness to anxious behavior rooted in personality (trait anxiety) and anxiety as a fleeting emotional state (state anxiety). The instrument is targeted to measure anxiety in upper elementary or junior high school students. It consists of two 20-item Likert scales. The STAIC S-Anxiety scale consists of 20 statements that ask children how they feel at a **particular moment in time**. The STAIC T-Anxiety scale also consists of 20 item statements, but children respond to these items by indicating how they **generally** feel. Examples from the state anxiety questionnaire include:

1. I feel	very relaxed	relaxed	not relaxed
2. I feel	very upset	upset	not upset

Age Range

While especially constructed to measure anxiety in 9- to 12-year-old children, the STAIC also may be used for younger children with average or above reading ability and for older children who are below average in ability.

Psychometric Properties of the STAIC

Studies have supported the validity and internal consistency of the STAIC. Normed scores are available for fourth-, fifth-, and sixth-grade elementary school children.

Ordering Information

The STAIC can be obtained from Mind Garden online at www.mindgarden.com/ or by calling 650-261-3550.

The State-Trait Anxiety Inventory for Adults
(C. D. Spielberger, et al.)

Description of the STAI

The STAI also differentiates between proneness to anxious behavior rooted in personality (trait anxiety) and anxiety as a fleeting emotional state (state anxiety). The instrument is targeted to measure anxiety in adults as well as in high school and college-age students. It consists of two 20-item Likert scales and can be administered in 10 minutes. The STAI S-Anxiety scale consists of 20 statements that ask individuals how they feel at a **particular moment in time**. The STAI T-Anxiety scale also consists of 20 item statements, but individuals respond to these items by indicating how they **generally** feel.

Examples from the state anxiety questionnaire include:

1	2	3	4
Almost Never	Sometimes	Often	Almost Always

	1	2	3	4
A. I feel at ease	1	2	3	4
B. I feel upset	1	2	3	4

Examples from the T-Anxiety scale include:

1	2	3	4
Almost Never	Sometimes	Often	Almost Always

	1	2	3	4
A. I am a steady person	1	2	3	4
B. I lack self-confidence	1	2	3	4

Age Range

Adults as well as high school and college-age students

Psychometric Properties

The STAI is a valid and highly reliable tool for measuring anxiety. Normed scores are available for adults as well as for high school and college students.

Ordering Information
Both of these scales can be obtained from
Mind Garden online at www.mindgarden.com/ or by calling 650-261-3550.

KySS Worries Questionnaire (Ages 10-21 years)
(Bernadette Mazurek Melnyk and Zendi Moldenhauer)

Description of the KySS Worries Questionnaire

The KySS Worries Questionnaire is a 15-item Likert-scale questionnaire that taps common worries in older school-age children and youth. A parent version of the scale also is available. The original scale consisted of 13 items. Since the original scale was created, two additional items (#14-weight and #15-level of activity/exercise) were added to the scale.

Age Range

The worries questionnaire is targeted for use with older school-age children and teens, between the ages of 10 and 21 years of age. A separate scale targets the worries of parents of school-age children and teens.

Psychometric Properties

Content validity was established by pediatric and mental health experts. Face validity was established by 15 parents as well as 15 children and teens, between 10 and 20 years of age. Cronbach's alpha with a sample of 621 school-age children and teens was .87 for the first 13 items on the scale. Cronbach's alpha with a sample of 603 parents was .90 for the first 13 items on the scale.

Use

These instruments are in the public domain and may be reproduced and used without permission from the authors.

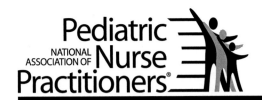

Please answer each of the following questions by circling your answers.

Do you worry about any of the following for yourself?

		Not at all	Sometimes	Often	Nearly always	Always
1)	Depression	1	2	3	4	5
2)	Anxiety	1	2	3	4	5
3)	Parents separating or divorcing	1	2	3	4	5
4)	Violence/being hurt	1	2	3	4	5
5)	Physical abuse/neglect	1	2	3	4	5
6)	Sexual abuse/rape	1	2	3	4	5
7)	Sexual activity	1	2	3	4	5
8)	Substance abuse	1	2	3	4	5
9)	Eating disorders	1	2	3	4	5
10)	Problems with your self-esteem	1	2	3	4	5
11)	Your relationship with your parents	1	2	3	4	5
12)	Knowing how to cope with things that stress you	1	2	3	4	5
13)	Being made fun of by your friends	1	2	3	4	5
14)	Your weight	1	2	3	4	5
15)	Your level of activity/exercise	1	2	3	4	5

16)   Do you have any other worries? If yes, please describe them.

_____

_____

17)   Do your worries interfere with your ability to do school work? ___ Yes ___No

18)   Do your worries affect your relationship with your friends?   ___ Yes ___ No

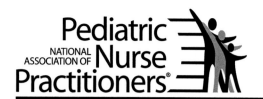

Please answer each of the following questions by circling your answers.

Do you worry about any of the following for child?

		Not at all	Sometimes	Often	Nearly always	Always
1)	Depression	1	2	3	4	5
2)	Anxiety	1	2	3	4	5
3)	Parents separating or divorcing	1	2	3	4	5
4)	Violence/being hurt	1	2	3	4	5
5)	Physical abuse/neglect	1	2	3	4	5
6)	Sexual abuse/rape	1	2	3	4	5
7)	Sexual activity	1	2	3	4	5
8)	Substance abuse	1	2	3	4	5
9)	Eating disorders	1	2	3	4	5
10)	Problems with your self-esteem	1	2	3	4	5
11)	Your relationship with your parents	1	2	3	4	5
12)	Knowing how to cope with things that stress you	1	2	3	4	5
13)	Being made fun of by your friends	1	2	3	4	5
14)	Your weight	1	2	3	4	5
15)	Your level of activity/exercise	1	2	3	4	5

16) Do you have any other worries about your child? If yes, please describe them.

_____

_____

17) Do your child's worries interfere with your ability to do school work? ___ Yes ___No

18) Do your child's worries affect your relationship with your friends? ___ Yes ___ No

Generalized Anxiety Disorder-7 and Generalized Anxiety Disorder-2 Scales

Description

The Generalized Anxiety Disorder 7 (GAD-7) is a self-reported screening questionnaire for anxiety, which has seven items that measure severity of various signs of generalized anxiety disorder according to reported response categories of "not at all," "several days," "more than half the days," and "nearly every day." Assessment is indicated by the total score, which is determined by adding together the scores for all seven items of the scale. Although originally developed to diagnose generalized anxiety disorder, the GAD-7 also has good sensitivity and specificity as a screening tool for panic, social anxiety, and post-traumatic stress disorder. It is available in many languages (see http://www.phqscreeners.com/).

The Generalized Anxiety Disorder 2 (GAD-2) scale consists of the first two questions from the GAD-7. Assessment is indicated by the total score on the two items.

Age Range

Although the majority of psychometric testing has been conducted with adults (Kroenke, 2010), the GAD-7 is being widely used with adolescents.

Psychometric Properties

Studies have supported the validity and reliability of the GAD-7 as a measure of anxiety in the general population (Kroenke, 2010; Lowe et al., 2008; Spitzer et al., 2006). The GAD-7 and GAD-2 (the shorter two-item questionnaire) has high sensitivity and specificity for generalized anxiety disorder and high specificity for panic disorder, social anxiety disorder, and post-traumatic stress disorder (Kroenke, 2007).

Scoring

Cut points of 5, 10, and 15 represent mild, moderate, and severe levels of anxiety. When screening for anxiety disorders, a recommended cut point for further evaluation is a score of 10 or greater. A total score on the GAD-2 of >3 suggests anxiety disorder or panic disorder (Spitzer, 2006).

Use

The GAD-7 and GAD-2 are in the public domain and no permission is required to reproduce, translate, display or distribute the tool.

GENERALIZED ANXITY DISORDER 7 Item (GAD-7) Scale

Over the last 2 weeks, how often have you been bothered by the following problems?	Not at all sure	Several days	Over half the days	Nearly every day
1. Feeling nervous, anxious, or on edge	0	1	2	3
2. Not being able to stop or control worrying	0	1	2	3
3. Worrying too much about different things	0	1	2	3
4. Trouble relaxing	0	1	2	3
5. Being so restless that it's hard to sit still	0	1	2	3
6. Becoming easily annoyed or irritable	0	1	2	3
7. Feeling afraid as if something awful might happen	0	1	2	3
Add the score for each column	+	+	+	
Total Score *(add your column scores)* =				

If you checked off any problems, how difficult have these made it for you to do your work, take care of things at home, or get along with other people?

Not difficult at all _____
Somewhat difficult _____
Very difficult _____
Extremely difficult _____

Source: Spitzer RL, Kroenke K, Williams JBW, Lowe B. A brief measure for assessing generalized anxiety disorder. *Arch Inern Med.* 2006;166:1092-1097.

Developed by Drs. Robert L. Spitzer, Janet B.W. Williams, Kurt Kroenke and colleagues, with an educational grant from Pfizer Inc. No permission required to reproduce, translate, display, or distribute.

Screen for Child Anxiety Related Disorders (SCARED)
Child Version and Parent Version

Description

The screen for child anxiety related disorders (SCARED) is a 41-item self-report questionnaire that taps anxiety related disorders. Children answer each of the 41 items (e.g., "When I feel frightened, it's hard to breathe"; "I get headaches when I am at school") on a 0 to 3 scale from "Not True or Hardly Ever True" or "Somewhat True or Sometimes True" or "Very True or Often True" to describe their mental state over the past 3 months.

Age

The scale is appropriate for use in 8- to 17-year-old children and teens, and their parents.

Psychometric Properties

The SCARED has established validity and excellent internal consistency reliability (Birmaher et al., 1997; Monga et al., 2000).

Scoring

A total score of ≥25 may indicate the presence of an anxiety disorder. Scores higher than 30 are more specific. Cut-off scores on specific items may indicate panic disorder, generalized anxiety disorder, separation anxiety, social anxiety disorder, and significant school avoidance (see the SCARED tool on the following pages for the items that are totaled for cut-off scores to determine the specific anxiety disorders that may exist).

Availability

Free for download on Website: http://www.psychiatry.pitt.edu/research/tools-research/assessment-instruments. At the end of the instrument, there is information regarding scoring the instrument.

Screen for Child Anxiety Related Disorders (SCARED)
CHILD Version—Page 1 of 2 (to be filled out by the CHILD)

Developed by Boris Birmaher, M.D., Suneeta Khetarpal, M.D., Marlane Cully, M.Ed., David Brent, M.D., and Sandra McKenzie, Ph.D., Western Psychiatric Institute and Clinic, University of Pittsburgh *(October, 1995). E-mail:* birmaherb@upmc.edu

See: Birmaher, B., Brent, D. A., Chiappetta, L., Bridge, J., Monga, S., & Baugher, M. (1999). Psychometric properties of the Screen for Child Anxiety Related Emotional Disorders (SCARED): a replication study. *Journal of the American Academy of Child and Adolescent Psychiatry, 38*(10), 1230–6.

Name: _____   Date: _____

Directions:
Below is a list of sentences that describe how people feel. Read each phrase and decide if it is "Not True or Hardly Ever True" or "Somewhat True or Sometimes True" or "Very True or Often True" for you. Then, for each sentence, fill in one circle that corresponds to the response that seems to describe you *for the last 3 months*.

	0 Not True or Hardly Ever True	1 Somewhat True or Sometimes True	2 Very True or Often True	
1. When I feel frightened, it is hard to breathe	O	O	O	PN
2. I get headaches when I am at school.	O	O	O	SH
3. I don't like to be with people I don't know well.	O	O	O	SC
4. I get scared if I sleep away from home.	O	O	O	SP
5. I worry about other people liking me.	O	O	O	GD
6. When I get frightened, I feel like passing out.	O	O	O	PN
7. I am nervous.	O	O	O	GD
8. I follow my mother or father wherever they go.	O	O	O	SP
9. People tell me that I look nervous.	O	O	O	PN
10. I feel nervous with people I don't know well.	O	O	O	SC
11. I get stomachaches at school.	O	O	O	SH
12. When I get frightened, I feel like I am going crazy.	O	O	O	PN
13. I worry about sleeping alone.	O	O	O	SP
14. I worry about being as good as other kids.	O	O	O	GD
15. When I get frightened, I feel like things are not real.	O	O	O	PN
16. I have nightmares about something bad happening to my parents.	O	O	O	SP
17. I worry about going to school.	O	O	O	SH
18. When I get frightened, my heart beats fast.	O	O	O	PN
19. I get shaky.	O	O	O	PN
20. I have nightmares about something bad happening to me.	O	O	O	SP

Used with permission

	0 Not True or Hardly Ever True	1 Somewhat True or Sometimes True	2 Very True or Often True	
21. I worry about things working out for me.	O	O	O	GD
22. When I get frightened, I sweat a lot.	O	O	O	PN
23. I am a worrier.	O	O	O	GD
24. I get really frightened for no reason at all.	O	O	O	PN
25. I am afraid to be alone in the house.	O	O	O	SP
26. It is hard for me to talk with people I don't know well.	O	O	O	SC
27. When I get frightened, I feel like I am choking.	O	O	O	PN
28. People tell me that I worry too much.	O	O	O	GD
29. I don't like to be away from my family.	O	O	O	SP
30. I am afraid of having anxiety (or panic) attacks.	O	O	O	PN
31. I worry that something bad might happen to my parents.	O	O	O	SP
32. I feel shy with people I don't know well.	O	O	O	SC
33. I worry about what is going to happen in the future.	O	O	O	GD
34. When I get frightened, I feel like throwing up.	O	O	O	PN
35. I worry about how well I do things.	O	O	O	GD
36. I am scared to go to school.	O	O	O	SH
37. I worry about things that have already happened.	O	O	O	GD
38. When I get frightened, I feel dizzy.	O	O	O	PN
39. I feel nervous when I am with other children or adults and I have to do something while they watch me (for example: read aloud, speak, play a game, play a sport).	O	O	O	SC
40. I feel nervous when I am going to parties, dances, or any place where there will be people that I don't know well.	O	O	O	SC
41. I am shy.	O	O	O	SC

SCORING:

A total score of ≥ **25** may indicate the presence of an **Anxiety Disorder**. Scores higher than 30 are more specific. **TOTAL =**

A score of **7** for items 1, 6, 9, 12, 15, 18, 19, 22, 24, 27, 30, 34, 38 may indicate **Panic Disorder** or **Significant Somatic Symptoms.** **PN =**

A score of **9** for items 5, 7, 14, 21, 23, 28, 33, 35, 37 may indicate **Generalized Anxiety Disorder.** **GD =**

A score of **5** for items 4, 8, 13, 16, 20, 25, 29, 31 may indicate **Separation Anxiety SOC.** **SP =**

A score of **8** for items 3, 10, 26, 32, 39, 40, 41 may indicate **Social Anxiety Disorder.** **SC =**

A score of **3** for items 2, 11, 17, 36 may indicate **Significant School Avoidance.** **SH =**

For children ages 8 to 11, it is recommended that the clinician explain all questions, or have the child answer the questionnaire sitting with an adult in case they have any questions.

The SCARED is available at no cost at www.wpic.pitt.edu/research under tools and assessments, or at www.pediatric bipolar.pitt.edu under instruments.

March 27, 2012

Screen for Child Anxiety Related Disorders (SCARED)
PARENT Version—Page 1 of 2 (to be filled out by the PARENT)

Developed by Boris Birmaher, M.D., Suneeta Khetarpal, M.D., Marlane Cully, M.Ed., David Brent, M.D., and Sandra McKenzie, Ph.D., Western Psychiatric Institute and Clinic, University of Pittsburgh *(October, 1995). E-mail:* birmaherb@upmc.edu

See: Birmaher, B., Brent, D. A., Chiappetta, L., Bridge, J., Monga, S., & Baugher, M. (1999). Psychometric properties of the Screen for Child Anxiety Related Emotional Disorders (SCARED): a replication study. *Journal of the American Academy of Child and Adolescent Psychiatry, 38*(10), 1230–6.

Name: _____   Date: _____

Directions:

Below is a list of sentences that describe how people feel. Read each phrase and decide if it is "Not True or Hardly Ever True" or "Somewhat True or Sometimes True" or "Very True or Often True" for your child. Then, for each statement, fill in one circle that corresponds to the response that seems to describe your child *for the last 3 months.* Please respond to all statements as well as you can, even if some do not seem to concern your child.

	0 Not True or Hardly Ever True	1 Somewhat True or Sometimes True	2 Very True or Often True	
1. When my child feels frightened, it is hard for him/her to breathe	O	O	O	PN
2. My child gets headaches when he/she am at school.	O	O	O	SH
3. My child doesn't like to be with people he/she does't know well.	O	O	O	SC
4. My child gets scared if he/she sleeps away from home.	O	O	O	SP
5. My child worries about other people liking him/her.	O	O	O	GD
6. When my child gets frightened, he/she fells like passing out.	O	O	O	PN
7. My child is nervous.	O	O	O	GD
8. My child follows me wherever I go.	O	O	O	SP
9. People tell me that my child looks nervous.	O	O	O	PN
10. My child feels nervous with people he/she doesn't know well.	O	O	O	SC
11. My child gets stomachaches at school.	O	O	O	SH
12. When my child gets frightened, he/she feels like he/she is going crazy.	O	O	O	PN
13. My child worries about sleeping alone.	O	O	O	SP
14. My child worries about being as good as other kids.	O	O	O	GD
15. When my child gets frightened, he/she feels like things are not real.	O	O	O	PN
16. My child has nightmares about something bad happening to his/her parents.	O	O	O	SP
17. My child worries about going to school.	O	O	O	SH
18. When my child gets frightened, his/her heart beats fast.	O	O	O	PN
19. He/she child gets shaky.	O	O	O	PN
20. My child has nightmares about something bad happening to him/her.	O	O	O	SP

Used with permission

	0 Not True or Hardly Ever True	1 Somewhat True or Sometimes True	2 Very True or Often True	
21. My child worries about things working out for him/her.	O	O	O	GD
22. When my child gets frightened, he/she sweats a lot.	O	O	O	PN
23. My child is a worrier.	O	O	O	GD
24. My child gets really frightened for no reason at all.	O	O	O	PN
25. My child is afraid to be alone in the house.	O	O	O	SP
26. It is hard for my child to talk with people he/she doesn't know well.	O	O	O	SC
27. When my child gets frightened, he/she feels like he/she is choking.	O	O	O	PN
28. People tell me that my child worries too much.	O	O	O	GD
29. My child doesn't like to be away from his/her family.	O	O	O	SP
30. My child is afraid of having anxiety (or panic) attacks.	O	O	O	PN
31. My child worries that something bad might happen to his/her parents.	O	O	O	SP
32. My child feels shy with people he/she doesn't know well.	O	O	O	SC
33. My child worries about what is going to happen in the future.	O	O	O	GD
34. When my child gets frightened, he/she feels like throwing up.	O	O	O	PN
35. My child worries about how well he/she does things.	O	O	O	GD
36. My child is scared to go to school.	O	O	O	SH
37. My child worries about things that have already happened.	O	O	O	GD
38. When my child gets frightened, he/she feels dizzy.	O	O	O	PN
39. My child feels nervous when he/she is with other children or adults and he/she has to do something while they watch him/her (for example: read aloud, speak, play a game, play a sport).	O	O	O	SC
40. My child feels nervous when he/she is going to parties, dances, or any place where there will be people that he/she doesn't know well.	O	O	O	SC
41. My child is shy.	O	O	O	SC

SCORING:

A total score of ≥ **25** may indicate the presence of an **Anxiety Disorder**. Scores higher than 30 are more specific. | TOTAL = |

A score of **7** for items 1, 6, 9, 12, 15, 18, 19, 22, 24, 27, 30, 34, 38 may indicate **Panic Disorder** or **Significant Somatic Symptoms**. | PN = |

A score of **9** for items 5, 7, 14, 21, 23, 28, 33, 35, 37 may indicate **Generalized Anxiety Disorder**. | GD = |

A score of **5** for items 4, 8, 13, 16, 20, 25, 29, 31 may indicate **Separation Anxiety SOC**. | SP = |

A score of **8** for items 3, 10, 26, 32, 39, 40, 41 may indicate **Social Anxiety Disorder**. | SC = |

A score of **3** for items 2, 11, 17, 36 may indicate **Significant School Avoidance**. | SH = |

The SCARED is available at no cost at www.wpic.pitt.edu/research under tools and assessments, or at www.pediatric bipolar.pitt.edu under instruments.

March 27, 2012

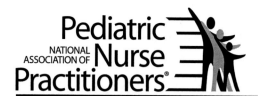

Information for Parents about Anxiety in Children and Teens

Fast Facts

- Fear and anxiety are a normal part of growing up, but they should not interfere with your child's daily activities.

- Anxiety disorders are among the most common mental health problems in children and teens.

- Children and teens with anxiety experience severe and persistent distress that interferes with their daily functioning; often these disorders are under-diagnosed.

- You might describe your child as a "worrier."

- Children and teens will often report physical complaints or describe "feeling sick" (e.g. stomach pain, headaches, chest pain, and fatigue).

- Many times, children with anxiety also are having problems with paying attention/staying focused at school; they may have problems being "moody."

- Many times, healthcare providers will mistake anxiety symptoms for attention deficit symptoms.

Common Signs of Anxiety for Kids and Teens:

Physical	Behavioral	Thoughts
Restlessness and irritability (very common in younger children) Headaches Stomachaches, nausea, vomiting, diarrhea Feeling tired Palpitations, increased heart rate, increased blood pressure Hyperventilation/shortness of breath Muscle tension Difficulty sleeping Dizziness, tingling fingers, weakness Tremors	Escape/avoidant behaviors Crying Clinging to/fear of separating from parents Speaking in a soft voice Variations in speech patterns Nail-biting Thumb-sucking Always "checking out" surroundings Freezing Regression (bedwetting, temper tantrums)	Worry about "what ifs…" Always thinking something terrible will happen Unreasonable, rigid thinking

Medical Problems That Mimic Anxiety Symptoms

- Low blood sugar
- Thyroid problems
- Seizures
- Irregular heart beat
- Migraine headaches
- Breathing problems

Medications/Drugs That May Cause Anxiety Symptoms

- Caffeine
- Nicotine
- Antihistamines (Benadryl)
- Medications for asthma
- Marijuana
- Nasal decongestants, such as pseudoephedrine
- Stimulant medication (e.g., Ritalin)
- Street drugs (e.g., cocaine)
- Steroids
- Prescribed medications to treat anxiety, when started, can cause effects that mimic anxiety symptoms, but these symptoms often subside after a few days.

Treatment

- Talk to your primary care provider if you have concerns; describe what you are noticing about your child.

- Ask your primary care provider for things to read or Web sites to visit to learn more about your child's symptoms.

- Therapy might be recommended to help treat your child's symptoms. It could involve individual, group, or family work.

- Consider what could be changed at home or in school to help your child deal with his or her worries (e.g., set a regular bedtime routine or think about which activities are stressful for your child and think about ways to handle them differently).

- Medication is often recommended as an alternative treatment if symptoms are disturbing your child's day-to-day activities. Your provider may recommend a class of medicines called "*SSRIs,* short for *Selective Serotonin Reuptake Inhibitors.*"

    o   Be sure to ask:
    - — What symptoms will the medication treat?
    - — How long will my child have to take this medication?
    - — How much medication will my child have to take, and how many times a day will he/she have to take it?
    - — How often will we see and/or talk to you about how my child is doing on the medication?
    - — What happens if my child misses a dose of medication?
    - — How do we stop the medication?

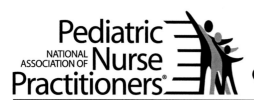

Information for Parents on
How to Help Your Child/Teen
Cope with Stressful Events or Uncertainty

The most important thing that you can do to help your child/teen cope with stressful events is to remain as calm as possible when you are with him or her. Children pick up on their parents' anxiety very quickly. If they sense you are anxious, they will be anxious as well. Therefore, if you are having difficulty coping with a stressful situation, it is a good idea to reach out to resources to help yourself, such as friends, family members, support groups, clergy, or healthcare professionals. Taking care of your own stress so that you are less anxious will help your child to stay calm.

Recognize Signs of Anxiety/Stress in Your Child

- Children and teens typically regress when stressed. That is, they go back to doing things they did when they were younger to help themselves feel more comfortable and secure. For instance, a preschool child may go back to sucking his/her thumb and a school-age child or teen may act more dependent upon the parents or have difficulty separating from them.

- Other common signs of anxiety in <u>young children</u> include: restlessness/hyperactivity, temper tantrums, nightmares, clinging behaviors, difficulty separating, and distress around new people.

- Common signs of anxiety in <u>older school age-children and teens</u> include: difficulty concentrating and sleeping, anger, restlessness/hyperactivity, worry, and physical complaints, such as stomachaches or headaches.

- At age 9 years, children realize that death is permanent. Fears of death or physical violence and harm are often common after this age.

- Signs and symptoms of anxiety such as these are usually healthy, temporary coping strategies that help your child to deal with stress. However, if these symptoms persist for several weeks or interfere with your child's functioning, talk to your child's primary healthcare provider about them. Your child's doctor or nurse practitioner will know what to do to help.

- Be honest and give age-appropriate and developmentally appropriate explanations about stressful events when they occur.

- For young children (under 8 years of age), only provide answers to questions they are asking and do not overwhelm them with too much detail. Use language that young children can understand. Do not expose young children to visual images in the newspapers or on television that may be terrifying.

- It may be easier for young children to express how they are feeling by asking them to talk about how their stuffed animals or dolls are feeling or thinking.

- Help children and teens to express how they are feeling about what they have seen or heard. If children have difficulty verbally expressing their feelings, ask them to make a drawing about how they are feeling. Older school-age children and teens can benefit from writing about how they feel.

- Ask your child/teen, "What is the scariest or worst thing about this event for you?" or "What is worrying you the most right now?" and take time to really listen to what he or she has to say.

- Reassure children that they did nothing wrong to cause what happened. Toddlers and preschool children, especially, feel guilty when stressful events happen.

- Tell children and teens that what they are feeling (e.g., anger, anxiety, and helplessness) is normal and that others feel the same way.

- Decrease anxiety in your child by reassuring him or her that you will get through this <u>together</u>. Emphasize that adults are doing everything possible to take care of the stressful situation and that he or she is not alone.

- Help your child/teen to release tension by encouraging daily physical exercise and activities.

- Continue to provide as much structure to your child's schedules and days as possible.

- Recognize that added stress/anxiety usually increases psychological or physical symptoms (e.g., headaches or abdominal pain) in children/teens that are already anxious or depressed.

- Young children who are depressed typically have different symptoms (e.g., restlessness, excessive motor activity) from those experienced by older school-age children or teens who are depressed (e.g., sad or withdrawn affect; anger, difficulty sleeping or eating; talking about feeling hopeless).

- Use this opportunity as a time to work with your child on their coping skills (e.g., relaxation techniques, positive reappraisal, and prayer). Children watch how their parents cope and often take on the same coping strategies. Therefore, showing your child that you use positive coping strategies to deal with stress will help him or her to develop healthy ways of coping.

- Be sure to have your child or teen seen by a healthcare provider or mental health professional for signs or symptoms of persistent anxiety, depression, recurrent pain, persistent behavioral changes, or if he or she has difficulty maintaining routine schedules.

- Remember that stressful times can be an opportunity to build future coping and life skills as well as to bring your family closer together.

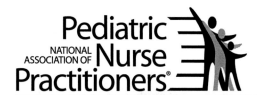

Information for Helping Children, Teens, and Their Families Cope with War and/or Terrorism

1. Be honest and give age-appropriate and developmentally appropriate explanations about the traumatic event.

   - For young children, in particular, only provide answers to questions they are asking and do not over-whelm them with too much detail.

   - Use language that young children can understand.

   - It may be easier for young children to express how they are feeling by asking them to talk about how their stuffed animals or dolls are feeling or thinking.

   - Help children and teens to express how they are feeling about what they have seen or heard. If children have difficulty verbally expressing their feelings, ask them to make a drawing about how they are feeling. Older school-age children and teens can benefit from writing about how they feel.

   - Ask children and teens, "What is the scariest or worst thing about this for you?" or "What is worrying you the most?"

2. Do not expose young children to visual images in the newspapers or on television that are potentially terrifying.

3. Reassure children that they did nothing wrong to cause what happened.

   - Toddlers and preschool children, especially, feel guilty when something tragic happens.

4. Tell children and teens that what they are feeling (e.g., anger, anxiety, and helplessness) is normal and that others feel the same way.

5. Alleviate some of their anxiety by reassuring children that we will get through this <u>together</u> and will be stronger as a result of what we have been through. Emphasize that adults will be there to help them through this and that they are not alone.

6. Spend some special time with your child every day, even if only 15 minutes.

7. Help children and teens to release their tension by encouraging daily physical exercise and activities.

8. Continue to provide structure to children's schedules and days.

9. Recognize that war or a tragic event could elevate psychological or physical symptoms (e.g., headaches, abdominal pain or chest pain, nightmares), especially in children and teens who are already depressed or anxious.

   - Remember that young children who are depressed typically have different symptoms (e.g., restlessness, excessive motor activity) from those experienced by older school-age children or teens who are depressed (e.g., sad or withdrawn affect; difficulty sleeping or eating; talking about feeling hopeless).

   - Anger can be a sign of anxiety in children and teens.

   - Children, even teens, who are stressed typically regress (e.g., revert to doing things that they did when they were younger, such as sucking their thumbs, bedwetting, or acting dependent upon their parents). This is a healthy temporary coping strategy. However, if these symptoms persist for several weeks, talk to your healthcare provider about them.

10. Use this opportunity as a time to work with children on their coping skills.

    • Use coping strategies that you know are typically helpful for your child, since each child copes in a way that is best for him or her (e.g., prayer, doing things to help other people, listening to music).

11. As a parent, remember that emotions are contagious. If you are highly upset or anxious, there is a good chance that your child also will feel the same way. If you are having difficulty coping with stress or with what is going on in the world around you, it is important to talk with someone who can help you to cope. You being calm will help your child to stay calm.

12. Be sure to have your child or teen seen by a healthcare provider or mental health professional for signs or symptoms of depression, persistent anxiety, recurrent pain, persistent behavioral changes, or if he or she has difficulty maintaining routine schedules.

13. Remember that this can be an opportunity to build future coping and life skills as well as to bring your family unit closer together.

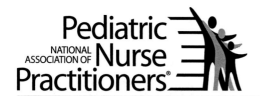

Information for Teens and School-Age Children About Stress and Anxiety

Fast Facts

- It is common for older children and teens to struggle with feelings of anxiety or stress and to worry about things (real or made up).

- These feelings can make it hard to go to school, talk with teachers, or hang out with friends.

- Your parents, teachers, and friends might describe you as a "worrier".

- Your body feels worry too. You might not feel good and may have headaches, stomachaches, or feel tired, especially when you have to do something that stresses you.

- Worry can make it hard to pay attention at school. It can even make you feel sad, angry/grumpy, or frustrated!

- Most people, at some time in their lives, need help to deal with stress. There is nothing to be ashamed of in asking for help with how you feel.

- There are many things you can do to help feel less stressed and worried.

- It is important to see a doctor or practitioner to talk about your worries and to undergo a check-up, as it is important to make sure that there is not a medical reason for why you are feeling the way that you do.

What You Can Do About Worry and Stress

- Talk to someone you trust about how you are feeling.

- If you have trouble talking, write down how you feel and then share it with someone.

- Try to do relaxing exercises (imagine being at your favorite place; take slow deep breaths and, when you breathe out, imagine all of your stress leaving you; listen to calming music).

- Do positive self-talk (e.g., "I am feeling calmer; I am going to handle this well").

- Stay focused in the present moment (try not to feel guilty about something that has happened in the past or worry about the future, because most things we worry about don't ever happen).

- Exercise for at least 30 minutes 3 to 4 days a week (this is a great way to release stress!).

- Don't take certain medications or drugs that can cause you to feel anxiety.
  These include caffeine, which is found in Pepsi, Mountain Dew, coffee, and tea; nicotine in cigarettes; marijuana; nasal decongestants (e.g., Sudafed); stimulant medication (e.g. Ritalin), or street drugs (e.g., cocaine).

When What You Are Doing Isn't Helping

- Talk to your parent(s), your doctor, or nurse practitioner if you think you worry too much about things. Describe how you think and feel.

- Ask your primary care provider for things to read or Web sites to visit so you and your parents can learn more about how you are feeling.

- Your doctor or practitioner might want you to meet with a counselor to help you with your worries. You might meet with the counselor alone, with your family, or in a group with other kids who have the same problems.

- Medication may help to stop your worry. Ask your doctor or practitioner how this could help.

Internet Resources

About Our Kids
www.aboutourkids.org

This Website contains a wealth of resources for families about child and adolescent mental health and parenting. Resources include science-based articles, newsletters, and manuals; a guide to common mental health problems; lists of recommended books, Websites, and organizations; a glossary of medical terms explained in an easy-to-understand format; and an ask-the-expert service. "About Our Kids" is presented by the New York University School of Medicine Child Study Center.

American Academy of Child and Adolescent Psychiatry
www.aacap.org

This Website is an excellent source of information on the assessment and treatment of child and adolescent mental health disorders. Handouts for use with families (i.e., Facts for Families) are available on a multitude of social and emotional problems, including anxiety disorders (#47 The Anxious Child). They are available in a variety of languages.

KidsHealth
www.kidshealth.org

This is an outstanding Website that contains health information for healthcare providers, parents, teens, and children. Many of the topics relate to emotions and behaviors (e.g., anxiety, fears, depression) and are developmentally sensitive to specific age groups. Physicians and other healthcare providers review all material before it is posted on this Website.

National Institute of Mental Health
www.nimh.nih.gov

This outstanding Website offers multiple educational handouts on a variety of mental health disorders, including anxiety disorders, and links to other informative Websites.

The REACH (REsource for Advancing Children's Health) Institute
http://www.thereachinstitute.org/about-REACH.html

The REACH Institute is dedicated to improving the mental health of American children and adolescents with emotional and behavioral challenges. Excellent resources at the Website are available for healthcare providers, agencies, and families.

REFERENCES

American Psychiatric Association (2013). *Diagnostic and Statistical Manual of Mental Disorders, Fifth Edition* (DSM-5). Washington, D.C.: APA.

Birmaher, B., Khetarpal, S., Brent, D., Cully, M., Balach, L., Kaufman, J., & Neer, S.M. (1997). The screen for child anxiety related emotional disorders (SCARED): Scale construction and psychometric characteristics. *Journal of the American Academy of Child and Adolescent Psychiatry*, 36(4), 545-553.

Ghalib, K.D., Vidair, H.B., Woodcome, H.A., Walkup, J.T., & Rynn, M.A. (2011). Assessment and treatment of child and adolescent anxiety disorders. In: Martin, A., Scahill, L., & Kratochvil, C.J. (Eds.), *Pediatric Psychopharmacology Principles and Practice 2nd ed*. New York: Oxford University Press, pp. 480-495.

Kroenke, K., Spitzer, R.L., Williams, J.B., et al. (2007). Anxiety disorders in primary care: prevalence, impairment, comorbidity, and detection. *Annals of Internal Medicine*, 146(5), 317-325.

Kroenke, K., Spitzer, R.L., Williams, J.B., & Lowe, B. (2010). The patient health questionnaire somatic, anxiety and depressive symptom scales: a systematic review. *General Hospital Psychiatry*, 32(4), 345-359.

Lowe, B., Decker, O., Muller, S., et al. (2008). Validation and standardization of the Generalized Anxiety Disorder Screener (GAD-7) in the general population. *Medical Care*, 46(3), 266-274.

Monga, S., Birmaher, B., Chiappetta, L., et al. (2000). Screen for child anxiety-related emotional disorders (SCARED): convergent and divergent validity. *Depression & Anxiety*, 12(2), 85-91.

Spitzer, R.L., Kroenke, K., Williams, J.B., & Lowe, B. (2006). A brief measure for assessing generalized anxiety disorder: The GAD-7. *Archives of Internal Medicine*, 166(10), 1092-1097.

Walkup, J.T., Albano, A.M., Piacentini, J., et al. (2008). Cognitive behavioral therapy, sertraline, or a combination in childhood anxiety. *The New England Journal of Medicine*, 359(26), 2753-2766.

SECTION 4
Holly Brown & Bernadette Mazurek Melnyk

Depressive Disorders

Fast Facts

- Depressive disorders include major depressive disorder (MDD), persistent depressive disorder (dysthymia), disruptive mood dysregulation disorder, premenstrual dysphoric disorder, substance/medication-induced depressive disorder, and depressive disorder due to another medical condition (DSM-5™, 2013).

- The common feature of depressive disorders is the presence of sad, empty, or irritable mood, which is associated with somatic and cognitive changes that interfere with functioning at home, in school, and/or with peers.

- An estimated 5% of children (males and females equally) and 10% to 20% of teens (females twice as often as males) are affected.

- The mean age of onset for an MDD is 14 years, and 8 years for dysthymia.

- Reoccurrence is as high as 60% to 70%; often reoccurs in adulthood.

- The risk in children/teens is increased if one or more parents is depressed.

- An estimated 40% to 70% of affected children/teens have mental health comorbidities (e.g., anxiety disorders, substance use, conduct disorders, ADHD).

- Detection is low, <20% of cases.

- Less than 25% of affected children and adolescents receive treatment.

- The average length of an untreated episode of MDD is 7-9 months.

- Depression is a risk factor for other high-risk behaviors and often precedes substance abuse by about 4 years.

- Depression is often misdiagnosed as ADHD in young children as they may present with inattention, impulsivity, and hyperactivity.

- The causes of depressive disorders can be multifactorial, including:
  - biological changes in chemistry of the brain, such as imbalances in serotonin, dopamine, and/or norepinephrine or excess cortisol

  - genetic

  - environmental (e.g., stressful situations)

  - depressogenic cognition (i.e., a negative pattern of thinking)

  - physical

  - drug related

Risk Factors for Depressive Disorders

- Parental depression or other family mental health problems
- Family dysfunction, including domestic violence and marital conflict
- Societal or family violence or abuse, physical or sexual abuse
- Acute or chronic illness
- Life stressors and changes, trauma and/or losses
- Low self-esteem
- Poor coping skills
- Attachment issues
- Lack of social or peer support/social isolation
- Substance abuse or other psychopathology
- Overweight/obesity

Depressive Disorders are a Major Risk Factor for Suicide

- Suicide is the third leading cause of death in teens (5% to 10% of high school students make attempts every year).
- Suicidality increases with age.
- The age group with the highest incidence of suicide is older male teens.
- Girls make more attempts at suicide, but males are more successful.

Predictors/Major Risk Factors for Suicide

- Degree of hopelessness (This is the #1 predictor of suicide.)
- Family history of suicide or recent suicide in school
- Method available (e.g., gun, medications)
- Prior history of self-harming behaviors or impulsivity
- Depression and/or a sudden change in mood
- Drug and alcohol abuse
- Inability to "contract for safety"
- Serious medical illness
- Family violence

Common Presentation Modes of Depressive Disorders by Age Group

- **Infants:** feeding difficulties, sleep disturbances, irritability, poor eye contact, irritable or apathetic
- **Toddlers and Preschoolers:** behavior problems, excessive tantrums, aggression, irritability, regression
- **School-age children:** sadness, irritability, impulsivity, crying spells, loss of pleasure or interest in activities, sleep problems, frequent complaints that no one likes me, somatic complaints (i.e., stomachaches or headaches), externalizing (i.e., acting out) behaviors
- **Adolescents:** sadness, hopelessness, self-hatred, withdrawn, loss of pleasure/interest in activities, neurovegetative symptoms (e.g., decrease in sleep, appetite, and concentration), drug and alcohol use (common), comorbidity with anxiety (common)

Screening for Depression

As with all mental health disorders, depression should not be diagnosed solely by a screening tool. Screening tools raise "red flags" that should be investigated further by sensitive clinical interviews.

The United States Preventive Services Task Force (USPSTF) recommends screening all adolescents (12-18 years of age) for MDD when systems are in place to ensure accurate diagnosis, psychotherapy (cognitive-behavioral or interpersonal) and follow-up (see **http://www.uspreventiveservicestaskforce.org/uspstf/uspschdepr.htm**)

Two questions recommended by the USPSTF for adults that are appropriate for older adolescents, especially if time is limited, include:

1. Over the past 2 weeks, have you ever felt down, depressed, or hopeless?
2. Over the past 2 weeks, have you felt little interest or pleasure in doing things?

Tools for depression screening that are free and in the public domain include:

- *The Center for Epidemiological Studies Depression Scale (CES-DC) for Children:* A valid and reliable instrument for depression screening in older school-age children and teens; 20 items on a 4-point Likert scale from 0 Not at All to 3 A Lot ("During the past week, I felt down and unhappy"); scores over 15 indicate significant levels of depression. This scale is free and in the public domain; it can be downloaded at www.brightfutures.org/mentalhealth/pdf/professionals/bridges/ces_dc.pdf. The older teen/young adult version of the CES-D can be downloaded for free at http://www.psych.uic.edu/csp/images/stories/physicians/rating%20scales/CES-DC.pdf. Further information about the scale's validity and reliability as well as a copy of it are included at the end of this section.

- *The Patient Health Questionnaire-9 (PHQ-9):* A 9-item depression scale for screening and monitoring depression, which has been found to be effective for screening adolescents as young as 13 years of age. The PHQ-9 is based directly on the diagnostic criteria for MDD in the DSM. Download at: http://www.depression-primarycare.org/clinicians/toolkits/materials/forms/phq9/. There also is a PHQ-9 modified version for adolescents.

- *The Patient Health Questionnaire- 2 (PHQ-2):* Uses the first 2 questions from the PHQ-9, including:

  (1) Over the past 2 weeks, how often have you been bothered by any of the following:

  (2) little interest or pleasure doing things

  (3) feeling down, depressed or hopeless
  Download at: **http://www.cqaimh.org/pdf/tool_phq2.pdf.**

Assessment of Depression

Consider

- Onset and development of symptoms; context in which symptoms occur/are sustained
- Biological/psychosocial stressors
- Comorbid psychopathology
- Impact of symptoms on activities of daily living and family
- Parent-child interactions
- Developmental history
- Coping behaviors and styles, sleep, and rhythmicity

Medical History
- Medical visits/hospitalizations (e.g., recurrent pain syndromes)
- Medical disorders (e.g., hypothyroidism, anemia, chronic illness) and medications

School History
- Academic, athletic, social, and behavioral functioning
- Potential versus actual achievements
- Pattern of attendance and school nurse visits

Social History
- Environmental stressors, separations, and losses
- Involvement with peers/withdrawal, giving away prized possessions

Family History
- Family mental health history (e.g., anxiety/mood disorders)
- Family medical history (e.g., headaches, chronic illness, recurrent pain)
- Parental responses to medications [e.g., Selective Serotonin Reuptake Inhibitors (SSRIs)]

Interviewing the Child/Adolescent
Consider
- The child's/adolescent's report of symptoms and sense of functional impairment

- Objective signs of depression (e.g., loss/gain of weight, hypo/hyperactivity)

- Depending on development, engage the child in play, drawing, or other artistic expression. Also, obtain history from collateral contacts.

Specific Assessment Questions for Children and Adolescents
- **Mood** ("Have you been feeling sad, down, blue or grouchy most of the day, more days than not?"; "Do you find yourself crying a lot?"; "Have you been getting into arguments more than usual?")
- **Anhedonia** ("Are you able to enjoy things you used to enjoy?"; "Do you feel bored or tired a lot of the time?")
- **Negative self-concept** ("How do you feel about yourself on a scale of 0 [meaning you do not feel good about yourself at all] to 10 [meaning you feel really good about yourself]?")
- **Guilt** ("Do you feel badly or guilty about things you have done?")
- **Relationships with friends** ("Do you have friends?"; "Are you liked by other kids?")
- **Neurovegetative signs** ("Do you have trouble falling asleep or staying asleep?"; "Do you have trouble concentrating in school?"; "How is your appetite -- are you eating more or less than usual?")
- **Somatic symptoms** ("Do you have a lot of headaches or stomachaches?")
- **Suicidal ideations** ("Do you ever wish you were dead?"; "Do you think about death or make plans to hurt yourself?"; "Have you ever hurt yourself?")
- **Current health and medications** (certain illnesses and medications can cause or present like mood disorders)
- **Alcohol and drug use** ("How much alcohol do you drink?"; "What drugs are you taking?"; "How often?")

Specific Assessment Questions for Parents
- Mood/affect: "How is your child's mood and emotions?"; "Is this a change from how he or she usually is?"

- Neurovegetative signs: "Is your child having trouble falling or staying asleep?"; "Has his or her appetite changed and, if yes, how?"
- Suicidal ideation: "Has your child ever talked about wanting to hurt him- or herself or die?"; "Is there a history of self-harm?"
- Impaired functioning at school or with peers: "Is there a change with how your child has been functioning at school, home, or with his or her peers?"

Special Assessment Findings With Bipolar Disorder
- Elevated, expansive, or irritable mood and abnormally and persistently increased goal-directed activity or energy, lasting at least 1 week and present most of the day, nearly every day (DSM-5™, 2013)
- Inflated self-esteem or grandiosity
- Decreased sleep
- More talkative than usual or pressure to keep talking
- Flight of ideas or racing thoughts
- Distractibility
- Increase in goal-directed activity (either socially, at work or school, or sexually) or psychomotor agitation
- Excessive involvement in activities that have a great potential for painful consequences (e.g., buying sprees, drug use, promiscuity).

Physical Diagnoses That Should Be Ruled Out With Depression If Suspected From History
- Hypothyroidism (obtain TSH, FT4)
- Anemia (obtain CBC with differential)
- Mononucleosis or chronic fatigue syndrome (obtain monospot)
- Eating disorders
- Substance use or withdrawal -- e.g., alcohol, cocaine, amphetamines, opiates (obtain toxicology screen)
- Premenstrual syndrome
- Diabetes (obtain fasting serum glucose)
- Head trauma or CNS lesions
- Cushing syndrome
- HIV/AIDS
- Mitral valve prolapse
- Systemic lupus erythematosus
- Developmental delay
- Failure to thrive
- Seizures
- Lead intoxication (obtain lead level)
- Medication side effects – e.g., benzodiazepines, beta-blockers, clonidine, corticosteroids, Accutane, oral contraceptives

Conditions That Should Be Ruled Out With a Bipolar Manic Episode If Suspected From History
- Hyperthyroidism
- Asthma medication
- Steroid use

Assess for Suicidal Ideation/Intent, Plan, and Means

If depression is suspected or patients make self-harming comments, **ALWAYS** ask about:

- Suicidal ideation

- Plan and means

- Intent

- **Suicide warning signs**: no hope for the future, change in behavior (giving away treasured items), mood (sudden upswing in mood), thinking (preoccupation with death), major life changes (major illness or death of a loved one)

Management of Suicidal Ideation

- Option if low-risk for suicide: Contract for safety and mobilize social supports (A safety contract is included in this guide.)

- Options if high-risk for suicide: Call 911; transport to the emergency department

- In-home crisis intervention programs

- Depending on severity, consider: outpatient counseling, inpatient hospitalization, or residential programs

Management of Depression

- Assess for suicidal ideation. Teach about suicide warning signs and contract for safety. Caution families to remove drugs, alcohol, and weapons from the home.

- Educate the family about the depressive condition, and support the child and family.

- Because of the gaps in guidelines that existed for primary care providers to manage adolescent depression, researchers from the United States and Canada established the Guidelines for Adolescent Depression-Primary Care (GLAD-PC) with clinical management flow charts (Cheung et al., 2007). Each of the following recommendations was graded on the level of supporting evidence based on the Oxford Centre for Evidence-Based Medicine grades of evidence (A-D) system (see.www.cebm.net/levels_of_evidence.asp). See the GLAD-PC tool kit for support materials at **www.glad-pc.org**.

    1. *Recommendation #1*: After diagnosis, in cases of mild depression, clinicians should consider a period of active support and monitoring (6 to 8 weeks of weekly or biweekly monitoring) before starting other evidence-based treatment.
    Grade of evidence: B
    Strength of recommendation: very strong

    2. *Recommendation #2:* If a primary care clinician identifies an adolescent with moderate or severe depression or complicating factors/conditions such as coexisting substance abuse or psychosis, consultation with a mental health specialist should be considered.
    Grade of evidence: C
    Strength of recommendation: strong

    3. *Recommendation #3*: Primary care clinicians should recommend scientifically tested and proven treatments (i.e., psychotherapies such as cognitive behavioral therapy (CBT) or interpersonal therapy (IPT) and/or antidepressant treatment, such as the SSRIs) whenever possible and appropriate to achieve the goals of the treatment plan.
    Grade of evidence: A
    Strength of recommendation: very strong

4. *Recommendation #4:* Primary care clinicians should monitor for the emergence of adverse events during antidepressant treatment (SSRIs). (Ideally, face to face contact with patients or their family members weekly during the first 4 weeks, then at biweekly visits for the next 4 weeks, then at 12 weeks, and as clinically indicated beyond 12 weeks. *Grade of evidence: B* *Strength of recommendation: very strong*

- Refer for psychotherapy or use one of the available cognitive behavioral skills building programs below (The Adolescent Coping with Depression Course or COPE). Do not force into therapy. The American Academy of Child and Adolescent Psychiatry recommends psychotherapy as the first treatment approach for depressed youth with mild to moderate depression. CBT, which teaches that how a person thinks affects how they feel and how they behave, and Interpersonal Therapy have been supported by research as effective treatments for depression, anxiety, and other mental health disorders (family therapy also may be indicated). Two manualized reproducible evidence-based intervention programs that are based on CBT include:

   1. The Adolescent Coping with Depression Course by G.N. Clarke and P.M. Lewinsohn; see http://www.kpchr.org/public/acwd/acwd.html) or

   2. COPE (Creating Opportunities for Personal Empowerment) for School-Age Children, Adolescents and Young Adults by Bernadette Mazurek Melnyk (Lusk & Melnyk, 2011; Lusk and Melnyk, 2013; Melnyk et al., 2009; Melnyk, Kelly & Lusk, in press; Melnyk et al., in press). Additional information about the COPE Program, a 7-session manualized program for depressed and anxious children, teens, and college students/ young adults, is provided in Section 18 on Brief Interventions. Contact Bernadette Melnyk at cope.melnyk@gmail.com

- Involve school and after-care personnel; interdisciplinary collaboration is important.

- Careful and regular follow-up with the family is crucial.

- Medications should be reserved for severe depression or moderate depression not responding to therapy, and should be prescribed in conjunction with counseling therapy.

- SSRIs (*Celexa, Effexor, Lexapro, Paxil, Prozac, Zoloft*) are the recommended first-line treatment (See Table 4.1). It is extremely important to start antidepressant medication at <u>LOW</u> doses in children and adolescents and increase dosage <u>SLOWLY</u>. A trial of 8 weeks is recommended; it usually takes 2 to 4 weeks to see an effect, sometimes longer. Families should be educated to observe for serotonin syndrome with the start of SSRIs, including insomnia and agitation. As a general rule of thumb, antidepressants should be used for 6 to 9 months after target symptoms are relieved, weaned slowly, and never stopped abruptly. Avoid tricyclic antidepressants (e.g., amitriptyline, nortriptyline) whenever possible, especially in patients with suicidal ideation due to the potential for cardiac toxicity with overdose. In one study (the Treatment for Adolescents With Depression Study), the group that received combined therapy of fluoxetine and individual cognitive-behavioral therapy showed a 71% response rate versus a 35% response in adolescents who were taking placebo and receiving weekly clinical monitoring (March et al., 2004).

Table 4.1 Prescribing Information for the Selective Serotonin Reuptake Inhibitors Used for the Treatment of Major Depressive Disorder

SSRI (recommended order of preference)	Usual Starting Dose (SD) and Target Dosage (TD) per day		Side Effects	Important Considerations for Use of SSRIs
– Fluoxetine (*Prozac*)	SD: TD:	5 – 10 mg 20 – 60 mg	**Common:** nausea, diarrhea, constipation, dry mouth, decreased or increased appetite, restlessness, diaphoresis, headaches, sleep changes (symptoms usually appear quickly but diminish over time) **Rare/Serious:** Prolonged QT interval, hyponatremia, seizures, serotonin syndrome, induction of mania, suicidality	*Prozac* is the only FDA-approved antidepressant for MDD in children aged 8 years or older; onset of therapeutic action typically takes 2 to 4 weeks (true for other SSRIs); consider increasing the dose if it is not improving symptoms in 6 to 8 weeks or switching to another SSRI. SSRIs can be stimulating in children and adolescents. **Use cautiously and observe for activation of known or unknown bipolar disorder and/or suicidal ideation.** If activating, have the medication taken in the morning to decrease insomnia. *Prozac* is contraindicated with the use of monoamine oxidase inhibitors (MAOIs) or within 2 weeks of MAOI use (true for all SSRIs). *Prozac* has a long half-life (13-15 days), which may potentiate interactions with another drug if introduced too early after discontinuation. **Monitor children/teens and their symptoms in person regularly on a weekly basis during the first 4 weeks of treatment.** Assess therapeutic levels when initiating and increasing dosage. Use with caution in patients with a history of seizures (true for all SSRIs). Tapering is usually not necessary due to the drug's long half-life.
– Citalopram (*Celexa*)	SD: TD:	5 – 10 mg 20 – 40 mg	**Common:** Similar to *Prozac, Celexa* also may cause flu-like rhinitis, abdominal pain, back pain, fatigue; less activating than *Prozac*. **Rare/Serious:** Same as those associated with *Prozac*	As with *Prozac*, tapering is usually not necessary, yet tapering is a prudent approach to avoid withdrawal symptoms.

SSRI (recommended order of preference)	Usual Starting Dose (SD) and Target Dosage (TD) per day		Side Effects	Important Considerations for Use of SSRIs
– Sertraline (*Zoloft*)	SD: TD:	12.5 – 25 mg 50 – 100 mg	**Common and Rare/ Serious:** Similar to those associated with *Prozac*	As with Prozac, taper to avoid withdrawal symptoms, such as dizziness, nausea, stomach cramps, and sweating. A good approach to tapering is a 50% reduction for 3 days, then another 50% reduction for 3 days, followed by discontinuation.
– Paroxetine (*Paxil*)	SD: TD:	5 – 10 mg 20 – 40 mg	**Common and Rare/ Serious:** Similar to those associated with *Prozac*; sedation is common; may be less activating than other SSRIs.	Not specifically approved for depression; however, preliminary evidence suggests efficacy for depressed children and adolescents. Often preferred for patients with depression and comorbid anxiety. Taper to avoid withdrawal effects.
–Fluvoxamine (*Luvox*)	SD: TD:	25 – mg 50-200 – mg	**Common and Rare/ Serious:** Same as those associated with Prozac, sedation is common	If sedating, advise to take at bedtime. Useful for patients with comorbid depression and anxiety. Divide doses above 50 mg/day into 2 doses and give the larger dose at bedtime. Taper to avoid withdrawal effects.
–Escitalopram (*Lexapro*)	SD: TD:	5-10 – mg 10-20 – mg	**Common and Rare/ Serious:** Same as those associated with Prozac; sedation is unusual	Well tolerated Useful for the treatment of depression and comorbid anxiety disorder Approved for treatment of depression in adolescents, starting at 12 years of age Tapering is not usually necessary, but it is helpful for many patients to avoid withdrawal symptoms.

Important Note: Caution must be exercised when prescribing SSRIs to children and adolescents (up to age 25 years) with psychiatric disorders as studies have shown an increased risk of suicidal thinking and behavior (suicidality) in the first few months of starting treatment. Patients started on SSRIs should be observed closely for worsening of symptoms, suicidality, or unusual changes in behavior. Families should be advised to monitor for these signs/symptoms and alert the provider if they are present.

WARNING: SSRIs MAY INCREASE SUICIDAL IDEATION IN CHILDREN AND ADOLESCENTS/YOUNG ADULTS.

- Refer when:

    1. There is poor or incomplete response to two interventions or no improvement with psychosocial interventions within 2 months

    2. There is an increase in symptoms despite treatment

    3. A recurrent episode occurs within 1 year of previous episode

    4. The patient or families request referral

Special Notes on the Management of Bipolar Disorder

- Manic episodes in children and adolescents are treated as they are in adults.

- Lithium is the only medication that is FDA-approved for manic episodes in teens, 12 years of age and older.

- Divalproex (Depakote) is commonly used as a mood stabilizer to treat bipolar disorder in children and adolescents.

- Atypical antipsychotic medications (e.g., olanzapine [Zyprexa]; risperidone [Risperdal], aripiprazole [Abilify]) are also used in combination with divalproex. Olanzapine is approved for use in manic/mixed episodes in teens, aged 13 years and older. Risperidone is approved for acute mania/mixed mania in children 10 years of age and older. Aripiprazole is approved for bipolar maintenance.

- Many atypical antipsychotic medications (e.g., olanzapine, risperidone) contribute to substantial weight gain in children and adolescents and, therefore, are often discontinued by individuals. Sedation also is common and may help if taken at bedtime. These medications also may increase risk for diabetes and dyslipidemia. Weight gain is less frequent and severe with aripiprazole.

- Due to multiple challenges in the management of children and adolescents with bipolar disorder, involvement of a psychiatric mental health provider is essential.

Special Notes on Postpartum Depression

- Postpartum depression (PPD) occurs in approximately 10% to 15% of women within 4 weeks after delivery of a child (specify postpartum onset).

- Of every 1000 women who give birth, one to two experience postpartum psychosis.

- When delusions are present, it often involves the infant (e.g., being possessed by the devil).

- PPD is often accompanied by severe anxiety and panic attacks.

- Many mothers go untreated.

- Routine screening in the first 4 weeks after delivery is important.

Postpartum Blues

- PPD must be differentiated from postpartum blues that typically occur 3 to 7 days after birth
- Affects 70% to 80% of women
- Peaks at 3 to 5 days
- Predominantly positive mood with labile and intense episodes of irritability
- Lasts from hours to several days
- Resolves without significant consequences
- May be related to hormonal shifts after delivery

Screening Tools for Postpartum Depression

- Edinburgh Postnatal depression (EPDS): quick screen with 10 items; in the public domain and available for free download at **http://www.dbpeds.org/media/edinburghscale.pdf.**
- Center for Epidemiologic Study Depression Scale (CES-D): in the public domain and available for free download at http://cooccurring.org/public/document/ces-d.pdf.

Parental Depression

- Has multiple negative adverse outcomes on children
- Ask parents if they are having difficulty in caring for their child/children
- Ask about support systems
- Ask about current stressors
- Ask about past depression and outcomes
- Ask permission to speak to other family members
- Assess risk for suicidal behavior
- Help parents plan for how to talk to their children and family members about their depression
- Assess how the child is dealing with the parent's depression
- Refer parent to a mental health provider

Resources for Families

- Depression and Bipolar Support Alliance

    http://www.dbsalliance.org/site/PageServer?pagename=home

- National Alliance for the Mentally Ill

    www.nami.org

- National Mental Health Association

    www.nmha.org; 703-684-7722;

DSM-5™ Diagnostic Criteria for Persistent Depressive Disorder (Dysthymia)

This disorder represents a consolidation of DSM-5™-defined chronic major depressive disorder and dysthymic disorder.

A. Depressed mood for most of the day, for more days than not, as indicated by either subjective account or observation by others, for at least 2 years.

   Note: In children and adolescents, mood can be irritable and duration must be at least 1 year.

B. Presence, while depressed, of two (or more) of the following:

   1. Poor appetite or overeating.

   2. Insomnia or hypersomnia.

   3. Low energy or fatigue.

   4. Low self-esteem.

   5. Poor concentration or difficulty making decisions.

   6. Feelings of hopelessness.

C. During the 2-year period (1 year for children or adolescents) of the disturbance, the individual has never been without the symptoms in Criteria A and B for more than 2 months at a time.

D. Criteria for a major depressive disorder may be continuously present for 2 years.

E. There has never been a manic episode or a hypomanic episode, and criteria have never been met for cyclothymic disorder.

F. The disturbance is not better explained by a persistent schizoaffective disorder, schizophrenia, delusional disorder, or other specified or unspecified schizophrenia spectrum and other psychotic disorder.

G. The symptoms are not attributable to the physiological effects of a substance (e.g., a drug of abuse, a medication) or another medical condition (e.g., hypothyroidism).

H. The symptoms cause clinically significant distress or impairment in social, occupational, or other important areas of functioning.

Note: Because the criteria for a major depressive episode include four symptoms that are absent from the symptom list for persistent depressive disorder (dysthymia), a very limited number of individuals will have depressive symptoms that have persisted longer than 2 years but will not meet criteria for persistent depressive disorder. If full criteria for a major depressive episode have been met at some point during the current episode of illness, they should be given a diagnosis of major depressive disorder. Otherwise, a diagnosis of other specified depressive disorder or unspecified depressive disorder is warranted.

Specify if:

With anxious distress

With mixed features

With melancholic features

With atypical features

With mood-congruent psychotic features

With mood-incongruent psychotic features

With peripartum onset

Specify if:

In partial remission

In full remission

Specify if:

Early onset: If onset is before age 21 years.

Late onset: If onset is at age 21 years or older.

Specify if (for most recent 2 years of persistent depressive disorder):

With pure dysthymic syndrome: Full criteria for a major depressive episode have not been met in at least the preceding 2 years.

With persistent major depressive episode: Full criteria for a major depressive episode have been met throughout the preceding 2-year period.

With intermittent major depressive episodes, with current episode: Full criteria for a major depressive episode are currently met, but there have been periods of at least 8 weeks in at least the preceding 2 years with symptoms below the threshold for a full major depressive episode.

With intermittent major depressive episodes, without current episode: Full criteria for a major depressive episode are not currently met, but there has been one or more major depressive episodes in at least the preceding 2 years.

Specify current severity:

Mild

Moderate

Severe

DSM-5™ Diagnostic Criteria for Major Depressive Disorder

A. Five (or more) of the following symptoms have been present during the same 2-week period and represent a change from previous functioning; at least one of the symptoms is either (1) depressed mood or (2) loss of interest or pleasure.

   Note: Do not include symptoms that are clearly attributable to another medical condition.

   1. Depressed mood most of the day, nearly every day, as indicated by either subjective report (e.g., feels sad, empty, hopeless) or observation made by others (e.g., appears tearful). (Note: In children and adolescents, can be irritable mood.)

   2. Markedly diminished interest or pleasure in all, or almost all, activities most of the day, nearly every day (as indicated by either subjective account or observation).

   3. Significant weight loss when not dieting or weight gain (e.g., a change of more than 5% of body weight in a month), or decrease or increase in appetite nearly every day. (Note: In children, consider failure to make expected weight gain.)

   4. Insomnia or hypersomnia nearly every day.

   5. Psychomotor agitation or retardation nearly every day (observable by others, not merely subjective feelings of restlessness or being slowed down).

   6. Fatigue or loss of energy nearly every day.

   7. Feelings of worthlessness or excessive or inappropriate guilt (which may be delusional) nearly every day (not merely self-reproach or guilt about being sick).

   8. Diminished ability to think or concentrate, or indecisiveness, nearly every day (either by subjective account or as observed by others).

   9. Recurrent thoughts of death (not just fear of dying), recurrent suicidal ideation without a specific plan, or a suicide attempt or a specific plan for committing suicide.

B. The symptoms cause clinically significant distress or impairment in social, occupational, or other important areas of functioning.

C. The episode is not attributable to the physiological effects of a substance or to another medical condition.
   Note: Criteria A–C represent a major depressive episode.
   Note: Responses to a significant loss (e.g., bereavement, financial ruin, losses from a natural disaster, a serious medical illness or disability) may include the feelings of intense sadness, rumination about the loss, insomnia, poor appetite, and weight loss noted in Criterion A, which may resemble a depressive episode. Although such symptoms may be understandable or considered appropriate to the loss, the presence of a major depressive episode in addition to the normal response to a significant loss should also be carefully considered. This decision inevitably requires the exercise of clinical judgment based on the individual's history and the cultural norms for the expression of distress in the context of loss.[1]

D. The occurrence of the major depressive episode is not better explained by schizoaffective disorder, schizophrenia, schizophreniform disorder, delusional disorder, or other specified and unspecified schizophrenia spectrum and other psychotic disorders.

E. There has never been a manic episode or a hypomanic episode.
   Note: This exclusion does not apply if all of the manic-like or hypomanic-like episodes are substance-induced or are attributable to the physiological effects of another medical condition.

Coding and Recording Procedures

The diagnosis code for major depressive disorder is based on whether this is a single or recurrent episode, current severity, presence of psychotic features, and remission status. Current severity and psychotic features are only indicated if full criteria are currently met for a major depressive episode. Remission specifiers are only indicated if the full criteria are not currently met for a major depressive episode. Codes are as follows:

Severity/course specifier	Single episode	Recurrent episode*
Mild (p. 188)	296.21 (F32.0)	296.31 (F33.0)
Moderate (p. 188)	296.22 (F32.1)	296.32 (F33.1)
Severe (p. 188)	296.23 (F32.2)	296.33 (F33.2)
With psychotic features** (p. 188)	296.24 (F32.3)	296.34 (F33.3)
In partial remission (p. 188)	296.25 (F32.4)	296.35 (F33.41)
In full remission (p. 188)	296.26 (F32.5)	296.36 (F33.42)
Unspecified	296.20 (F32.9)	296.30 (F33.9)

*For an episode to be considered recurrent, there must be an interval of at least 2 consecutive months between separate episodes in which criteria are not met for a major depressive episode. The definitions of specifiers are found on the indicated pages.

**If psychotic features are present, code the "with psychotic features" specifier irrespective of episode severity.

In recording the name of a diagnosis, terms should be listed in the following order: major depressive order, single or recurrent episode, severity/psychotic/remission specifiers, followed by as many of the following specifiers without codes that apply to the current episode.

Specify:

With anxious distress

With mixed features

With melancholic features

With atypical features

With mood-congruent psychotic features

With mood-incongruent psychotic features

With catatonia; Coding note: Use additional code 293.89 (F06.1)

With peripartum onset

With seasonal pattern (recurrent episode only)

[1] In distinguishing grief from a major depressive episode (MDE), it is useful to consider that in grief the predominant affect is feelings of emptiness and loss, while in MDE it is persistent depressed mood and the inability to anticipate happiness or pleasure. The dysphoria in grief is likely to decrease in intensity over days to weeks and occurs in waves, the so-called pangs of grief. These waves tend to be associated with thoughts or reminders of the deceased. The depressed mood of a MDE is more persistent and not tied to specific thoughts or preoccupations. The pain of grief may be accompanied by positive emotions and humor that are uncharacteristic of the pervasive unhappiness and misery characteristic of a major depressive episode. The thought content associated with grief generally features a preoccupation with thoughts and memories of the deceased, rather than the self-critical or pessimistic ruminations seen in a MDE. In grief, self-esteem is generally preserved, whereas in a MDE, feelings of worthlessness and self-loathing are common. If self-derogatory ideation is present in grief, it typically involves perceived failings vis-à-vis the deceased (e.g., not visiting frequently enough, not telling the deceased how much he or she was loved). If a bereaved individual thinks about death and dying, such thoughts are generally focused on the deceased and possibly about "joining" the deceased, whereas in a major depressive episode such thoughts are focused on ending one's own life because of feeling worthless, undeserving of life, or unable to cope with the pain of depression.

Reprinted with permission from the Diagnostic and Statistical Manual of Mental Disorders, Fifth Edition, (Copyright ©2013). American Psychiatric Association. All Rights Reserved.

DSM-5™ Diagnostic Criteria for Bipolar I Disorder

For a diagnosis of bipolar I disorder, it is necessary to meet the following criteria for a manic episode. The manic episode may have been preceded by and may be followed by hypomanic or major depressive episodes.

Manic Episode

A. A distinct period of abnormally and persistently elevated, expansive, or irritable mood and abnormally and persistently increased goal-directed activity or energy, lasting at least 1 week and present most of the day, nearly every day (or any duration if hospitalization is necessary).

B. During the period of mood disturbance and increased energy or activity, three (or more) of the following symptoms (four if the mood is only irritable) are present to a significant degree and represent a noticeable change from unusual behavior:

   1. Inflated self-esteem or grandiosity.

   2. Decreased need for sleep (e.g., feels rested after only 3 hours of sleep).

   3. More talkative than usual or pressure to keep talking.

   4. Flight of ideas or subjective experience that thoughts are racing.

   5. Distractibility (i.e., attention too easily drawn to unimportant or irrelevant external stimuli), as reported or observed.

   6. Increase in goal-directed activity (either socially, at work or school, or sexually) or psychomotor agitation (i.e., purposeless non-goal-directed activity).

   7. Excessive involvement in activities that have a high potential for painful consequences (e.g., engaging in unrestrained buying sprees, sexual indiscretions, or foolish business investments).

C. The mood disturbance is sufficiently severe to cause marked impairment in social or occupational functioning or to necessitate hospitalization to prevent harm to self or others, or there are psychotic features.

D. The episode is not attributable to the physiological effects of a substance (e.g., a drug of abuse, a medication, other treatment) or to another medical condition. **Note:** A full manic episode that emerges during antidepressant treatment (e.g., medication, electroconvulsive therapy) but persists at a fully syndromal level beyond the physiological effect of that treatment is sufficient evidence for a manic episode and, therefore, a bipolar I diagnosis.

Note: Criteria A-D constitute a manic episode. At least one lifetime manic episode is required for the diagnosis of bipolar I disorder.

Hypomanic Episode

A. A distinct period of abnormally and persistently elevated, expansive, or irritable mood and abnormally and persistently increased activity or energy, lasting at least 4 consecutive days and present most of the day, nearly every day.

B. During the period of mood disturbance and increased energy and activity, three (or more) of the following symptoms (four if the mood is only irritable) have persisted, represent a noticeable change from usual behavior, and have been present to a significant degree:

   1. Inflated self-esteem or grandiosity.

   2. Decreased need for sleep (e.g., feels rested after only 3 hours of sleep).

   3. More talkative than usual or pressure to keep talking.

   4. Flight of ideas or subjective experience that thoughts are racing.

   5. Distractibility (i.e., attention too easily drawn to unimportant or irrelevant external stimuli), as re ported or observed.

   6. Increase in goal-directed activity (either socially, at work or school, or sexually) or psychomotor agitation (i.e., purposeless non-goal-directed activity).

   7. Excessive involvement in activities that have a high potential for painful consequences (e.g., engaging in unrestrained buying sprees, sexual indiscretions, or foolish business investments).

C. The episode is associated with an unequivocal change in functioning that is uncharacteristic of the individual when not symptomatic.

D. The disturbance in mood and the change in functioning are observable by others.

E. The episode is not severe enough to cause marked impairment in social or occupational functioning or to necessitate hospitalization. If there are psychotic features, the episode is, by definition, manic.

F. The episode is not attributable to the physiological effects of a substance (e.g., a drug of abuse, a medication, other treatment). **Note:** A full hypomanic episode that emerges during antidepressant treatment (e.g., medications, electroconvulsive therapy) but persists at a fully syndromal level beyond the physiological effect of that treatment is sufficient evidence for a hypomanic episode diagnosis. However, caution is indicated so that one or two symptoms (particularly increased irritability, edginess, or agitation following antidepressant use) are not taken as sufficient for diagnosis of a hypomanic episode, nor necessarily indicative of a bipolar diathesis.

Note: Criteria A-F constitute a hypomanic episode. Hypomanic episodes are common in bipolar I disorder but are not required for the diagnosis of bipolar I disorder.

Major Depressive Episode

A. Five (or more) of the following symptoms have been present during the same 2-week period and represent a change from previous functioning: at least one of the symptoms is either (1) depressed mood or (2) loss of interest or pleasure.

   Note: Do not include symptoms that are clearly attributable to another medical condition.

   1. Depressed mood most of the day, nearly every day, as indicated by either subjective report (e.g., feels sad, empty, or hopeless) or observation made by others (e.g., appears tearful). (**Note:** In children and adolescents, can be irritable mood.)

   2. Markedly diminished interest or pleasure in all, or almost all, activities most of the day, nearly every day (as indicated by wither subjective account or observation).

3. Significant weight loss when not dieting or weight gain (e.g., a change of more than 5% of body weight in a month), or decrease or increase in appetite nearly every day. (**Note:** In children, consider failure to make expected weight gain.)

4. Insomnia or hypersomnia nearly every day.

5. Psychomotor agitation or retardation nearly every day (observable by others; not merely subjective feelings of restlessness or being slowed down).

6. Fatigue or loss of energy nearly every day.

7. Feelings of worthlessness or excessive or inappropriate guilt (which may be delusional) nearly every day (not merely self-reproach or guilt about being sick).

8. Diminished ability to think or concentrate, or indecisiveness, nearly every day (either by subjective account or as observed by others).

9. Recurrent thoughts of death (not just fear of dying), recurrent suicidal ideation without a specific plan, or a suicide attempt or a specific plan for committing suicide.

B. The symptoms cause clinically significant distress or impairment in social, occupational, or other important areas of functioning.

C. The episode is not attributable to the physiological effects of a substance or another medical condition.

Note: Criteria A–C constitute a major depressive episode. Major depressive episodes are common in bipolar I disorder but are not required for the diagnosis of bipolar I disorder.

Note: Responses to a significant loss (e.g., bereavement, financial ruin, losses from natural disaster, a serious medical illness or disability) may include feelings of intense sadness, rumination about the loss, insomnia, poor appetite, and weight loss noted in Criterion A, which may resemble a depressive episode. Although such symptoms may be understandable or considered appropriate to the loss, the presence of major depressive episode in addition to the normal response to a significant loss should also be carefully considered. This decision inevitably requires the exercise of clinical judgment based on the individual's history and the cultural norms for the expression of distress in the context of loss.[1]

Bipolar I Disorder

A. Criteria have been met for at least one manic episode (Criteria A–D under "Manic Episode" above).

B. The occurrence of the manic and major depressive episode(s) is not better explained by schizoaffective disorder, schizophrenia, schizophreniform disorder, delusional disorder, or other specified or unspecified schizophrenia spectrum and other psychotic disorder.

Coding and Recording Procedures

The diagnostic code for bipolar I disorder is based on type of current or most recent episode and its status with respect to current severity, presence of psychotic features, and remission status. Current severity and psychotic features are only indicated if full criteria are currently met for a manic or major depressive episode. Remission specifiers are only indicated if the full criteria are not currently met for a manic, hypomanic, or major depressive episode. Codes are as follows:

Bipolar I disorder	Current or most recent episode manic	Current or most recent episode hypomanic*	Current or most recent episode depressed	Current or most recent episode unspecified**
Mild (p. 154)	296.41 (F31.11)	NA	296.51 (F31.31)	NA
Moderate (p. 154)	296.42 (F31.12)	NA	296.52 (F31.32)	NA
Severe (p. 154)	296.43 (F31.13)	NA	296.53 (F31.4)	NA

[1] In distinguishing grief from a major depressive episode (MDE), it is useful to consider that in grief the predominant affect is feelings of emptiness and loss, while in MDE it is persistent depressed mood and the inability to anticipate happiness or pleasure. The dysphoria in grief is likely to decrease in intensity over days to weeks and occurs in waves, the so-called pangs of grief. These waves tend to be associated with thoughts or reminders of the deceased. The depressed mood of a MDE is more persistent and not tied to specific thoughts or preoccupations. The pain of grief may be accompanied by positive emotions and humor that are uncharacteristic of the pervasive unhappiness and misery characteristic of a major depressive episode. The thought content associated with grief generally features a preoccupation with thoughts and memories of the deceased, rather than the self-critical or pessimistic ruminations seen in a MDE. In grief, self-esteem is generally preserved, whereas in a MDE, feelings of worthlessness and self-loathing are common. If self-derogatory ideation is present in grief, it typically involves perceived failings vis-à-vis the deceased (e.g., not visiting frequently enough, not telling the deceased how much he or she was loved). If a bereaved individual thinks about death and dying, such thoughts are generally focused on the deceased and possibly about "joining" the deceased, whereas in a major depressive episode such thoughts are focused on ending one's own life because of feeling worthless, undeserving of life, or unable to cope with the pain of depression.

Bipolar I disorder	Current or most recent episode manic	Current or most recent episode hypomanic*	Current or most recent episode depressed	Current or most recent episode unspecified**
With psychotic features*** (p. 152)	296.44 (F31.2)	NA	296.54 (F31.5)	NA
In partial remission (p. 154)	296.45 (F31.73)	296.45 (F31.73)	296.55 (F31.75)	NA
In full remission (p. 154)	296.46 (F31.74)	296.46 (F31.74)	296.56 (F31.76)	NA
Unspecified	296.40 (F31.9)	296.40 (F31.9)	296.50 (F31.9)	NA

*Severity and psychotic specifiers do not apply; code 296.40 (F31.0) for cases not in remission.
**Severity, psychotic, and remission specifiers do not apply. Code 296.7 (F31.9).
***If psychotic features are present, code the "with psychotic features" specifier irrespective of episode severity.

In recording the name of a diagnosis, terms should be listed in the following order: bipolar I disorder, type of current or most recent episode, severity/psychotic/remission specifiers, followed by as many specifiers without codes as apply to the current or most recent episode.

Specify:

With anxious distress	With mood-congruent psychotic features
With mixed features	With mood-incongruent psychotic features
With rapid cycling	With catatonia; Coding note: Use additional code 293.89 (F06.1).
With melancholic features	With peripartum onset
With atypical features	With seasonal pattern

DSM-5™ Diagnostic Criteria for Bipolar II Disorder

For a diagnosis of bipolar II disorder, it is necessary to meet the following criteria for a current or past hypomanic episode and the following criteria for a current or past major depressive episode:

Hypomanic Episode

   A. A distinct period of abnormally and persistently elevated, expansive, or irritable mood and abnormally and persistently increased activity or energy, lasting at least 4 consecutive days and present most of the day, nearly every day.

   B. During the period of mood disturbance and increased energy and activity, three (or more) of the following symptoms (four if the mood is only irritable) have persisted, represent a noticeable change from usual behavior, and have been present to a significant degree:

   1. Inflated self-esteem or grandiosity.

   2. Decreased need for sleep (e.g., feels rested after only 3 hours of sleep).

   3. More talkative than usual or pressure to keep talking.

   4. Flight of ideas or subjective experience that thoughts are racing.

   5. Distractibility (i.e., attention too easily drawn to unimportant or irrelevant external stimuli), as reported or observed.

   6. Increase in goal-directed activity (either socially, at work or school, or sexually) or psychomotor agitation (i.e., purposeless non-goal-directed activity).

   7. Excessive involvement in activities that have a high potential for painful consequences (e.g., engaging in unrestrained buying sprees, sexual indiscretions, or foolish business investments).

   C. The episode is associated with an unequivocal change in functioning that is uncharacteristic of the individual when not symptomatic.

   D. The disturbance in mood and the change in functioning are observable by others.

   E. The episode is not severe enough to cause marked impairment in social or occupational functioning or to necessitate hospitalization. If there are psychotic features, the episode is, by definition, manic.

   F. The episode is not attributable to the physiological effects of a substance (e.g., a drug of abuse, a medication, other treatment).

Note: A full hypomanic episode that emerges during antidepressant treatment (e.g., medications, electroconvulsive therapy) but persists at a fully syndromal level beyond the physiological effect of that treatment is sufficient evidence for a hypomanic episode diagnosis. However, caution is indicated so that one or two symptoms (particularly increased irritability, edginess, or agitation following antidepressant use) are not taken as sufficient for diagnosis of a hypomanic episode, nor necessarily indicative of a bipolar diathesis.

Major Depressive Episode

A. Five (or more) of the following symptoms have been present during the same 2-week period and represent a change from previous functioning: at least one of the symptoms is either (1) depressed mood or (2) loss of interest or pleasure.
Note: Do not include symptoms that are clearly attributable to another medical condition.

1. Depressed mood most of the day, nearly every day, as indicated by either subjective report (e.g., feels sad, empty, or hopeless) or observation made by others (e.g., appears tearful). (**Note**: In children and adolescents, can be irritable mood.)

2. Markedly diminished interest or pleasure in all, or almost all, activities most of the day, nearly every day (as indicated by either subjective account or observation).

3. Significant weight loss when not dieting or weight gain (e.g., a change of more than 5% of body weight in a month), or decrease or increase in appetite nearly every day. (**Note:** In children, consider failure to make expected weight gain.)

4. Insomnia or hypersomnia nearly every day.

5. Psychomotor agitation or retardation nearly every day (observable by others; not merely subjective feelings of restlessness or being slowed down).

6. Fatigue or loss of energy nearly every day.

7. Feelings of worthlessness or excessive or inappropriate guilt (which may be delusional) nearly every day (not merely self-reproach or guilt about being sick).

8. Diminished ability to think or concentrate, or indecisiveness, nearly every day (either by subjective account or as observed by others).

9. Recurrent thoughts of death (not just fear of dying), recurrent suicidal ideation without a specific plan, or a suicide attempt or a specific plan for committing suicide.

B. The symptoms cause clinically significant distress or impairment in social, occupational, or other important areas of functioning.

C. The episode is not attributable to the physiological effects of a substance or another medical condition.

Note: Criteria A-C constitute a major depressive episode.

Note: Responses to a significant loss (e.g., bereavement, financial ruin, losses from natural disaster, a serious medical illness or disability) may include feelings of intense sadness, rumination about the loss, insomnia, poor appetite, and weight loss noted in Criterion A, which may resemble a depressive episode. Although such symptoms may be understandable or considered appropriate to the loss, the presence of major depressive episode in addition to the normal response to a significant loss should also be carefully considered. This decision inevitably requires the exercise of clinical judgment based on the individual's history and the cultural norms for the expression of distress in the context of loss.[1]

Bipolar II Disorder

A. Criteria have been met for at least one hypomanic episode (Criteria A-F under "Hypomanic Episode" above) and at least one major depressive episode (Criteria A-C under "Major Depressive Episode" above).

B. There has never been a manic episode.

C. The occurrence of the hypomanic episode(s) and major depressive episode(s) is not better explained by schizoaffective disorder, schizophrenia, schizophreniform disorder, delusional disorder, or other specified or unspecified schizophrenia spectrum and other psychotic disorder.

D. The symptoms of depression or the unpredictability caused by frequent alternation between periods of depression and hypomania causes clinically significant distress or impairment in social, occupational, or other important areas of functioning.

Coding and Recording Procedures

Bipolar II disorder has one diagnostic code: 296.89 (F31.81). Its status with respect to current severity, presence of psychotic features, course, and other specifiers cannot be coded but should be indicated in writing (e.g., 296.89 [F31.81] bipolar II disorder, current episode depressed, moderate severity, with mixed features; 296.89 [F31.81] bipolar II disorder, most recent episode depressed, in partial remission).

Specify current or most recent episode:

Hypomanic   **Depressed**

Specify if:

With anxious distress

With mixed features

With rapid cycling

With mood-congruent psychotic features

With mood-incongruent psychotic features

With catatonia; Coding note: Use additional code 293.89 (F06.1).

With peripartum onset

With seasonal pattern: Applies only to the pattern of major depressive episodes.

Specify course if full criteria for a mood episode are not currently met:

In partial remission   **In full remission**

Specify severity if full criteria for a mood episode are currently met:

Mild   **Moderate**   **Severe**

---

[1] In distinguishing grief from a major depressive episode (MDE), it is useful to consider that in grief the predominant affect is feelings of emptiness and loss, while in MDE it is persistent depressed mood and the inability to anticipate happiness or pleasure. The dysphoria in grief is likely to decrease in intensity over days to weeks and occurs in waves, the so-called pangs of grief. These waves tend to be associated with thoughts or reminders of the deceased. The depressed mood of a MDE is more persistent and not tied to specific thoughts or preoccupations. The pain of grief may be accompanied by positive emotions and humor that are uncharacteristic of the pervasive unhappiness and misery characteristic of a major depressive episode. The thought content associated with grief generally features a preoccupation with thoughts and memories of the deceased, rather than the self-critical or pessimistic ruminations seen in a MDE. In grief, self-esteem is generally preserved, whereas in a MDE, feelings of worthlessness and self-loathing are common. If self-derogatory ideation is present in grief, it typically involves perceived failings vis-à-vis the deceased (e.g., not visiting frequently enough, not telling the deceased how much he or she was loved). If a bereaved individual thinks about death and dying, such thoughts are generally focused on the deceased and possibly about "joining" the deceased, whereas in a major depressive episode such thoughts are focused on ending one's own life because of feeling worthless, undeserving of life, or unable to cope with the pain of depression.

Section 4 - Depressive Disorders

Screening Tools for Child and Adolescent Depression

As with other disorders, depression should not be diagnosed solely by a screening tool. Further evaluation in the form of a clinical interview is necessary for children and adolescents identified as depressed through a screening process. Further evaluation also is warranted for children or adolescents who exhibit depressive symptoms but who do not screen positive.

There are a few valid and reliable depression screening tools for children and adolescents.

The USPSTF recommends screening all adolescents (12-18 years of age) for MDD when systems are in place to ensure accurate diagnosis, psychotherapy (cognitive-behavioral or interpersonal) and follow-up, and concludes that the evidence is insufficient to assess the balance of benefits and harms of screening of children (7-11 years of age) (see **http://www.uspreventiveservicestaskforce.org/uspstf/ uspschdepr.htm**).

The USPSTF recommends asking adults the following two questions, which may be as effective as using longer screening instruments. These questions also may be indicated when interviewing teens, especially if time is limited for the use of longer screening instruments.

1. Over the past 2 weeks, have you ever felt down, depressed, or hopeless?

2. Over the past 2 weeks, have you felt little interest or pleasure in doing things?

Center for Epidemiological Studies Depression Scale for Children (CES-DC)
(L.S. Radloff)

Description

The Center for Epidemiological Studies Depression Scale for Children (CES-DC) (see the instrument on the following page) is a 20-item self-report depression inventory with possible scores ranging from 0 to 60. Each response to an item is scored as follows:

> 0 = "Not At All"
>
> 1 = "A Little"
>
> 2 = "Some"
>
> 3 = "A Lot"

However, items 4, 8, 12, and 16 are phrased positively, and thus are scored in the opposite order:

> 3 = "Not At All"
>
> 2 = "A Little"
>
> 1 = "Some"
>
> 0 = "A Lot"

Higher CES-DC scores indicate increasing levels of depression. Weissman and colleagues (1980), the developers of the CES-DC, have used the cut-off score of 15 as being suggestive of depressive symptoms in children and adolescents. That is, scores over 15 can be indicative of significant levels of depressive symptoms.

Psychometric Properties

The CES-DC has been found to be a valid and reliable tool for depression screening in older school-age children and adolescents.

References

Faulstich, M.E., Carey, M.P., Ruggiero, L., et al. (1986). Assessment of depression in childhood and adolescence: an evaluation of the Center for Epidemiological Studies Depression Scale for Children (CES-DC). American Journal of Psychiatry, 143(8), 1024-1027.

Weissman, M.M., Orvaschel, H., Padian, N. (1980). Children's symptom and social functioning self-report scales: comparison of mothers' and children's reports. Journal of Nervous Mental Disorders, 168(12), 736-740.

Number _____

Score _____

INSTRUCTIONS

Below is a list of the ways you might have felt or acted. Please check how *much* you have felt this way during the *past week*.

DURING THE PAST WEEK	Not At All	A Little	Some	A Lot
1. I was bothered by things that usually don't bother me.				
2. I did not feel like eating, I wasn't very hungry.				
3. I wasn't able to feel happy, even when my family or friends tried to help me feel better.				
4. I felt like I was just as good as other kids.				
5. I felt like I couldn't pay attention to what I was doing.				

DURING THE PAST WEEK	Not At All	A Little	Some	A Lot
6. I felt down and unhappy.				
7. I felt like I was too tired to do things.				
8. I felt like something good was going to happen.				
9. I felt like things I did before didn't work out right.				
10. I felt scared.				

DURING THE PAST WEEK	Not At All	A Little	Some	A Lot
11. I didn't sleep as well as I usually sleep.				
12. I was happy.				
13. I was more quiet than usual.				
14. I felt lonely, like I didn't have any friends.				
15. I felt like kids I know were not friendly or that they didn't want to be with me.				

DURING THE PAST WEEK	Not At All	A Little	Some	A Lot
16. I had a good time.				
17. I felt like crying.				
18. I felt sad.				
19. I felt people didn't like me.				
20. It was hard to get started doing things.				

From: Bright Futures at Georgetown University, available at www.brightfutures.org; in the public domain.

Patient Health Questionniare-9 (PHQ-9) and PHQ-9 Modified for Teens

The Patient Health Questionnaire-9 (PHQ-9) assists clinicians in identifying individuals who may be affected by depression. It is available in the public domain and free for use in multiple languages at **http://www.phqscreeners.com/overview.aspx**. The instrument has been modified for use with adolescents 12-18 years of age (i.e., PHQ-9 Modified for Teens).

Description

These 9-item self-report instruments can be administered in less than 5 minutes. The tools are used as a brief screen for depression; they identify adults and adolescents at risk for depression so that healthcare providers can conduct a clinical interview for definitive diagnosis and treatment.

Psychometric Properties

The PHQ-9 has been established as valid and reliable across culturally diverse populations and a variety of medical conditions. In a recent study with 442 adolescents 13 to 17 years of age, a **PHQ-9** score of 11 or higher had a sensitivity of 89.5% and a specificity of 77.5% for detecting youth who met the *Diagnostic and Statistical Manual of Mental Disorders* criteria for major depression. Increasing **PHQ-9** scores were significantly correlated with increasing levels of functional impairment as well as reports of psychosocial problems by the teens' parents (Richardson et al., 2010).

Scoring

Item scores are summed. Total scores of 11 or higher is a positive screen. Regardless of the total score on the 9 items, endorsement of serious suicidal ideation or past suicide attempt (questions 12 and 13) should be interpreted as a positive screen.

1-4:	Minimal depression
5-9:	Mild depression
10-14:	Moderate depression ($\geq$11 positive score)
15-19:	Moderately severe depression
20-27:	Severe depression

Coding for Reimbursement

The following codes can be used for mental health screening:

96110- Mental health screening

99420- Health risk assessment

PATIENT HEALTH QUESTIONNAIRE- 9
(PHQ-9)

Over the last 2 weeks, how often have you been bothered by any of the following problems?

(Use " ✓ " to indicate your answer)	Not At All	Several days	More than half the days	Nearly Everyday
1. Little interest or pleasure in doing things	0	1	2	3
2. Feeling down, depressed, or hopeless	0	1	2	3
3. Trouble falling or staying asleep, or sleeping too much	0	1	2	3
4. Feeling tried or having little enerrgy	0	1	2	3
5. Poor appetite or overeating	0	1	2	3
6. Feeling bad about yourself – or that you are a failure or have let yourself or your family down	0	1	2	3
7. Trouble concentrating on things, such as reading the newspaper or watching television	0	1	2	3
8. Moving or speaking slowly that other people could have notice? Or the opposite – being so fidgety or restless that you have been moving around a lot more than usual	0	1	2	3
9. Thoughts that you would be better off dead or of hurting yourself in some way	0	1	2	3

FOR OFFICE CODING ___0___ + _____ + ____ + _____
=Total Score: ___

If you checked off <u>any</u> problems, how <u>difficult</u> have these problems made it for you to do your work, take care of things at home, or get along with other people?

Not difficult at all   Somewhat difficult   Very difficult   Extremely difficult

Office use only   Severity score:

Developed by Drs. Robert L. Spitzer, Janet B.W. Williams, Kurt Kroenke and colleagues, with an educational grant from Pfizer Inc. No permission required to reproduce, translate, display or distribute.

(PHQ-9) MODIFIED FOR

How often have you been bothered by each of the following symptoms during the past two weeks?

Name:_____ Clinician:_____ Date:_____

For each symptom put an "X" in the box beneath the answer that best describes how you have been feeling.

(Use " **X** " to indicate your answer)	Not at all	Several days	More than half the days	Nearly Everyday
1. Feeling down, depressed, irritable, or hopeless?				
2. Little interest or pleasure in doing things?				
3. Trouble falling asleep, staying asleep, or sleeping too much?				
4. Poor appetite, weight loss, or overeating?				
5. Feeling tired, or having little energy?				
6. Feeling bad about yourself – or feeling that you are a failure, or that you have let yourself or your family down?				
7. Trouble concentrating on things like school work, reading or watching TV?				
8. Moving or speaking so slowly that other people could have noticed? Or the opposite – being so fidgety or restless that you were moving around a lot more than usual?				
9. Thoughts that you would be better off dead, or of hurting yourself in some way?				

In the <u>past year</u> have you felt depressed or sad most days, even if you felt okay some days?

[ ] Yes   [ ] No

If you are experiencing any of the problems on this form, how difficult have these problems made it for you to do your work, take care of things at home or get along with other people?

[ ] Not difficult at all   [ ] Somewhat difficult   [ ] Very difficult   [ ] Extremely difficult

Has there been a time in the <u>past month</u> when you have had serious thoughts about ending your life?

[ ] Yes   [ ] No

Have you <u>EVER</u>, in your WHOLE LIFE, tried to kill yourself or made a suicide attempt?

[ ] Yes   [ ] No

**If you have had thoughts that you would be better off dead or of hurting yourself in some way, please discuss this with your Health Care Clinician, go to a hospital emergency room or call 911.

Office use only   **Severity score:**

Modified with permission by the GLAD-PC team from the PHQ-9 (Spitzer, Williams & Kroenke, 1999), Revised PHQ-A (Johnson 2002), and the CDS (DISC Development Group, 2000).

Edinburgh Postnatal Depression Scale

The Edinburgh *Postnatal Depression Scale (EPDS)* assists clinicians in identifying mothers suffering from postpartum depression early and easily. It is in the public domain and free for use in clinical settings.

Description

This 10-item, widely used self-report instrument can be administered in less than 5 minutes. Used as a brief screening tool, the EPDS identifies women who are at high risk for postpartum depression so that healthcare professionals can then refer them for definitive diagnosis and treatment. Mothers respond using a 4-point Likert scale to the items, which tap various clinical depression symptoms, such as guilt, sleep disturbance, low energy, and suicidal ideation. The EPDS is available in multiple languages and also can be used for depression screening during pregnancy.

Psychometric Properties

Multiple studies have supported the scale's validity and excellent reliability.

Administration and Scoring

The EPDS can be used across various specialties, including obstetrics, pediatrics, psychiatry, psychology, and social work.

Response categories are scored 0, 1, 2, and 3 according to increased severity of the symptom. Items 3, 5-10 are reverse scored (i.e., 3, 2, 1, and 0). The total score is calculated by adding together the scores for each of the 10 items. Mothers who score above 13 are likely to be suffering from a depressive illness of varying severity.

Edinburgh Postnatal Depression Scale[1] (EPDS)

Name: _____   Address: _____

Your Date of Birth: _____   _____

Baby's Date of Birth: _____   Phone: _____

As you are pregnant or have recently had a baby, we would like to know how you are feeling. Please check the answer that comes closest to how you have felt **IN THE PAST 7 DAYS**, not just how you feel today.

Here is an example, already completed.

I have felt happy:
- ☐ Yes, all the time
- ☒ Yes, most of the time   This would mean: "I have felt happy most of the time" during the past week.
- ☐ No, not very often   Please complete the other questions in the same way.
- ☐ No, not at all

In the past 7 days:

1. I have been able to laugh and see the funny side of things
   - ☐ As much as I always could
   - ☐ Not quite so much now
   - ☐ Definitely not so much now
   - ☐ Not at all

2. I have looked forward with enjoyment to things
   - ☐ As much as I ever did
   - ☐ Rather less than I used to
   - ☐ Definitely less than I used to
   - ☐ Hardly at all

*3. I have blamed myself unnecessarily when things went wrong
   - ☐ Yes, most of the time
   - ☐ Yes, some of the time
   - ☐ Not very often
   - ☐ No, never

4. I have been anxious or worried for no good reason
   - ☐ No, not at all
   - ☐ Hardly ever
   - ☐ Yes, sometimes
   - ☐ Yes, very often

*5 I have felt scared or panicky for no very good reason
   - ☐ Yes, quite a lot
   - ☐ Yes, sometimes
   - ☐ No, not much
   - ☐ No, not at all

*6. Things have been getting on top of me
   - ☐ Yes, most of the time I haven't been able to cope at all
   - ☐ Yes, sometimes I haven't been coping as well as usual
   - ☐ No, most of the time I have coped quite well
   - ☐ No, I have been coping as well as ever

*7 I have been so unhappy that I have had difficulty sleeping
   - ☐ Yes, most of the time
   - ☐ Yes, sometimes
   - ☐ Not very often
   - ☐ No, not at all

*8 I have felt sad or miserable
   - ☐ Yes, most of the time
   - ☐ Yes, quite often
   - ☐ Not very often
   - ☐ No, not at all

*9 I have been so unhappy that I have been crying
   - ☐ Yes, most of the time
   - ☐ Yes, quite often
   - ☐ Only occasionally
   - ☐ No, never

*10 The thought of harming myself has occurred to me
   - ☐ Yes, quite often
   - ☐ Sometimes
   - ☐ Hardly ever
   - ☐ Never

Administered/Reviewed by _____   Date _____

[1]Source: Cox, J.L., Holden, J.M., and Sagovsky, R. 1987. Detection of postnatal depression: Development of the 10-item Edinburgh Postnatal Depression Scale.   *British Journal of Psychiatry* 150:782-786 .

[2]Source: K. L. Wisner, B. L. Parry, C. M. Piontek, Postpartum Depression N Engl J Med vol. 347, No 3, July 18, 2002, 194-199

Users may reproduce the scale without further permission providing they respect copyright by quoting the names of the authors, the title and the source of the paper in all reproduced copies.

Edinburgh Postnatal Depression Scale[1] (EPDS)

Postpartum depression is the most common complication of childbearing.[2] The 10-question EPDS is a valuable and efficient way of identifying patients at risk for "perinatal" depression. The EPDS is easy to administer and has proven to be an effective screening tool.

Mothers who score above 13 are likely to be suffering from a depressive illness of varying severity. The EPDS score should not override clinical judgment. A careful clinical assessment should be carried out to confirm the diagnosis. The scale indicates how the mother has felt *during the previous week*. In doubtful cases it may be useful to repeat the tool after 2 weeks. The scale will not detect mothers with anxiety neuroses, phobias, or personality disorders.

Women with postpartum depression need not feel alone. They may find useful information on the Websites of the National Women's Health Information Center (www.4women.gov) and from groups such as Postpartum Support International (www.chss.iup.edu/postpartum) and Depression after Delivery (www.depressionafterdelivery.com).

SCORING

QUESTIONS 1, 2, & 4 (without an *)

Are scored 0, 1, 2 or 3 with top box scored as 0 and the bottom box scored as 3.

w 3, 510 (marked with an *)

Are reverse scored, with the top box scored as a 3 and the bottom box scored as 0.

Maximum score: 30
Possible Depression: 10 or greater
Always look at item 10 (suicidal thoughts)

Users may reproduce the scale without further permission, providing they respect copyright by quoting the names of the authors, the title, and the source of the paper in all reproduced copies.

Instructions for using the Edinburgh Postnatal Depression Scale:

1. The mother is asked to check the response that comes closest to how she has been feeling in the previous 7 days.

2. All the items must be completed.

3. Care should be taken to avoid the possibility of the mother discussing her answers with others. (Answers come from the mother or pregnant woman.)

4. The mother should complete the scale herself, unless she has limited command of the English language or has difficulty with reading.

[1]Source: Cox, J. L., Holden, J. M., and Sagovsky, R. 1987. Detection of postnatal depression: Development of the 10-item Edinburgh Postnatal Depression Scale. British Journal of Psychiatry, 150:782-786.

[2]Source: K. L. Wisner, B. L. Parry, C. M. Piontek, Postpartum Depression N Engl J Med vol. 347, No 3, July 18, 2002, 194-199.

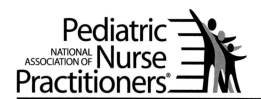

What Is Depression?

Depression is an unhappy mood that affects daily functioning, including thoughts, feelings, behavior, and overall health. When depression is too severe or lasts too long, it is considered an illness that can be treated. Left untreated, depression can take the joy out of life and even take away the desire to live. Everyone experiences minor upsets, but this does not mean that everyone is depressed. To have true depression, the symptoms must be present for at least 2 weeks.

How Common Is Depression?

Depression in children and teens is far more common than most people realize and affects school-age girls and boys equally. After puberty, girls are twice as likely as boys to be depressed. Ten out of 100 teens get seriously depressed each year, and many more have mild levels of sadness or the blues. About 1 in 10 children without known problems has suicidal thoughts.

What Are the Signs of Depression?

The most important signs to look for are feelings of sadness and hopelessness. While every child or teen is sad some of the time, no child should feel sad all of the time. If you notice that your child is unhappy and can't seem to have fun, think of this as a sign of depression. To be hopeless or without hope means to feel that nothing can go right, that nothing will change, and that no one can help.

Poor self-esteem is another important sign of depression. This is the teen's or child's attitude toward himself. If your child's self-esteem is poor, he or she may feel stupid, ugly, or worthless. Another sign is a change in school performance. If your child was a good student and now wants to stay home, or if his/her grades suddenly fall, he/she may be depressed. Other signs include sleep problems, appetite changes, irritability, anger, crying, and aches and pains, such as headaches or stomachaches.

What would your child say if he or she is depressed? Don't expect your child to say much, because you can't count on him/her telling you how he/she feels. While your child may talk of being unhappy, he or she probably won't say, "I'm depressed" the way an adult will. So, you want to be aware of the signs.

What If My Child Should Mention Suicide?

Sometimes a child mentions that he or she does not want to live. If your child mentions suicide: Take it seriously. Talk to your child. Ask if he or she has made a plan for suicide. If so, it is more serious. If suicide is mentioned or if an attempt is made, seek professional help immediately. Do not assume your child is just looking for attention. Don't ever dare a youngster who mentions suicide to "go ahead." You may think it's a bluff, but he or she may take the dare.

How Can a Parent Help?

You can be very helpful to your depressed child. Some suggestions include: Be supportive -- listen to what your child has to say. Encourage him or her to keep talking. If your child can't talk well with you, perhaps he or she can talk with a sibling, aunt, friend, teacher, or healthcare provider. Encourage your child to describe or write down how he or she feels. Don't get angry if he/she describes unhappy feelings. **If the problem is severe, worrisome, or lasts more than 2 weeks, get professional help. Talk to your child's healthcare provider if you have any concern that your child may be depressed.**

What Are the Causes of Depression in Children?

There is no single answer to the cause of depression. It is probable that several factors combine to create the condition. The child's environment, especially if it is unhappy and stressful, is often a major cause. Depression also may be triggered by difficult situations, such as a death or divorce in the family or abuse. Another possible contributing factor is heredity. Studies show that depression frequently runs in families, so genetics may play a part in the depression of some children. Yet other reasons are a lack of a certain chemical in the brain, called serotonin, and a negative pattern of thinking (e.g., I can't do anything right; everything is bad).

What Are the Treatments for Depression?

- Treatment is possible and helpful. The choice of treatment depends on the cause of the problem, the severity of the depression, and whether suicidal thoughts are present. Psychotherapy, such as cognitive behavior therapy, is the primary treatment. By meeting regularly with a therapist, your child can find out the causes of his/her depression, and then learn ways to help deal with it. It is usually good for the family to become involved in the treatment.

- Medication can be an effective part of treatment. Antidepressants have few side effects and are not habit-forming or addictive.

- Finally, you should not feel guilty if your child is depressed. The important point is to realize that there is a problem and to get help for it. If you are concerned, be sure to talk to your child's healthcare provider. Remember, depression in children and teens is treatable.

What Can I Do to Prevent or Help My Child with Depression?

- Stay involved in your child's life. Spend time with your child regularly, even if it's only a family dinner. Too often, parents respond to growing teenagers' wishes for independence by withdrawing from their teens' lives. The most important thing for parents to do is to be aware of and involved in their teen's life.

- Support positive relationships by encouraging your teen to get involved in school, clubs, or community events. Help your teen find interests and activities where he or she can connect with other teens. Also, know where your teen is and what he/she is doing when they go out.

- Talk to your teen, and listen when he/she talks to you! Parents should talk to their children as often as possible so teens can talk about their problems and worries. Ask your teen about school and friends. Listen to his/her troubles and help find solutions.

- Teach your child coping and problem-solving skills; it also is important for you to role model positive ways of coping and dealing with stress.

- Know the warning signs of depression and be aware if your child shows any of these signs while talking to you, especially if he or she mentions suicide. Praise your teen's accomplishments rather than finding fault with things he/she does. Teens need to feel that their parents care about them and that what they are doing is recognized.

- It is mainly your job to make sure that your child receives the treatment he or she needs. Make sure that your teen takes his/her medication and goes to counseling. Be supportive.

- For more information about depression, contact the school counselor, psychologist, or social worker at your child's school, or contact your child's doctor or nurse practitioner.

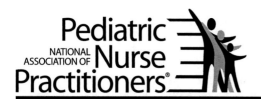

Information on Depression for Teens

What Is Depression?

Depression is a common and serious condition that can affect your thoughts, feelings, behavior, and overall health. Ten out of 100 teens get seriously depressed each year, and many more have mild levels of sadness or the blues. There is hope for teens with depression because it can be treated.

When You're Depressed, You Might Think, Feel or Act in Some of These Ways

- You feel sad or cry a lot and it doesn't go away.
- You feel guilty easily; you feel like you are no good; you've lost your confidence.
- Life seems empty or like nothing good is ever going to happen again.
- You tend to think negatively, like believing that you can't do anything right.
- You have a negative attitude a lot of the time, or it seems like you have no feelings.
- You don't feel like doing a lot of the things you used to enjoy -- like playing music, sports, being with friends, going out -- and you want to be left alone most of the time.
- It's hard to make up your mind. You forget lots of things, and it's hard to concentrate.
- You get angry often. Little things make you lose your temper; you overreact.
- Your sleep pattern changes; you start sleeping a lot more or you have trouble falling asleep at night. Or, you wake up really early most mornings and can't get back to sleep.
- Your eating habits change; you've lost your appetite or you eat a lot more.
- You feel restless and tired most of the time.
- You think about death, or feel like you're dying, or have thoughts about hurting yourself or committing suicide.

Some teens who are depressed also can get "manic" at times, which may be a sign of bipolar disorder. When you're manic, you may feel or act in some of these ways

- You feel high as a kite... like you're "on top of the world."
- You get unreal ideas about the great things you can do- things that you really can't do.
- Thoughts go racing through your head and you talk a lot.
- You're a nonstop party, constantly running around.
- You do too many wild or risky things, like reckless driving, spending money, and having sex with multiple partners.
- You're so "up" that you don't need much sleep.
- You're rebellious or irritable and can't get along at home or school, or with your friends.

If you think you're depressed... TALK TO SOMEONE!

If you have had some of these symptoms and they have lasted a couple of weeks or have caused a big change in your routine, you should talk to someone who can help, like a psychologist, nurse or doctor, or your school counselor!

Treatment for Depression

Having depression doesn't mean that a person is weak, or a failure, or isn't really trying... it means they need TREATMENT. Most people with depression can be helped with counseling, and some are helped with counseling and medicine.

COUNSELING means talking about feelings with a special healthcare provider who can help you with the relationships, thoughts, or behaviors that are causing the depression. Don't wait; ask your parents or your school counselor for help today. MEDICINE is used to treat more serious depression. These medications are not "uppers" and are not addictive. When depression is so bad that you can't focus on anything else, when it interferes with your life, medication might be necessary along with counseling. But most often, counseling alone works. With treatment, most depressed people start to feel better in just a few weeks.

What about Suicide?

Most people who are depressed do not commit suicide. But, depression increases the risk for suicide or suicide attempts. It is NOT true that people who talk about suicide do not attempt it. Suicidal thoughts, remarks, or attempts are ALWAYS SERIOUS... if any of these happen to you or a friend, you must tell a responsible adult IMMEDIATELY.... It's better to be safe than sorry.

Why Do People Get Depressed?

Sometimes people get seriously depressed after something like a divorce in the family, major money problems, the death of someone they love, a messed-up home life, or breaking up with a boyfriend or girlfriend. Other times, depression just happens. Often, teens react to the pain of depression by getting into trouble: trouble with alcohol, drugs, or sex; trouble with school or bad grades; problems with family or friends. This is another reason why it's important to get treatment for depression before it leads to other trouble.

Myths about Depression

- **MYTH:** It's normal for teens to be moody; Teens don't suffer from "real" depression.

- **FACT:** Depression is more than just being moody; and it affects people at any age.

- **MYTH:** Telling an adult that a friend might be depressed is betraying a trust. If someone wants help, he or she will get it.

- **FACT:** Depression, which saps energy and self-esteem, interferes with a person's ability or wish to get help. It is an act of true friendship to share your concerns with an adult who can help. No matter what you "promised" to keep secret, your friend's life is more important than a promise.

- **MYTH:** Talking about depression only makes it worse.

- **FACT:** Talking about your feelings to someone who can help, like a psychologist or nurse practitioner, is the first step toward beating depression. Talking to a close friend also can provide you with the support and encouragement you need to talk to your parents or school counselor about getting help for depression.

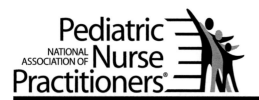

CONTRACT FOR SELF SAFETY

I _____ , promise to keep myself safe.
If I am thinking about hurting myself, I will tell my parent,
another close adult, or my nurse practitioner or doctor.

_____   _____
Signature of Adolescent   Signature of Provider or
                                                  Parent/Guardian

_____
Date

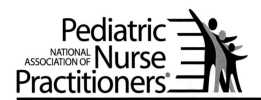

CONTRACT FOR OTHERS' SAFETY

I _____ , promise to keep others around me safe from harm. If I am thinking about hurting anyone, I will tell my parent, another close adult, or my nurse practitioner or doctor.

_____
Signature of Adolescent

_____
Signature of Provider or
Parent/Guardian

_____
Date

Resources for Child and Adolescent Depressive Disorders

KidsHealth
www.kidshealth.org

This Website contains a wealth of resources for families about child and adolescent mental health and parenting. Resources include science-based articles, newsletters, and manuals; a guide to common mental health problems; lists of recommended books, Websites, and organizations; a glossary of medical terms explained in an easy-to-understand format; and an ask-the-expert service. "About Our Kids" is presented by the New York University School of Medicine Child Study Center.

American Academy of Child and Adolescent Psychiatry (AACAP)
www.aacap.org

This Website contains information about research, legislative activities, and meetings regarding child and adolescent mental health; policy statements; clinical practice guidelines; and a directory of child and adolescent psychiatrists. It also offers a set of Fact Sheets for families in English, Spanish, and several other languages on a variety of topics that include ADHD, bullying, depression, and suicide.

COPE (Creating Opportunities for Personal Empowerment) for Children, Adolescents and Young Adults

The COPE Program is an evidence-based, 7-session, manualized, reproducible, cognitive-behavioral skills building intervention program, based on the 12 key components of CBT, which can be used for depression and anxiety disorders with children, adolescents, and young adults in primary care, specialty clinics, school-based settings and hospitals (Lusk & Melnyk, 2011; Lusk & Melnyk, 2013; Melnyk, Kelly & Lusk, in press). A 15-session program also is available, which contains the 7 CBT skills building sessions along with sessions on nutrition and physical activity for delivery by teachers or other professionals in school-based settings (Melnyk et al., 2009; Melnyk et al., in press). An on-line version of the 7-session program is available for adolescents. Contact Bernadette Melnyk at cope.melnyk@gmail.com.

National Institute of Mental Health
www.nimh.nih.gov
This outstanding Website offers multiple educational handouts on a variety of mental health disorders, including mood disorders, and links to other informative Websites.

The REACH (REsource for Advancing Children's Health) Institute
http://www.thereachinstitute.org/about-REACH.html

The REACH Institute is dedicated to improving the mental health of American children and adolescents with emotional and behavioral challenges. It provides workshops for healthcare providers that teach the best evidence-based therapies, from psychotherapy to pharmacology, to improve the mental health of children and teens. Excellent resources at the Website are available for healthcare providers, agencies, and families.

United States Preventive Services Task Force (USPSTF)
http://www.ahrq.gov/clinic/uspstfix.htm

The USPSTF is an independent group of national experts in prevention and evidence-based practice that works to improve the health of all Americans by making evidence-based recommendations about clinical preventive services such as screenings, counseling services, or preventive medications. The USPSTF is made up of 16 volunteer members from the fields of preventive medicine and primary care, including internal medicine, family medicine, pediatrics, behavioral health, obstetrics/gynecology, and nursing. Every year, the USPSTF updates the Guide to Clinical Preventive Services, which contains evidence-based recommendations for a variety of topics, including screening for depression and obesity in children and adolescents.

Youth Depression Treatment and Prevention Programs
http://www.kpchr.org/public/acwd/acwd.html.

The following downloadable evidenced-based cognitive-behavioral intervention programs for adolescents, developed by Lewinsohn, Clark, and colleagues, are available free of charge. These programs were developed for use by mental health professionals with groups of adolescents who are depressed or at risk for future depression.

- The Adolescent Coping with Depression [CWD-A] Course. This is an evidence-based treatment intervention for actively depressed adolescents. The program also includes a separate intervention for the parents of these depressed adolescents.

- The Adolescent Coping with Stress Course [CWS] Course. This is an evidence-based group prevention intervention for youth at risk for future depression.

- A brief, individual treatment program (5 to 9 sessions) for depressed youth who also are receiving SSRI antidepressant medication is available.

REFERENCES

American Psychiatric Association (2013). *Diagnostic and Statistical Manual of Mental Disorders. Fourth Edition* (DSM-V). Washington, DC: APA.

Cheung, A.H., Zuckerbrot, R.A., Jensen, P.S. et al (2007). Guidelines for adolescent depression in primary care (GLAD-PC): II. Treatment and ongoing management. *Pediatrics*, 120(5), e1313-e1326.

Jellinek, M., Patel, B.P., & Froehle, M. (2002). *Bright Futures in Practice: Mental Health- Vol I. Practice Guide.* Arlington, VA: National Center for Education in Maternal and Child Health.

Jellinek, M., Patel, B.P., & Froehle, M. (2002). *Bright Futures in Practice: Mental Health- Vol II. Tool Kit.* Arlington, VA: National Center for Education in Maternal and Child Health.

Lusk, P. & Melnyk, B.M. (2011). The brief cognitive-behavioral COPE intervention for depressed adolescents: outcomes and feasibility of delivery in 30-minute outpatient visits. Journal of the American Psychiatric Nurses Association, 17(3), 226-236.

Lusk, P. & Melnyk, B.M. (2013). COPE for depressed and anxious teens: a brief cognitive-behavioral skills building intervention to increase access to timely, evidence-based treatment. *Journal of Child and Adolescent Psychiatric Nursing,* 26(1), 23-31.

March, J., Silva, S., Petrycki, S., et al. (2004). Fluoxetine, cognitive-behavioral therapy, and their combination for adolescents with depression: Treatment for Adolescents with Depression Study (TADS) randomized controlled trial. *Journal of the American Medical Association*, 292(7), 807-820.

Melnyk, B.M., Jacobson, D., Kelly, S., et al. (in press). Promoting healthy lifestyles in high school adolescents. A randomized controlled trial. *American Journal of Preventive Medicine*.

Melnyk, B.M., Jacobson, D., Kelly, S., O'Haver, J., Small, L., & Mays, M.Z. (2009). Improving the mental health, healthy lifestyle choices and physical health of Hispanic adolescents: a randomized controlled pilot study. *Journal of School Health.* 79(12), 575-584.

Melnyk, B.M., Kelly, S., & Lusk, P. (in press). Outcomes and feasibility of a manualized cognitive-behavioral skills building intervention: group COPE for depressed and anxious adolescents. *Journal of Child and Adolescent Psychiatric Nursing.* Melnyk, B.M., & Moldenhauer, Z. (2006). *The KySS Guide to Child and Adolescent Mental Health Screening, Early Intervention and Health Promotion.* Cherry Hill, New Jersey: National Association of Pediatric Nurse Practitioners (NAPNAP) and NAPNAP Foundation.

Richardson, L.P., McCauley, E., Grossman, D.C., et al. (2010). Evaluation of the Patient Health Questionnaire-9 Item for detecting major depression among adolescents. *Pediatrics*, 126(6), 1117-1123.

Sadock, B.J., & Sadock, V.A. (2009). Kaplan & Sadock's Concise Textbook of *Child and Adolescent Psychiatry.* Philadelphia, Pennsylvania: Wolters Kluwer/Lippincott Williams & Wilkins.

Stahl, S.M. (2011). *Stahl's Essential Psychopharmacology. The Prescriber's Guide (4th edition)* New York, NY: Cambridge University Press.

SECTION 5
Ann Guthery

Attention-Deficit/Hyperactivity Disorder (ADHD)

Fast Facts

- ADHD is the most common behavior disorder in children.
- ADHD is present in 4%-12% of school-age children.
- ADHD is more common in males than in females (3-6:1).
- It typically presents during early childhood, before 7 years of age, although changes in the DSM-5™ have noted that most lifetime cases are captured with an onset of age 12-14.
- The disorder involves a persistent pattern of inattention, impulsiveness, or both.
- Children with ADHD often have comorbid disorders (e.g., anxiety disorders, depressive disorders, learning disorders, oppositional defiant disorder).

Comorbidities Important for Assessment

- Specific learning disabilities (10%-40%)
- Oppositional defiant disorder (30%-60%)
- Depression/anxiety disorders
- Bipolar disorder
- Fetal alcohol syndrome
- Tourette's syndrome
- Psychosocial morbidities

Mimics of ADHD

- Language disorder
- Learning disability
- Anxiety/obsessive compulsive disorder
- Depressive and bipolar disorders
- Oppositional defiant disorder
- Iron deficiency anemia
- Malnutrition
- Side effects of medication
- Substance abuse
- Sleep disorder
- Child abuse/neglect
- Stressful home environment
- Parenting problem
- Parental psychopathology
- Inadequate educational setting

Medical Conditions Associated With ADHD

- Seizure disorder

- Thyroid disorder

- Traumatic brain injury

- Fetal alcohol syndrome

- Lead poisoning

Testing That Must Be Considered

- Vision

- Hearing

- CBC with differential (to rule out anemia)

- TSH, FT4 (to rule out thyroid disorders)

- Lead screen

- Genetic screen

- Toxicology screen

Rating Scales

Rating scales (e.g., the Vanderbilt, the Clinical Attention Profile, and the SNAP IV) can be a useful adjunct in the diagnosis of ADHD and in the monitoring of response to treatment. Other helpful tools for ADHD can be downloaded as part of the National Initiative for Children's Healthcare Quality and the American Academy of Pediatrics' toolkit at www.nichq.org/resources/toolkit.

Multiple Sources of Information

Information from parents, the child, teachers, primary care providers, and other caretakers is important for diagnostic consideration.

Referral and Collaboration

It is important to refer a child with ADHD to a mental health provider when the condition has not improved in 3 months or if other comorbid conditions exist (e.g., anxiety disorder, oppositional defiant disorder).

Psycho-education and Follow-up

Psycho-education with the child, parents, and teachers is important as part of the management strategy. Careful follow-up is imperative, especially in monitoring initial response to medication therapy.

DSM-5™ Diagnostic Criteria for Attention-Deficit/Hyperactivity Disorder

A. A persistent pattern of inattention and/or hyperactivity-impulsivity that interferes with functioning or development, as characterized by (1) and/or (2):

1. **Inattention:** Six (or more) of the following symptoms have persisted for at least 6 months to a degree that is inconsistent with developmental level and that negatively impacts directly on social and academic/occupational activities:

   Note: The symptoms are not solely a manifestation of oppositional behavior, defiance, hostility, or failure to understand tasks or instructions. For older adolescents and adults (age 17 and older), at least five symptoms are required.

   a. Often fails to give close attention to details or makes careless mistakes in schoolwork, at work, or during other activities (e.g., overlooks or misses details, work is inaccurate).

   b. Often has difficulty sustaining attention in tasks or play activities (e.g., has difficulty remaining focused during lectures, conversations, or lengthy reading).

   c. Often does not seem to listen when spoken to directly (e.g., mind seems elsewhere, even in the absence of any obvious distraction).

   d. Often does not follow through on instructions and fails to finish schoolwork, chores, or duties in the workplace (e.g., starts tasks but quickly loses focus and is easily sidetracked).

   e. Often has difficulty organizing tasks and activities (e.g., difficulty managing sequential tasks; difficulty keeping materials and belongings in order; messy, disorganized work; has poor time management; fails to meet deadlines).

   f. Often avoids, dislikes, or is reluctant to engage in tasks that require sustained mental effort (e.g., schoolwork or homework; for older adolescents and adults, preparing reports, completing forms, reviewing lengthy papers).

   g. Often loses things necessary for tasks or activities (e.g., school materials, pencils, books, tools, wallets, keys, paperwork, eyeglasses, mobile telephones).

   h. Is often easily distracted by extraneous stimuli (for older adolescents and adults, may include unrelated thoughts).

   i. Is often forgetful in daily activities (e.g., doing chores, running errands; for older adolescents and adults, returning calls, paying bills, keeping appointments).

2. **Hyperactivity and impulsivity:** Six (or more) of the following symptoms have persisted for at least 6 months to a degree that is inconsistent with developmental level and that negatively impacts directly on social and academic/occupational activities:

   Note: The symptoms are not solely a manifestation of oppositional behavior, defiance, hostility, or a failure to understand tasks or instructions. For older adolescents and adults (age 17 and older), at least five symptoms are required.

a. Often fidgets with or taps hands or feet or squirms in seat.

b. Often leaves seat in situations when remaining seated is expected (e.g., leaves his or her place in the classroom, in the office or other workplace, or in other situations that require remaining in place).

c. Often runs about or climbs in situations where it is inappropriate. (Note: In adolescents or adults, may be limited to feeling restless).

d. Often unable to play or engage in leisure activities quietly.

e. Is often "on the go," acting as if "driven by a motor" (e.g., is unable to be or uncomfortable being still for extended time, as in restaurants, meetings; may be experienced by others as being restless or difficult to keep up with).

f. Often talks excessively.

g. Often blurts out an answer before a question has been completed (e.g., completes people's sentences; cannot wait for turn in conversation).

h. Often has difficulty waiting his or her turn (e.g., while waiting in line).

i. Often interrupts or intrudes on others (e.g., butts into conversations, games, or activities; may start using other people's things without asking or receiving permission; for adolescents and adults, may intrude into or take over what others are doing).

A. Several inattentive or hyperactive-impulsive symptoms were present prior to age 12 years.

B. Several inattentive or hyperactive-impulsive symptoms are present in two or more settings (e.g., at home, school, or work; with friends or relatives; in other activities).

C. There is clear evidence that the symptoms interfere with, or reduce the quality of, social, academic, or occupational functioning.

D. The symptoms do not occur exclusively during the course of schizophrenia or another psychotic disorder and are not better explained by another mental disorder (e.g., mood disorder, anxiety disorder, dissociative disorder, personality disorder, substance intoxication or withdrawal).

Specify whether:

314.01 (F90.2) Combined presentation: If both Criterion A1 (inattention) and Criterion A2 (hyperactivity-impulsivity) are met for the past 6 months.

314.00 (F90.0) Predominately inattentive presentation: If Criterion A1 (inattention) is met but Criterion A2 (hyperactivity-impulsivity) is not met for the past 6 months.

314.01 (F90.1) Predominately hyperactive/impulsive presentation: If Criterion A2 (hyperactivity-impulsivity) is met and Criterion A1 (inattention) is not met for the past 6 months.

Specify if:

In partial remission: When full criteria were previously met, fewer than the full criteria have been met for the past 6 months, and the symptoms still result in impairment in social, academic, or occupational functioning.

Specify current severity:

Mild: Few, if any, symptoms in excess of those required to make the diagnosis are present, and symptoms result in no more than minor impairments in social or occupational functioning.

Moderate: Symptoms or functional impairment between "mild" and "severe" are present.

Severe: Many symptoms in excess of those required to make the diagnosis, or several symptoms that are particularly severe, are present, or the symptoms result in marked impairment in social or occupational functioning.

Changes in ADHD in the DSM-5™

1. Change the age of onset from onset of impairing symptoms by age 7 to onset of symptoms by age 12.

2. Change the three subtypes to three current presentations.

3. Add a fourth presentation for restrictive inattentive.

4. Change the examples in the items, without changing the exact wording of the DSM-IV items, to accommodate a life span relevance of each symptom and to improve clarity.

5. Remove pervasive developmental disorder (PDD) from the exclusion criteria.

6. Modify the Pre-amble A1 and A2 to indicate that information must be obtained from the two different informants (parents and teachers for children and third party/significant other for adults) whenever possible.

7. Still under consideration: adjust the cut point for diagnosis in adults.

Table 5.1 Pharmacotherapy Treatments for Children and Adolescents With ADHD: Initial Dose, Kinetics, and Side Effects

Drug	Dose	Kinetics	Side Effects/Comments
Methylphenidate HCl – short acting *(Ritalin/Methylin)* 5-, 10-, 20-mg tablets	Start: 0.3 mg/kg/dose or 2.5-5 mg before 8:00 AM and 12:00 noon. May increase by 0.1 mg/kg/dose weekly up to 0.3 until 1.0 mg/kg/dose is reached. Maximum dose is 2 mg/kg/24 hrs or 80 mg/24 hrs. Not recommended for children <5 years.	Onset: 30 min Peak: 1.9 hrs Duration: 4-6 hrs	Nervousness, insomnia, anorexia, weight loss, decreased height velocity, tics, stomachaches, headaches. Use with caution with underlying seizure disorder. Contraindicated: monoamine oxidase inhibitors. Monitor height, weight, blood pressure. Avoid caffeine and decongestants. Avoid doses after 4:00 PM. Consider drug holidays.
Methylphenidate HCl – intermediate acting *(Ritalin*-SR, *Metadate* ER, *Methylin* ER) 10-, 20-mg tablets	Starting dose: 10 mg QD Maximum dose: 80 mg/day	Onset: 30-90 min Peak: 4.7 hrs Duration: 8 hrs	Do not crush or chew tablets. See comments for methylphenidate.
Methylphenidate HCl – long acting (*Metadate* CD, 20-mg tablets) (*Concerta*, 18-, 36-, 54-mg tablets) (*Daytrana* patch, 10mg, 15 mg 20 mg, 30 mg) *Quillivant* XR liquid 25 mg/5 mL)	Starting dose: 20 mg QD or 18 mg for Concerta Maximum dose: 80 mg/day of Metadate or 54 mg/day of Concerta Starting dose for Daytrana is 10 mg and max. dose is 30 mg Quillavant can start at 2 ml = 10 mg to max. dose of 12 ml = 60 mg per day.	Onset: 30-90 min Peak: 4.7 hrs Duration: 8-12 hrs. Leave patch on for 9 hours and it will still work up to 12 hours.	Do not crush or chew tablets. See comments for methylphenidate. Adhesive may cause skin irritation with the patch, use of olive oil to remove adhesive or use of a cortisone cream can help with irritation.
Dextroamphetamine – short acting (*Dexedrine, Dextrostat*) 5-, 10-, 15-mg tablets, 5 mg/mL elixir	3-5 years: 2.5 mg/24 hrs every morning. Increase by 2.5 mg/24 hrs weekly. 6 yrs: 5 mg/24 hrs every morning Increase by 5 mg/24 hrs at weekly intervals. Max. dose: 40 mg/24 hrs	Onset: 20-60 min Peak: 2 hrs Duration: 4-6 hrs	See comments for methylphenidate. Medication should generally not be used in children <5 yrs because ADHD diagnosis should be made only with specialist consultation.
Dextroamphetamine – intermediate acting (*Adderall, Dexedrine Spansule*) 5-, 10-, 15-, 20-mg tablets	3-5 years: 2.5-5 mg QD or 0.3 mg/kg/dose Increase by 2.5-5 mg every week. >6 years: 5 mg/24 hrs QD or 0.3 mg/kg/dose Max. dose: 40 mg/24 hrs	Onset: 30-90 min Peak: 6-8 hrs	See comments for methylphenidate.
Dextroamphetamine – long acting *Adderall* XR 5,10, 15, 20, 25, 30 mg *Vyvanse* 20, 30, 40, 50, 60, 70 mg	>6 years Starting dose: 5 mg QD for Adderall XR or 0.3 mg/kg/dose. Max. dose: 40 mg/24 hrs For *Vyvanse*, starting dose is 20 mg to max. of 70 mg.	Onset: 30-90 min Duration: >8 hrs Often *Vyvanse* can last for 12-13 hours.	See comments for methylphenidate. Adderall XR has long- and short-acting beads in the capsule. *Vyvanse* is a pro-drug and is not active until L-lysine interacts with it in the intestinal tract.

Note: Stimulants work best when given regularly. Adjust dose of stimulant medication as the child grows. There is a risk of abuse with stimulants.

Caution: Use stimulants cautiously in children with marked anxiety, tension, or agitation since these symptoms may be aggravated. Stimulants are contraindicated in children with motor tics or with a family history of diagnosis of Tourette's syndrome, although comorbid diagnosis of ADHD and Tourette's syndrome is rare. Avoid giving nasal decongestants with stimulants.

Adapted from:
- Green, S.M. (Ed.) (2003). Tarascon Pocket Pharmacopoeia Deluxe Download. Lompoc, California: Tarascon Publishing.
- Robertson, J., & Shikofski, N. (Eds.) (2005). *Harriet Lane Handbook: A Manual for Pediatric House Officers (17th Edition)*. St. Louis, Missouri: C.V. Mosby.
- Werry, J. S., & Aman, M.G. (Eds.) (1998). *Practitioner's Guide to Psychoactive Drugs for Children and Adolescents (2nd Edition)*, New York, NY: Plenum Publishing Corporation
- Stahl, S.M. (2009). *Essential Psychophamacology Prescribers Guide*. Cambridge, Massachusetts: Cambridge University Press.

Non-Stimulants Used to Treat ADHD

Strattera (Atomoxetine HCl)

Doses: 10, 18, 25, 40, 60, 80 and 100 mg. Starting dose is 0.5 mg/kg/day; titrate upwards 1.5mg/kg/day
Can take 2-4 weeks to see results

Common side effects include upset stomach, decreased appetite, nausea or vomiting, dizziness, tiredness, and mood swings.
If a patient has serious heart problems, Strattera should be avoided as it could make increases in heart rate and blood pressure worse.
Strattera can cause liver injury in some patients.
There is a black box warning stating: In some children and teens, *Strattera* increased the risk of suicidal thoughts or actions. Results from *Strattera* clinical studies with over 2200 child or teenage ADHD patients suggest that some children and teenagers may have a higher chance of having suicidal thoughts or actions. Although no suicides occurred in these studies, 4 out of every 1000 patients developed suicidal thoughts.

Intuniv (Guanfacine)

Doses: 1, 2, 3, 4 mg. Starting dose is 1 mg to a maximum dose of 4 mg.

Intuniv should be swallowed whole with liquid, without crushing, chewing, or breaking the tablet. Intuniv should not be taken with a high-fat meal. Regular checks of the child's blood pressure and heart rate are recommended.

Serious side effects can include low blood pressure and low heart rate. Medicine needs to be tapered as withdrawal symptoms could occur including increased blood pressure, headache, increased heart rate, and lightheadedness.

Common side effects include sleepiness, tiredness, trouble sleeping, low blood pressure, nausea, stomach pain, and dizziness.

Intuniv can be used alone or in combination with a stimulant. One 9-week study included 455 children who were on a stable stimulant dose for at least 4 weeks and had some improvement, but still had ADHD symptoms. These children then took either Intuniv or a placebo with their stimulant. Researchers saw a 30% improvement in the ADHD symptoms when Intuniv was added as compared to placebo.

Kapvay (Clonidine HCl)
Doses: 0.1, 0.2 mg. Starting dose is 0.1mg QHS; titrate to 0.1 mg BID to a maximum dose of 0.1 mg QAM and 0.2 mg QHS.

Kapvay should be swallowed whole with liquid, without crushing, chewing, or breaking the tablet. Regular checks of the child's blood pressure and heart rate are recommended. It can be taken with and without food.

Serious side effects include low blood pressure and low heart rate.

Common side effects include sleepiness, tiredness, cough, sneezing, runny nose, sore throat, stuffy nose, irritability, trouble sleeping, nightmares, change in mood, constipation, increased body temperature, dry mouth, ear pain.

Suddenly stopping *Kapvay* may cause withdrawal symptoms including increased blood pressure, headache, increased heart rate, lightheadedness, tightness in the chest, and nervousness.

Adapted from information from Eli Lilly and Company, Shire Inc., and Shionogi, Inc.

The National Initiative for Children's Healthcare Quality (NICHQ) Vanderbilt Assessment Scale for ADHD-Parent Informant

Description

The National Initiative for Children's Healthcare Quality (NICHQ) and the American Academy of Pediatrics (AAP) have sponsored a set of tools for evaluating children with ADHD developed at Vanderbilt University. The initial evaluation scale monitors 57 symptoms for ADHD and other disorders and school performance as reported by the parent(s).

NICHQ Vanderbilt Assessment Scale: Parent Informant

Today's Date: _____

Child's Name: _____

Child's Date of Birth: _____

Parent's Name: _____

Parent's Phone Number: _____

Directions: Each rating should be considered in the context of what is appropriate for the age of your child. When completing this form, please think about your child's behaviors in the past 6 months.

Is this evaluation based on a time when the child

☐ **was on medication**   ☐ **was not on medication**   ☐ **not sure?**

Symptoms	Never	Occasionally	Often	Very Often
1. Does not pay attention to details or makes careless mistakes with, for example, homework	0	1	2	3
2. Has difficulty keeping attention to what needs to be done	0	1	2	3
3. Does not seem to listen when spoken to directly	0	1	2	3
4. Does not follow through when given directions and fails to finish activities (not due to refusal or failure to understand)	0	1	2	3
5. Has difficulty organizing tasks and activities	0	1	2	3
6. Avoids, dislikes, or does not want to start tasks that require ongoing mental effort	0	1	2	3
7. Loses things necessary for tasks or activities (toys, assignments, pencils, books)	0	1	2	3
8. Is easily distracted by noises or other stimuli	0	1	2	3
9. Is forgetful in daily activities	0	1	2	3

For Office Use Only ____/9

Symptoms	Never	Occasionally	Often	Very Often
10. Fidgets with hands or feet or squirms in seat	0	1	2	3
11. Leaves seat when remaining seated is expected	0	1	2	3
12. Runs about or climbs too much when remaining seated is expected	0	1	2	3
13. Has difficulty playing or beginning quiet play activities	0	1	2	3
14. Is "on the go" or often acts as if "driven by a motor"	0	1	2	3
15. Talks too much	0	1	2	3
16. Blurts out answers before questions have been completed	0	1	2	3
17. Has difficulty waiting his or her turn	0	1	2	3
18. Interrupts or intrudes in on others' conversations and/or activities	0	1	2	3

For Office Use Only ____/9

Symptoms (continued)

	Never	Occasionally	Often	Very Often
19. Argues with adults	0	1	2	3
20. Loses temper	0	1	2	3
21. Actively defies or refuses to go along with adults' requests or rules	0	1	2	3
22. Deliberately annoys people	0	1	2	3
23. Blames others for his or her mistakes or misbehaviors	0	1	2	3
24. Is touchy or easily annoyed by others	0	1	2	3
25. Is angry or resentful	0	1	2	3
26. Is spiteful and wants to get even	0	1	2	3

For Office Use Only ____ /8

	Never	Occasionally	Often	Very Often
27. Bullies, threatens, or intimidates others	0	1	2	3
28. Starts physical fights	0	1	2	3
29. Lies to get out of trouble or to avoid obligations (ie, "cons" others)	0	1	2	3
30. Is truant from school (skips school) without permission	0	1	2	3
31. Is physically cruel to people	0	1	2	3
32. Has stolen things that have value	0	1	2	3
33. Deliberately destroys others' property	0	1	2	3
34. Has used a weapon that can cause serious harm (bat, knife, brick, gun)	0	1	2	3
35. Is physically cruel to animals	0	1	2	3
36. Has deliberately set fires to cause damage	0	1	2	3
37. Has broken into someone else's home, business, or car	0	1	2	3
38. Has stayed out at night without permission	0	1	2	3
39. Has run away from home overnight	0	1	2	3
40. Has forced someone into sexual activity	0	1	2	3

For Office Use Only ____ /14

	Never	Occasionally	Often	Very Often
41. Is fearful, anxious, or worried	0	1	2	3
42. Is afraid to try new things for fear of making mistakes	0	1	2	3
43. Feels worthless or inferior	0	1	2	3
44. Blames self for problems, feels guilty	0	1	2	3
45. Feels lonely, unwanted, or unloved; complains that "no one loves him or her"	0	1	2	3
46. Is sad, unhappy, or depressed	0	1	2	3
47. Is self-conscious or easily embarrassed	0	1	2	3

For Office Use Only ____ /7

Performance	Excellent	Above Average	Average	Somewhat of a Problem	Problematic
48. Reading	1	2	3	4	5
49. Writing	1	2	3	4	5
50. Mathematics	1	2	3	4	5

For Office Use Only 4s: ____ /3
For Office Use Only 5s: ____ /3

	Excellent	Above Average	Average	Somewhat of a Problem	Problematic
51. Relationship with parents	1	2	3	4	5
52. Relationship with siblings	1	2	3	4	5
53. Relationship with peers	1	2	3	4	5
54. Participation in organized activities (eg, teams)	1	2	3	4	5

For Office Use Only 4s: ____ /4
For Office Use Only 5s: ____ /4

Section 5 - Attention-Deficit/Hyperactivity Disorder (ADHD)   149

Other Conditions

Tic Behaviors: To the best of your knowledge, please indicate if this child displays the following behaviors:

1. **Motor Tics:** Rapid, repetitive movements such as eye blinking, grimacing, nose twitching, head jerks, shoulder shrugs, arm jerks, body jerks, or rapid kicks.

   ☐ No tics present.   ☐ Yes, they occur nearly every day but go unnoticed by most people.   ☐ Yes, noticeable tics occur nearly every day.

2. **Phonic (Vocal) Tics:** Repetitive noises including but not limited to throat clearing, coughing, whistling, sniffing, snorting, screeching, barking, grunting, or repetition of words or short phrases.

   ☐ No tics present.   ☐ Yes, they occur nearly every day but go unnoticed by most people.   ☐ Yes, noticeable tics occur nearly every day.

3. If **YES** to 1 or 2, do these tics interfere with the child's activities (like reading, writing, walking, talking, or eating)?   ☐ No   ☐ Yes

Previous Diagnosis and Treatment: To the best of your knowledge, please answer the following questions:

1. Has your child been diagnosed with a tic disorder or Tourette syndrome?	☐ No	☐ Yes
2. Is your child on medication for a tic disorder or Tourette syndrome?	☐ No	☐ Yes
3. Has your child been diagnosed with depression?	☐ No	☐ Yes
4. Is your child on medication for depression?	☐ No	☐ Yes
5. Has your child been diagnosed with an anxiety disorder?	☐ No	☐ Yes
6. Is your child on medication for an anxiety disorder?	☐ No	☐ Yes
7. Has your child been diagnosed with a learning or language disorder?	☐ No	☐ Yes

Comments:

For Office Use Only

Total number of questions scored 2 or 3 in questions 1–9: _____

Total number of questions scored 2 or 3 in questions 10–18: _____

Total number of questions scored 2 or 3 in questions 19–26: _____

Total number of questions scored 2 or 3 in questions 27–40: _____

Total number of questions scored 2 or 3 in questions 41–47: _____

Total number of questions scored 4 in questions 48–50: _____

Total number of questions scored 5 in questions 48–50: _____

Total number of questions scored 4 in questions 51–54: _____

Total number of questions scored 5 in questions 51–54: _____

Adapted from the Vanderbilt Rating Scales developed by Mark L. Wolraich, MD.

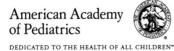

American Academy
of Pediatrics
DEDICATED TO THE HEALTH OF ALL CHILDREN™

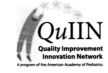

QuIIN
Quality Improvement
Innovation Network
A program of the American Academy of Pediatrics

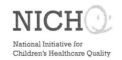

NICHQ
National Initiative for
Children's Healthcare Quality

Scoring Instructions for NICHQ Vanderbilt Assessment Scales

The validation studies for the NICHQ Vanderbilt Assessment Scales were for the 6- to 12-year-old age group. However, to the extent that they collect information to establish *Diagnostic and Statistical Manual of Mental Disorders, Fourth Edition (DSM-IV)* criteria, they are applicable to other groups, particularly preschoolers, where they have identified that *DSM-IV* criteria are still appropriate.

These scales should *not* be used alone to make a diagnosis of ADHD without confirming and elaborating the information with interviews with at least the primary caregivers (usually parents) and patients. You must take into consideration information from multiple sources. Scores of 2 or 3 on a single symptom question reflect *often-occurring* behaviors. Scores of 4 or 5 on performance questions reflect problems in performance.

The initial assessment scales, parent and teacher, have 2 components: symptom assessment and impairment in performance. On both parent and teacher initial scales, the symptom assessment screens for symptoms that meet criteria for inattentive (items 1-9) and hyperactive (items 10-18) attention-deficit/hyperactivity disorder (ADHD).

To meet *DSM-IV* criteria for the diagnosis, one must have at least 6 positive responses to the inattentive 9 or hyperactive 9 core symptoms, or both. A positive response is a 2 or 3 (often, very often) (you could draw a line straight down the page and count the positive answers in each subsegment). There is a place to record the number of positives in each subsegment.

The initial scales have symptom screens for 3 other comorbidities: oppositional-defiant disorder, conduct disorder, and anxiety/depression. (The initial teacher scale also screens for learning disabilities.) These are screened by the number of positive responses in each of the segments. The specific item sets and numbers of positives required for each comorbid symptom screen set are detailed below and on the next page.

The second section of the scale has a set of performance measures, scored 1 to 5, with 4 and 5 being somewhat of a problem/problematic. To meet criteria for ADHD there must be at least 2 items of the performance set in which the child scores a 4, or 1 item of the performance set in which the child scores a 5; ie, there must be impairment, not just symptoms, to meet diagnostic criteria. The sheet has a place to record the number of positives (4s, 5s).

Parent Assessment Scale	Teacher Assessment Scale
Predominantly Inattentive subtype • Must score a 2 or 3 on 6 out of 9 items on questions 1–9. AND • Score a 4 on at least 2, or 5 on at least 1, of the performance questions 48–54.	**Predominantly Inattentive subtype** • Must score a 2 or 3 on 6 out of 9 items on questions 1–9. AND • Score a 4 on at least 2, or 5 on at least 1, of the performance questions 36–43.
Predominantly Hyperactive/Impulsive subtype • Must score a 2 or 3 on 6 out of 9 items on questions 10–18. AND • Score a 4 on at least 2, or 5 on at least 1, of the performance questions 48–54.	**Predominantly Hyperactive/Impulsive subtype** • Must score a 2 or 3 on 6 out of 9 items on questions 10–18. AND • Score a 4 on at least 2, or 5 on at least 1, of the performance questions 36–43.
ADHD Combined Inattention/Hyperactivity • Requires the criteria on Inattentive AND Hyperactive/Impulsive subtypes	**ADHD Combined Inattention/Hyperactivity** • Requires the criteria on Inattentive AND Hyperactive/Impulsive subtypes
Oppositional-Defiant Disorder • Must score a 2 or 3 on 4 out of 8 behaviors on questions 19–26. AND • Score a 4 on at least 2, or 5 on at least 1, of the performance questions 48–54.	**Oppositional-Defiant/Conduct Disorder** • Must score a 2 or 3 on 3 out of 10 items on questions 19–28. AND • Score a 4 on at least 2, or 5 on at least 1, of the performance questions 36–43.
Conduct Disorder • Must score a 2 or 3 on 3 out of 14 behaviors on questions 27–40. AND • Score a 4 on at least 2, or 5 on at least 1, of the performance questions 48–54.	

Parent Assessment Scale	Teacher Assessment Scale
Anxiety/Depression • Must score a 2 or 3 on 3 out of 7 behaviors on questions 41–47. AND • Score a 4 on at least 2, or 5 on at least 1, of the performance questions 48–54.	**Anxiety/Depression** • Must score a 2 or 3 on 3 out of 7 items on questions 29–35. AND • Score a 4 on at least 2, or 5 on at least 1, of the performance questions 36–43.
	Learning Disabilities • Must score a 4 on both, or 5 on 1, of questions 36 and 38.

The parent and teacher follow-up scales have the first 18 core ADHD symptoms and the comorbid symptoms oppositional-defiant (parent) and oppositional-defiant/conduct (teacher) disorders. The Performance section has the same performance items and impairment assessment as the initial scales; it is followed by a side-effect reporting scale that can be used to assess and monitor the presence of adverse reactions to prescribed medications, if any.

Scoring the follow-up scales involves tracking inattentive (items 1–9) and hyperactive (items 10–18) ADHD, as well as the aforementioned comorbidities, as measures of improvement over time with treatment.

Parent Assessment Scale	Teacher Assessment Scale
Predominantly Inattentive subtype • Must score a 2 or 3 on 6 out of 9 items on questions 1–9. AND • Score a 4 on at least 2, or 5 on at least 1, of the performance questions 27–33.	**Predominantly Inattentive subtype** • Must score a 2 or 3 on 6 out of 9 items on questions 1–9. AND • Score a 4 on at least 2, or 5 on at least 1, of the performance questions 29–36.
Predominantly Hyperactive/Impulsive subtype • Must score a 2 or 3 on 6 out of 9 items on questions 10–18. AND • Score a 4 on at least 2, or 5 on at least 1, of the performance questions 27–33.	**Predominantly Hyperactive/Impulsive subtype** • Must score a 2 or 3 on 6 out of 9 items on questions 10–18. AND • Score a 4 on at least 2, or 5 on at least 1, of the performance questions 29–36.
ADHD Combined Inattention/Hyperactivity • Requires the criteria on Inattentive AND Hyperactive/Impulsive subtypes	**ADHD Combined Inattention/Hyperactivity** • Requires the criteria on Inattentive AND Hyperactive/Impulsive subtypes
Oppositional-Defiant Disorder • Must score a 2 or 3 on 4 out of 8 behaviors on questions 19–26. AND • Score a 4 on at least 2, or 5 on at least 1, of the performance questions 27–33.	**Oppositional-Defiant/Conduct Disorder** • Must score a 2 or 3 on 3 out of 10 items on questions 19–28. AND • Score a 4 on at least 2, or 5 on at least 1, of the performance questions 29–36.

Used with permission of the American Academy of Pediatrics. Caring for Children with ADHD: A Resource Toolkit for Clinicians [CD-ROM]. 2nd ed. Elk Grove Village, IL: American Academy of Pediatrics; 2012.

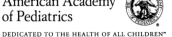

American Academy of Pediatrics
DEDICATED TO THE HEALTH OF ALL CHILDREN™

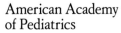

QuIIN
Quality Improvement Innovation Network
A program of the American Academy of Pediatrics

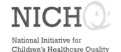

NICHQ
National Initiative for Children's Healthcare Quality

Swanson, Nolan and Pelham (SNAP-IV-C)
(Swanson et al)

James M. Swanson, PhD, University of California, Irvine, CA 92715

The Swanson, Nolan and Pelham Scales-IV Revised (SNAP IV-C) is an instrument that uses observer ratings and self-report ratings to help assess ADHD and evaluate problem behavior in children and adolescents. The CRS-R instruments are used for routine screenings in schools, mental health clinics, residential treatment centers, pediatric offices, juvenile detention facilities, child protective agencies, and outpatient settings.

Instrument(s) Description
Snap IV- Teacher and Parent Rating Scale

The SNAP IV-C contains 90 items. It is typically used with teachers and parents or caregivers when comprehensive information and DSM-IV consideration are required.

Scales include:
- Oppositional defiant disorder
- Conduct disorder
- Intermittent explosive disorder
- Stereotypic movement disorder
- Cognitive problems/inattention
- Hyperactivity
- Anxious-shy
- Posttraumatic stress disorder
- Obsessive-compulsive disorder
- Perfectionism
- Narcolepsy
- Personality disorders (histrionic, narcissistic, and borderline)
- Social problems
- Adjustment disorder
- Psychosomatic disorder
- Depression
- Dysthymia
- Mania
- Conners' Global Index
- DSM-IV Symptom Subscales
- ADHD Index

Sample Items

The SNAP-IV-C provides a series of statements that the parent or teacher responds to regarding the child's behavior for the past month. The response is in a Likert-type format, using the following categories:

- Not true at all (Never, Seldom)
- Just a little true (Occasionally)
- Pretty much true (Often, Quite a bit)
- Very much true (Very often, Very frequent)

Scoring

The first nine items for the SNAP-IV-C cover inattention symptoms of ADHD. Examples of questions are listed below. A score of 18 or higher shows inattention.

1. Makes careless mistakes
2. Can't pay attention
3. Doesn't listen
4. Fails to finish work
5. Disorganized
6. Can't concentrate
7. Loses things
8. Distractible
9. Forgetful

The next 9 questions focus on hyperactivity and impulsivity. A Score of 18 or higher shows hyperactivity.

Questions 19-26 focus on oppositional defiant disorder, and a score of 18 or higher shows ODD symptoms.

The remainder of the questions are designed to let you know if there may be comorbid issues along with ADHD that should be explored. For example, if Questions 66-73 were scored 2 or higher, there may be symptoms of depression. Or if Questions 51-56 were scored 2 or higher, then there may be anxiety.

Validity/Norms

The SNAP was originally developed with the DSM III and has been revised with the DSM IV and has been used in numerous ADHD and genetic clinical trials. It has shown excellent internal consistency, but data on norms for age and gender have been sparse. One study (Bussing et al, 2008) looked at over 12,000 kindergarten to 5th grade students in a north central Florida public school district during the 1998-1999 school year. The SNAP was given to both teachers and parents. Reliability for parent ratings and teacher ratings showed statistical significance at $p<.001$. The findings did not suggest a difference based on age, gender, or race, but did state that this school district was known for high poverty rates and limited diversity.

Administer to:

For the *SNAP-IV-C*: parents and teachers of children and adolescents ages 5-17

The SNAP-IV Teacher and Parent Rating Scale

James M. Swanson, Ph.D., University of California, Irvine, CA 92715

Name:_____ Gender:_____ Age:_____ Grade:_____

Ethnicity (circle one which best applies):   African-American   Asian   Caucasian   Hispanic   Other_____

Completed by:_____ Type of Class:_____ Class size:_____

For each item, check the column which best describes this child:	Not At All	Just A Little	Quite A Bit	Very Much
1. Often fails to give close attention to details or makes careless mistakes in schoolwork or tasks	_____	_____	_____	_____
2. Often has difficulty sustaining attention in tasks or play activities	_____	_____	_____	_____
3. Often does not seem to listen when spoken to directly	_____	_____	_____	_____
4. Often does not follow through on instructions and fails to finish schoolwork, chores, or duties	_____	_____	_____	_____
5. Often has difficulty organizing tasks and activities	_____	_____	_____	_____
6. Often avoids, dislikes, or reluctantly engages in tasks requiring sustained mental effort	_____	_____	_____	_____
7. Often loses things necessary for activities (e.g., toys, school assignments, pencils, or books)	_____	_____	_____	_____
8. Often is distracted by extraneous stimuli	_____	_____	_____	_____
9. Often is forgetful in daily activities	_____	_____	_____	_____
10. Often has difficulty maintaining alertness, orienting to requests, or executing directions	_____	_____	_____	_____
11. Often fidgets with hands or feet or squirms in seat	_____	_____	_____	_____
12. Often leaves seat in classroom or in other situations in which remaining seated is expected	_____	_____	_____	_____
13. Often runs about or climbs excessively in situations in which it is inappropriate	_____	_____	_____	_____
14. Often has difficulty playing or engaging in leisure activities quietly	_____	_____	_____	_____
15. Often is "on the go" or often acts as if "driven by a motor"	_____	_____	_____	_____
16. Often talks excessively	_____	_____	_____	_____
17. Often blurts out answers before questions have been completed	_____	_____	_____	_____
18. Often has difficulty awaiting turn	_____	_____	_____	_____
19. Often interrupts or intrudes on others (e.g., butts into conversations/games)	_____	_____	_____	_____
20. Often has difficulty sitting still, being quiet, or inhibiting impulses in the classroom or at home	_____	_____	_____	_____
21. Often loses temper	_____	_____	_____	_____
22. Often argues with adults	_____	_____	_____	_____
23. Often actively defies or refuses adult requests or rules	_____	_____	_____	_____
24. Often deliberately does things that annoy other people	_____	_____	_____	_____
25. Often blames others for his or her mistakes or misbehavior	_____	_____	_____	_____
26. Often touchy or easily annoyed by others	_____	_____	_____	_____
27 Often is angry and resentful	_____	_____	_____	_____
28. Often is spiteful or vindictive	_____	_____	_____	_____
29. Often is quarrelsome	_____	_____	_____	_____
30. Often is negative, defiant, disobedient, or hostile toward authority figures	_____	_____	_____	_____
31. Often makes noises (e.g., humming or odd sounds)	_____	_____	_____	_____
32. Often is excitable, impulsive	_____	_____	_____	_____
33. Often cries easily	_____	_____	_____	_____
34. Often is uncooperative	_____	_____	_____	_____
35. Often acts "smart"	_____	_____	_____	_____
36. Often is restless or overactive	_____	_____	_____	_____
37. Often disturbs other children	_____	_____	_____	_____
38. Often changes mood quickly and drastically	_____	_____	_____	_____
39. Often easily frustrated if demand are not met immediately	_____	_____	_____	_____
40. Often teases other children and interferes with their activities	_____	_____	_____	_____

Section 5 - Attention-Deficit/Hyperactivity Disorder (ADHD)

Check the column which best describes this child:

	Not At All	Just A Little	Quite A Bit	Very Much
41. Often is aggressive to other children (e.g., picks fights or bullies)	____	____	____	____
42. Often is destructive with property of others (e.g., vandalism)	____	____	____	____
43. Often is deceitful (e.g., steals, lies, forges, copies the work of others, or "cons" others)	____	____	____	____
44. Often and seriously violates rules (e.g., is truant, runs away, or completely ignores class rules)	____	____	____	____
45. Has persistent pattern of violating the basic rights of others or major societal norms	____	____	____	____
46. Has episodes of failure to resist aggressive impulses (to assault others or to destroy property)	____	____	____	____
47. Has motor or verbal tics (sudden, rapid, recurrent, nonrhythmic motor or verbal activity)	____	____	____	____
48. Has repetitive motor behavior (e.g., hand waving, body rocking, or picking at skin)	____	____	____	____
49. Has obsessions (persistent and intrusive inappropriate ideas, thoughts, or impulses)	____	____	____	____
50. Has compulsions (repetitive behaviors or mental acts to reduce anxiety or distress)	____	____	____	____
51. Often is restless or seems keyed up or on edge	____	____	____	____
52. Often is easily fatigued	____	____	____	____
53. Often has difficulty concentrating (mind goes blank)	____	____	____	____
54. Often is irritable	____	____	____	____
55. Often has muscle tension	____	____	____	____
56. Often has excessive anxiety and worry (e.g., apprehensive expectation)	____	____	____	____
57. Often has daytime sleepiness (unintended sleeping in inappropriate situations)	____	____	____	____
58. Often has excessive emotionality and attention-seeking behavior	____	____	____	____
59. Often has need for undue admiration, grandiose behavior, or lack of empathy	____	____	____	____
60. Often has instability in relationships with others, reactive mood, and impulsivity	____	____	____	____
61 Sometimes for at least a week has inflated self esteem or grandiosity	____	____	____	____
62. Sometimes for at least a week is more talkative than usual or seems pressured to keep talking	____	____	____	____
63. Sometimes for at least a week has flight of ideas or says that thoughts are racing	____	____	____	____
64. Sometimes for at least a week has elevated, expansive or euphoric mood	____	____	____	____
65. Sometimes for at least a week is excessively involved in pleasurable but risky activities	____	____	____	____
66. Sometimes for at least 2 weeks has depressed mood (sad, hopeless, discouraged)	____	____	____	____
67. Sometimes for at least 2 weeks has irritable or cranky mood (not just when frustrated)	____	____	____	____
68. Sometimes for at least 2 weeks has markedly diminished interest or pleasure in most activities	____	____	____	____
69. Sometimes for at least 2 weeks has psychomotor agitation (even more active than usual)	____	____	____	____
70. Sometimes for at least 2 weeks has psychomotor retardation (slowed down in most activities)	____	____	____	____
71. Sometimes for at least 2 weeks is fatigued or has loss of energy	____	____	____	____
72. Sometimes for at least 2 weeks has feelings of worthlessness or excessive, inappropriate guilt	____	____	____	____
73. Sometimes for at least 2 weeks has diminished ability to think or concentrate	____	____	____	____
74. Chronic low self-esteem most of the time for at least a year	____	____	____	____
75. Chronic poor concentration or difficulty making decisions most of the time for at least a year	____	____	____	____
76. Chronic feelings of hopelessness most of the time for at least a year	____	____	____	____
77. Currently is hypervigilant (overly watchful or alert) or has exaggerated startle response	____	____	____	____
78. Currently is irritable, has anger outbursts, or has difficulty concentrating	____	____	____	____
79. Currently has an emotional (e.g., nervous, worried, hopeless, tearful) response to stress	____	____	____	____
80. Currently has a behavioral (e.g., fighting, vandalism, truancy) response to stress	____	____	____	____
81. Has difficulty getting started on classroom assignments	____	____	____	____
82. Has difficulty staying on task for an entire classroom period	____	____	____	____
83. Has problems in completion of work on classroom assignments	____	____	____	____
84. Has problems in accuracy or neatness of written work in the classroom	____	____	____	____
85. Has difficulty attending to a group classroom activity or discussion	____	____	____	____
86. Has difficulty making transitions to the next topic or classroom period	____	____	____	____
87. Has problems in interactions with peers in the classroom	____	____	____	____
88. Has problems in interactions with staff (teacher or aide)	____	____	____	____
89. Has difficulty remaining quiet according to classroom rules	____	____	____	____
90. Has difficulty staying seated according to classroom rules	____	____	____	____

Used with permission from James M. Swanson, PhD.

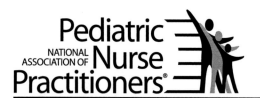

What Is ADHD?

ADHD is the name of a group of behaviors found in many children and adults. People with ADHD have trouble paying attention in school, at home, or at work. They may be much more active and/or impulsive than what is usual for their age. These behaviors contribute to significant problems in relationships, learning, and behavior. For this reason, children with ADHD are sometimes seen as being "difficult" or as having behavior problems. ADHD is common, affecting 4 to 12% of school-age children. It is more common in boys than in girls.

What Are the Symptoms of ADHD?

The child with ADHD who is inattentive will have 6 or more of the following symptoms:

- Difficulty following instructions
- Difficulty keeping attention on work or play activities at school and at home
- Loses things needed for activities at school and at home
- Appears not to listen
- Doesn't pay close attention to details
- Seems disorganized
- Has trouble with tasks that require planning ahead
- Forgets things
- Is easily distracted

The child with ADHD who is hyperactive/impulsive will have at least 6 symptoms:

- Runs or climbs inappropriately
- Is fidgety
- Can't play quietly
- Blurts out answers
- Interrupts people
- Can't stay in seat
- Talks too much
- Is always on the go
- Has trouble waiting his or her turn

What Causes ADHD?

Children with ADHD do not make enough chemicals in key areas in the brain that are responsible for organizing thought. Without enough of these chemicals, the organizing centers of the brain don't work well. This causes the symptoms in children with ADHD. Often there is a family history of ADHD. Things that *don't* cause ADHD: poor parenting (although a disorganized home life and school environment can make symptoms worse); too much or too little sugar, Aspartame, food additives or colorings; lack of vitamins; food allergies or other allergies; fluorescent lights; video games; or too much TV.

What Can I Do to Help My Child With ADHD?

A team effort, with parents, teachers, and doctors working together, is the best way to help your child. Children with ADHD tend to need more structure and clearer expectations. Families may benefit from talking with a specialist in managing ADHD-related behavior and learning problems. Medicine also helps many children. Talk with your doctor or nurse practitioner about treatments he/she recommends.

What Medicines Are Used to Treat ADHD?

Some of the medicines for ADHD are methylphenidate, dextroamphetamine, atomoxetine, guanfacine, and clonidine. These medicines improve attention/concentration and decrease impulsive and overactive behaviors.

What Can I Do at Home to Help My Child?

Children with ADHD may be challenging to parent. They may have trouble understanding directions. Children with ADHD are often in a constant state of activity. This can be challenging. You may need to change your home life a bit to help your child. Here are some things you can do to help:

- **Make a schedule**. Set specific times for waking up, eating, playing, doing homework, doing chores, watching TV or playing video games, and going to bed. Post the schedule where your child will always see it. Explain any changes to the routine in advance.

- **Make simple house rules**. It's important to explain what will happen when the rules are obeyed and when they are broken.

- **Make sure your directions are understood**. Get your child's attention and look directly into his or her eyes. Then tell your child in a clear, calm voice specifically what you want. Keep directions simple and short. Ask your child to repeat the directions back to you.

- **Reward good behavior**. Congratulate your child when he/she completes each step of a task.

- **Make sure your child is well supervised**. Because they are impulsive, children with ADHD may need more adult supervision than other children their age.

- **Watch your child around his or her friends**. It's sometimes hard for children with ADHD to learn social skills. Reward good play behaviors.

- **Set a homework routine**. Pick a regular place for homework, away from distractions such as other people, TV, and video games. Break homework time into small parts and allocate frequent breaks.

- **Focus on effort, not grades**. Reward your child when he or she tries to finish school work, not just for good grades. You can give extra rewards for earning better grades.

- **Talk with your child's teachers**. Find out how your child is doing at school -- in class, at playtime, at lunchtime. Ask for daily or weekly progress notes from the teacher.

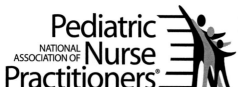

Information for Children and Teens About Attention-Deficit/Hyperactivity Disorder (ADHD)

"You're not paying attention." "Don't you know where you put your lunch money?" "Stop fidgeting!" "Don't interrupt." Can you imagine what it would be like to hear people talk to you this way every single day? If you can imagine it, or if it sounds just like what you're used to hearing, then you know what it's like to have attention-deficit/hyperactivity disorder or ADHD for short.

Children and teens who have ADHD are not "bad," "lazy," or "stupid." They have a behavior disorder, which means they may have problems paying attention or have trouble sitting still in their seats. They can also act on impulse -- this means doing things without thinking about them first. Children and teens with ADHD may spend a lot of time in the principal's office. They also might change their friends a lot.

Who Gets ADHD?

On average, 5 out of 100 kids have ADHD. That means that if your school has 500 kids, 25 may have ADHD – that's like one whole class! Children and teens who have ADHD usually start having problems before they are 7 years old. Sometimes the problems begin when they start going to school. Boys have ADHD more often than girls, but no one knows why.

In fact, no one is sure why anyone has ADHD, although scientists think that it probably has to do with different levels of brain activity. No one gets ADHD on purpose, so it isn't ever anyone's fault. And, ADHD isn't contagious – you can't catch it from someone like the flu. Someone might have a bigger chance of developing ADHD if one of his relatives already has ADHD.

What is ADHD?

ADHD stands for attention-deficit/hyperactivity disorder. ADHD is a disorder that affects the brain. It causes people to behave differently from others. People with ADHD have problems in 1 or 2 major ways. The first is that they may have trouble focusing on tasks or subjects. The second is that they may act on impulse (without thinking), which can lead to negative consequences. That's why ADHD gets a bad rap.

Symptoms and Signs of ADHD

The first type of ADHD includes problems with paying attention, staying organized, remembering things, problems completing work at school or home, difficulty following instructions, losing or forgetting things (e.g., homework). This type used to be called attention-deficit disorder, or ADD.

The second type involves hyperactivity and impulsivity and includes fidgeting, feelings of restlessness, difficulty awaiting your turn, and interrupting others.

The third type, which is the most common, involves a combination of the other two types. If you have ADHD, you may not be aware that you are behaving in a way that's different from others; you're just doing what comes naturally. But, you might notice that it's hard for you to pay attention. You might feel bored or frustrated in class. You may have a hard time getting started on assignments and finishing your work. Homework may take you much longer to complete.

ADHD can affect social situations, too. For example, you might react to someone by just saying what's on your mind -- what comes naturally -- and then you may get the feeling that you've shocked or offended the person or don't understand why people get mad at you. Some of the symptoms of ADHD can be difficult to deal with and can make a teen experience many different emotions. The more you understand about ADHD, the more involved you can be in your own treatment.

What Medicines Are Used to Treat ADHD?

Some medicines used to treat ADHD are called psychostimulants. They can help people with ADHD to better focus their attention on things.

School Tips for Helping Yourself With ADHD

If you have a study hall available to you during one class period or after school, use it and take advantage of a quiet time to study and complete homework.

Take notes during class. This can help to keep you focused on the material being taught.

Use your assignment book to keep lists of things to do. Don't make lists on scraps of paper -- you may end up losing them or forgetting about them. Get into the habit of completing a list of things to do each evening for what you want to accomplish the next day.

Talk to your teachers about your ADHD and how it affects your work. Ask for their assistance in areas you are experiencing problems. They will be more willing to help if they understand that you are trying to overcome these problems rather than making excuses.

Sit in front of the classroom. This will help you to focus on the lesson and will enable you to pay attention and will minimize distractions.

Be prepared. If you are constantly going to class unprepared, buy a box of pens and keep them in your locker. Buy several small pocket-size notebooks. Each morning, if you find you don't have a pen and paper, use a small pocket-size notebook, and take a pen from your locker.

If you end up each day at home without the books needed to complete your assignments, use different methods to remember which books to bring home. Ask the school about bringing home an extra set of books. You will not need to carry your books back and forth and will never forget your books at home or school.

Find a partner to help you. Find someone you trust and work well with to help you stay focused during the day. Have a special signal they can give you if they see you have lost your focus.

Clean out your locker every Friday. Get into the habit of bringing home all loose papers in your locker each Friday. When you get home, you can sort through to see what you need and organize the papers. Having a clean locker will help you to stay organized and be prepared.

Believe in yourself and your abilities. You can succeed in what you do.

Check out this helpful Website for children, teens, and adults with ADHD: National Resource Center for ADHD, available at **www.chadd.org**.

Internet Resources

American Academy of Child and Adolescent Psychiatry (AACAP)
www.aacap.org

This Website is an excellent source of information on the assessment and treatment of child and adolescent mental health disorders. Handouts for use with families (i.e., Facts for Families) are available on a multitude of problems, including ADHD.

American Academy of Pediatrics (AAP)
www.aap.org

This Website has excellent information for healthcare providers and parents on a variety of mental health topics, including ADHD. The AAP worked with the National Initiative for Children's Healthcare Quality to develop an evidence-based ADHD toolkit to assist practitioners in providing comprehensive care for children with this disorder.

Children and Adults with Attention-Deficit/Hyperactivity Disorder (CHADD)
www.chadd.org

This national nonprofit organization was founded in 1987 in response to the frustration and sense of isolation experienced by parents and their children with ADHD.

National Initiative for Children's Healthcare Quality (NICHQ)
www.nichq.org/resources/toolkit

The NICHQ works with experts to identify and categorize resources to assist clinicians to care for children with ADHQ. The ADHD toolkit can be downloaded at this Website.

National Institute of Mental Health
www.nimh.gov

This outstanding Website has multiple educational handouts on a variety of mental health disorders, including ADHD, and links to informative Websites.

National Resource Center on ADHD
http://www.help4ADHD.org/

This resource center is a program of CHADD, funded through a cooperative agreement with the Centers for Disease Control and Prevention.

REFERENCES

Bussing, R, Fernandez, M., Harwood, M., Hou, W. Garvan, C. W., Eyberg, S. M. (2008). Parent and teacher SNAP-IV ratings of attention deficit hyperactivity disorder symptoms: psychometric properties and normative ratings from a school district sample. *Assessment*, 15(3), 317-328.

Cosme Cruz, R.M., Clark, C.M., & Shin, L. (2012). A 10-year-old boy with ADHD symptoms. *Pediatric Annals*, 41(11), 456-458.

Magyary, D., & Brandt P (2002). A decision tree and clinical paths for the assessment and management of children with ADHD. *Issues in Mental Health Nursing*, 23(6), 553-566.

Olson, B.G., Rosenbaum P.F., Dosa N.P., et al (2005). Improving guideline adherence for the diagnosis of ADHD in an ambulatory pediatric setting. *Ambulatory Pediatrics*, 5(3), 138-142.

Shier, A.C., Reichenbacher, T., Ghuman, H.S., & Ghuman, J.K. Pharmacological treatment of attention deficit hyperactivity disorder in children and adolescents: clinical strategies. *Journal of Central Nervous System Disorders*, 20(5), 1-17.

SECTION 6
Mary Lynn Dell and John V. Campo

Somatoform Disorders

Fast Facts

- This DSM-5™ group of disorders replaces the somatoform disorders category in previous versions of the *Diagnostic and Statistical Manual*. This change is intended to simplify and lessen confusion compared to previous DSM disorders.

- These disorders often first present in general medical or non-psychiatric settings.

- Diagnostic criteria apply across the life span, so it is important to consider the child's or adolescent's developmental level during assessment and diagnosis.

- These disorders may or may not overlap or be comorbid with other medical disorders, such as irritable bowel syndrome, abdominal pain, fibromyalgia, headaches, or chronic pain.

- These disorders may or may not overlap or be comorbid with other psychiatric disorders that may have physiological symptoms, such as anxiety and depressive disorders.

- *Somatization* is a key concept. It refers to the subjective experience of physical symptoms for which clear pathology or injury is lacking or not diagnosable by standard-of-care methods, or when level of distress or disability exceeds what is typically associated with clinical findings.

- Due to complexities in the diagnosis of somatoform disorders historically, the term *medically unexplained symptoms* (MUS) often has been used to describe features of the somatic symptom disorders.

- Studies report that MUS range from 2% to 20% of children in various community and pediatric clinic settings.

- Somatic symptom disorders are associated with high healthcare costs and expenditures.

- Very minimal data exist at this time regarding new DSM-5™ somatic symptom disorders in children and adolescents.

Four Disorders Particularly Relevant to Children and Adolescents

1. **Somatic Symptom Disorder**

DSM-5™ Diagnostic Criteria for Somatic Symptom Disorder

A. One or more somatic symptoms that are distressing or result in significant disruption of daily life.

B. Excessive thoughts, feelings, or behaviors related to the somatic symptoms or associated health concerns as manifested by at least one of the following:

   1. Disproportionate and persistent thoughts about the seriousness of one's symptoms.

   2. Persistently high level of anxiety about health or symptoms.

   3. Excessive time and energy devoted to these symptoms or health concerns.

C. Although any one somatic symptom may not be continuously present, the state of being symptomatic is persistent (typically more than 6 months).

Specify if:

   With predominant pain (previously pain disorder): This specifier is for individuals whose somatic symptoms predominantly involve pain.

Specify if:

   Persistent: A persistent course is characterized by severe symptoms, marked impairment, and long duration (more than 6 months).

Specify current severity:

   Mild: Only one of the symptoms specified in Criterion B is fulfilled.

   Moderate: Two or more of the symptoms specified in Criterion B are fulfilled.

   Severe: Two or more of the symptoms specified in Criterion B are fulfilled, plus there are multiple somatic complaints (or one very severe somatic symptom).

Reprinted with permission from the Diagnostic and Statistical Manual of Mental Disorders, Fifth Edition, (Copyright ©2013). American Psychiatric Association. All Rights Reserved.

- A combination of distressing, often multiple, symptoms, to which the patient responds in excessive or maladaptive ways, resulting in significant disruption of daily life or impairment in functioning

- At least two of the following: 1) persistent, disproportionate worries about the medical seriousness of symptoms; 2) excessive anxiety about the symptoms; and 3) excessive time and energy spent concerned with the symptoms or health issues

- The youth must experience the distressing symptoms as described for at least 6 months.

- Subtypes include: 1) predominant somatic complaints (formerly the DSM-IV-TR Somatization Disorder); 2) predominant health anxiety (formerly the DSM-IV-TR Hypochondriasis); and 3) predominant pain (formerly the DSM-IV-TR Pain Disorder)

2. Other Specified Somatic Symptom and Related Disorders

- One or more somatic symptoms that the youth experiences as distressing or that interferes significantly with daily life

- Symptoms similar to those of Somatic Symptom Disorder above, but do not meet full diagnostic criteria in that category. Examples include Brief Somatic Symptom Disorder and Brief Illness Disorder, with duration of symptoms less than 6 months

3. Illness Anxiety Disorder

DSM-5™ Diagnostic Criteria for Illness Anxiety Disorder

A. Preoccupation with having or acquiring a serious illness.

B. Somatic symptoms are not present or, if present, are only mild in intensity. If another medical condition is present or there is a high risk for developing a medical condition (e.g., strong family history is present), the preoccupation is clearly excessive or disproportionate.

C. There is a high level of anxiety about health, and the individual is easily alarmed about personal health status.

D. The individual performs excessive health-related behaviors (e.g., repeatedly checks his or her body for signs of illness) or exhibits maladaptive avoidance (e.g., avoids doctor appointments and hospitals).

E. Illness preoccupation has been present for at least 6 months, but the specific illness that is feared may change over that period of time.

F. The illness-related preoccupation is not better explained by another mental disorder, such as a somatic symptom disorder, panic disorder, generalized anxiety disorder, body dysmorphic disorder, obsessive-compulsive disorder, or delusional disorder, somatic type.

Specify whether:

Care-seeking type: Medical care, including physician visits or undergoing tests and procedures, is frequently used.

Care-avoidant type: Medical care is rarely used.

- Somatic symptoms are not present or mild in severity
- Preoccupation with having or acquiring a serious illness; focused on an underlying medical diagnosis
- High level of anxiety about health and/or illness
- Performs health-related excessive behaviors or has maladaptive avoidance behaviors due to health concerns
- Symptoms present for at least 6 months
- Presentation is not better explained by another mental disorder.
- Similar to the DSM-IV-TR diagnosis of hypochondriasis

4. **Conversion Disorder (Functional Neurological Symptom Disorder)**
   - Known as "conversion disorder" in previous DSMs
   - Symptoms affect voluntary motor or sensory functions or cause loss of consciousness.
   - Symptoms are not due to general medical condition, substances, or cultural phenomena.
   - Symptoms may be inconsistent with known medical disorders.
   - A relevant psychological stressor is often present but not required.
   - Common symptoms include gait disturbances, tremors, shaking, jerking; weakness, numbness, tingling (often inconsistent with dermatomal patterns); vision or hearing deficits.
   - Psychodynamic explanations emphasize primary and secondary gain.

Risk Factors
- Family members with somatization symptoms
- Emotional and physical abuse or neglect
- Sexual abuse

Common Presenting Complaints
- Headache
- Abdominal pain
- Nausea, vomiting
- Fatigue
- Muscle aches and soreness
- Back pain
- Blurry vision
- Diarrhea
- Dyspnea
- Vocal cord dysfunction

Screening
- Thorough clinical history, with close attention to current stressors
- Children's Somatization Inventory – 35 items
- Functional Disability Inventory – 15 items, emphasizes past 2 weeks, school attendance

Assessment

- Thorough medical and psychiatric histories
- Thorough physical examination
- Appropriate laboratory, imaging, and other diagnostic testing, always balancing thoroughness with possible unintended harm from medical procedures
- Inquire about symptom models in relatives and significant others
- Inquire about academic history
- Inquire about peer relationships
- Review early childhood education and other early experiences when separated from caregiver
- Be alert to possible secondary gains

Management

- Based primarily on accumulated clinical experience due to relative lack of evidence-based treatment literature
- Often require multidisciplinary care from several types of healthcare professionals
- Emphasize collaboration and shared goals between patient, family, caregivers.
- Reassure patients and families that these symptoms are not fatal.
- Address anxiety directly.
- Cognitive-behavioral interventions – successful for abdominal pain, has addressed school absences and pain complaints
- Emphasize coping and minimizing sick role behaviors.
- Behavioral and operant interventions to reinforce healthy, adaptive behaviors and decrease incentives and reinforcements for maladaptive behaviors
- Parent training in basic behavioral and operant interventions is very helpful, often essential.
- Biofeedback, hypnosis, guided imagery, and relaxation techniques can be helpful. Imagery and relaxation are especially advantageous because patients can be taught to administer themselves.
- Family therapy – reinforce healthy attitudes and behaviors, cope with symptoms, address underlying conflicts.
- Communication with other professionals – medical, psychological, school, clergy, others
- Treat comorbid psychiatric disorders aggressively.
- Pharmacological interventions – refer to Table 6.1
- Monitor treatment outcomes, with particular attention to goals of school attendance, and healthy, fulfilling interpersonal, family, academic, and psychosocial functioning.

TABLE 6.1: Pharmacological Interventions in Somatic Symptom and Related Disorders

• No randomized controlled trials of psychoactive medications in pediatric somatic symptom disorders
• Use of psychoactive medications primarily based on case reports or extrapolated from adult populations with medical and psychiatric diagnoses
• Psychopharmacologic treatment most appropriately considered in the presence of comorbid anxiety or depression, especially when non-medication treatments have not been helpful.
Examples:
1. Recurrent abdominal pain – may start citalopram or fluoxetine at low dose (10 mg per day), increase to therapeutic dose of 20 mg daily over the next week, with maximum dose of 40 mg daily after 4 weeks
2. Low-dose benzodiazepines may be helpful short-term if symptoms are accompanied by severe anxiety – for instance, clonazepam 0.25 mg at bedtime gradually increased to maximum of 0.5 mg twice daily, or lorazepam 0.5 mg 3 times a day, gradually increased to 1.0 mg 3 times a day
• If medications are used, obtain informed consent, carefully explaining side effects, FDA black box warnings for antidepressants, and suicidality for those 24 years of age and under. Also, monitor for serotonin syndrome if the child is on more than one serotonergic agent, regardless of drug class.

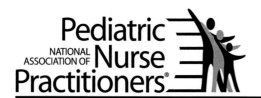

What is a somatic symptom disorder?

Somatic symptom disorders are conditions in which individuals experience physical symptoms that are not fully explained by the presence of a general medical condition after standard-of-care evaluations and diagnostic tests. In some patients, there may be a known medical condition or injury, but the amount of distress, worry about the condition, and disturbance in daily life is greater than what medical professionals and parents/caregivers would expect given the actual severity of the medical condition or injury.

Are the symptoms real?

Most definitely, yes! The symptoms your child is experiencing, whether abdominal pain, headache, muscle weakness or tingling, are very real, but medically unexplained. Telling your loved one that their symptoms are not real, or that they are "faking" or "making it up" just because the medical work-up cannot explain the cause almost never helps the symptoms go away.

What symptoms are most commonly involved?

Children and adolescents with this disorder may experience headaches, abdominal pain, nausea, vomiting, bloating, fatigue, muscle aches and soreness, back pain, diarrhea, vocal cord or voice problems, numbness, tingling, blurry vision, inability to walk or move a limb, and other issues. People of all ages have occasional aches and pains that come and go without an obvious explanation. In this instance, however, the severity of the symptoms intrudes on and disrupts functioning in daily life at home, school, and in other activities.

What other problems are seen with these disorders?

Sometimes disabling somatic symptoms may begin after a physical illness, infection, or injury. Examples include prolonged abdominal pain after a viral illness has cleared up, or numbness or tingling of the leg after being kicked in soccer practice. The somatic symptoms seem to "take on a life of their own" after the initial problem should have healed or resolved. Youth with somatic symptom disorders also have higher rates of depression and anxiety than general pediatric populations.

Are there other risk factors?

Physical and emotional abuse or neglect and sexual abuse are known risk factors for medically unexplained symptoms. Also, having other family members or significant others with unexplained medical symptoms may predispose a child to symptom expression, particularly during stressful life events.

How serious is this?

Somatic symptoms disorders are not fatal, but they can be serious if they interfere with a child's normal growth and development, including learning and academic achievement, peer and family relationships. Occasionally a child may be harmed if concerns about illness lead to prolonged physical inactivity and loss of healthy muscle tone. Children may also be harmed if clinicians order unnecessary tests, procedures, and treatments. Consequently, it is critical to avoid the temptation to request unnecessary medical testing or treatments that put the child at risk for complications and adverse effects.

How is the diagnosis made?

There is no single test or procedure for somatic symptom disorders. The diagnosis is made from a thorough clinical history, physical examination, and laboratory, imaging, and diagnostic tests appropriate for the concerns and problems the child is experiencing. Children should also be assessed for depression, anxiety, and the possibility of abuse or other traumatic experiences.

How are somatic treatment disorders treated or managed?

There is no single quick and easy procedure or medication for this. Treatment is based primarily on accumulated clinical wisdom and experience.

First of all, children and families should be assured that appropriate medical monitoring will be done for new or changing symptoms. In the meantime, many types of healthcare professionals may be involved in your child's care, including pediatric subspecialists, psychiatrists, nurses, physical and occupational therapists, teachers, and others. Families and the treatment team should establish and collaborate to achieve shared goals.

Specific treatment modalities often helpful include:

- Cognitive behavioral therapy – a particular type or school of therapy helpful in addressing stresses and behaviors that may be exacerbating the symptoms, as well as accompanying symptoms of depression and anxiety; encouraging a "rehabilitative" mindset that emphasizes the child's fundamental strengths and relative health is often critical.

- Behavioral therapies and parent training – assist parents with addressing illness behaviors and reinforcing healthy habits at home

- Family therapy – helps the patient and the entire family deal with the effects of the illness on everyone, as well as factors at home that might be contributing to the symptoms

- Many children and adolescents benefit from relaxation techniques, guided imagery, biofeedback, and hypnosis for symptom management

- Psychotropic medications for accompanying depression, anxiety, or other psychiatric disorders can sometimes be very helpful

- Communication with significant others in the youth's life is essential, including teachers, counselors, primary care doctors, therapists, clergy, and coaches

Resources for Somatoform Disorders

American Psychosomatic Society (APS)
http://www.psychosomatic.org/about/index.cfm

The mission of the American Psychosomatic Society is to promote and advance the scientific understanding and multidisciplinary integration of biological, psychological, behavioral, and social factors in human health and disease, and to foster the dissemination and application of this understanding in education and healthcare.

American Academy of Child and Adolescent Psychiatry (AACAP)
www.aacap.org

This Website contains information about research, legislative activities, and meetings regarding child and adolescent mental health; policy statements; clinical practice guidelines; and a directory of child and adolescent psychiatrists. It also offers a set of Fact Sheets for families in English, Spanish, and several other languages on a variety of topics that include ADHD, bullying, depression, and suicide.

The REACH (REsource for Advancing Children's Health) Institute
http://www.thereachinstitute.org/about-REACH.html

The REACH Institute is dedicated to improving the mental health of American children and adolescents with emotional and behavioral challenges. It provides workshops for healthcare providers that teach the best evidence-based therapies, from psychotherapy to pharmacology, to improve the mental health of children and teens. Excellent resources at the Website are available for healthcare providers, agencies, and families.

REFERENCES

American Psychiatric Association. (2000). *Diagnostic and Statistical Manual of Mental Disorders, Fourth Edition, Text Revision.* (DSM-IV-TR). Washington, DC: American Psychiatric Association.

American Psychiatric Association. (2011) DSM-V Somatic Symptom Disorders, Draft.

Campo, J.V. (2008). Disorders primarily seen in general medical settings. In R.L. Findling, (Ed.), *Clinical Manual of Child and Adolescent Psychopharmacology* (pp. 375-423). Arlington, VA: American Psychiatric Publishing, Inc.

Campo, J.V., Bridge J, Ehmann, M., et al. (2004). Recurrent abdominal pain, anxiety, and depression in primary care. *Pediatrics*, 113(4), 817-824.

Campo, J.V. & Fritz, G. (2001). A management model for pediatric somatization. *Psychosomatics*, 42(6), 467-476.

Dell, M.L. & Campo, J.V. (2011). Somatoform disorders in children and adolescents. *Psychiatric Clinics of North America*, 34(3), 643-660.

Fritz, G.K., Fritsch, S., & Hagino, O. (1997). Somatization disorders in children and adolescents: a review of the past 10 years. *Journal of the American Academy of Child and Adolescent Psychiatry*, 36(10), 1329-1338.

Looper, K.J. & Kirmayer, L.J. (2002). Behavioral medicine approaches to somatoform disorders. *Journal of Consulting and Clinical Psychology*, 70(3), 810-827.

Sanders, M.R., Shepherd, R.W., & Cleghorn, G., et al. (1994). The treatment of recurrent abdominal pain in children: a controlled comparison of cognitive-behavioral family intervention and standard pediatric care. *Journal of Consulting and Clinical Psychology*, 62(2), 306-314.

Schulman, J.L. (1988). Use of a coping approach in the management of children with conversion reactions. *Journal of the American Academy of Child and Adolescent Psychiatry*, 27(6), 785-788.

Stone, J., LaFrance, W.C., Levenson, J.L., & Sharpe, M. (2010). Issues for DSM-5: conversion disorder. *American Journal of Psychiatry*, 167(6), 626-627.

Walker, L.S., Garber, J., & Greene, J.W. (1993). Psychosocial correlates of recurrent childhood pain: a comparison of pediatric patients with recurrent abdominal pain, organic illness, and psychiatric disorders. *Journal of Abnormal Psychology*, 102(2), 248-258.

Walker, L.S. & Greene, J.W. (1991). The functional disability inventory: measuring a neglected dimension of child health status. *Journal of Pediatric Psychology*, 16(1), 39-58.

Witek, M.W., Rojas V., Alonso, C., et al. (2005). Review of benzodiazepine use in children and adolescents. *Psychiatric Quarterly*, 76(3) 283-296.

Wood, B.L. (2001). Physically manifested illness in children and adolescents: a biobehavioral family approach. *Child and Adolescent Psychiatric Clinics of North America*, 10(3), 543-562.

SECTION 7
Pamela Lusk

Disruptive Behaviors in Children and Adolescents

Fast Facts

- All children are oppositional from time to time, particularly when tired, hungry, stressed or upset. They may argue, talk back, disobey, and defy parents, teachers, and other adults in authority.

- Openly uncooperative and angry/hostile behavior becomes a concern when it is so frequent and consistent that it stands out when compared to other children of the same age and developmental level and when it affects the child's home, school, and social life (AACAP – 2011 Facts for Families).

- The child with disruptive behaviors may have ADHD or the "externalizing behaviors" (i.e., acting out behaviors) may be the symptoms of anxiety or depression. They may meet DSM-5™ criteria for a Trauma and Stressor-Related disorder, such as Adjustment Disorder with Disturbance of Emotions and Conduct, or that child may meet criteria for a DSM-5™ Disruptive, Impulse-Control, and Conduct Disorder, such as Oppositional Defiant Disorder (ODD) or Conduct Disorder.

- Symptoms of ADHD that present as disruptive behaviors include impulsivity, not following directions, intruding in others' activities, and not listening. These behaviors cause difficulties at home, in school, and in social situations.

- The first rule-out diagnosis will be ADHD if there is a possibility that the child's behaviors may meet the criteria for the disorder. Screening with the Vanderbilt Parent Assessment Scale or Conner's' Parent Rating Scale can be started in the office. These scales also have Oppositional Defiant subscales.

- In addition to the significant overlap between ADHD and ODD, the two conditions are often comorbid. Current evidence-based guidelines for treating ODD recommend treating the ADHD symptoms first as the best initial approach.

- Children with Disruptive Behavior disorders have difficulty with 1) flexibility, 2) frustration tolerance, and 3) problem solving.

- Oppositional behavior is sometimes used by the child to manage anxiety in the face of overwhelming demands. Irritable, antagonistic behaviors in youth are commonly found in anxiety disorders and depression.

- Children are barometers of family and environmental stress. When a child who has been functioning well presents with disruptive behaviors, a thorough exploration of what is going on in that child's life is warranted. They may meet Acute Stress Disorder or Adjustment Disorder criteria.

- Additional appointments can be scheduled to leverage the positive relationship the child has with the primary care provider (PCP) to explore the child's worries (e.g., the possibility of family distress, loss of a job by parent, uncertainty and instability about where the family lives, abuse – physical or sexual – to that child or someone they care about, neglect due to parent illness/ substance use, bullying/aggressive peers at school).

- Parenting factors can play a significant role in problem behaviors. There may be incentive for the behavior (e.g., gaining attention from the parent).

- Sometimes it is the provider that identifies a behavior, such as talking back to authority, as a significant problem. Physicians and nurse practitioners are more comfortable initiating a conversation about their observations of a child's behavioral, emotional or developmental issues with a parent they have known over a period of time.

- Some parents hold overly permissive, child-centered views of parenting. Following the long tradition of anticipatory guidance, parents are reminded that firm discipline combined with love is an important part of parenting. Discipline is a way of teaching a child how to live comfortably and successfully in a world that will make requests and have rules and expectations.

- Parents will bring their concerns about their child to the trusted expert – the pediatric healthcare provider; however, there are barriers to parent disclosure about disruptive behaviors. These include cultural beliefs and norms about normal and abnormal behavior, stigma, family conflict or dysfunction, being uninsured or underinsured, or not knowing where to go for mental health services (Foy &AAP Task Force on Mental Health, 2010).

- The pediatric practitioner can help parents "reframe" their understanding of the well child visit as not only physical, but also a place where behavioral and emotional concerns are assessed. An office equipped with prepared screening tools, handouts, books, DVDs, and audio CDs for families reinforces this message.

- Oppositional Defiant Disorder is found in 3% - 4% of children whose disruptive behaviors persist over months or years, occur across many situations, and result in pronounced impairment in their functioning in home, school, and peer settings. These children's anger is usually directed at authority figures. These children show extreme levels of argumentativeness, disobedience, stubbornness, negativity, and provocation of others.

- The more serious symptoms of Conduct Disorder, also included in DSM-5™ Disruptive, Impulse-Control, and Conduct Disorder, will be covered in the next section. Conduct disorder focuses largely on poorly controlled behaviors that violate the rights of others.

- Aggressive children underutilize pertinent social cues, misattribute hostile intent to peers, and generate fewer solutions to problems.

- An evidence-based approach to the child with disruptive behavior is empathy for the child and parents, and a reminder that **"Children do well if they can"** (Collaborative Problem Solving Approach, Explosive Child).

- Children with behavioral problems and irritable, fussy temperaments are at higher risk of being abused. Abuse may be triggered by the child's oppositional behaviors (Melnyk & Moldenhauer, 2006).

- Hope is instilled when the provider puts in place a plan to work with that child so he/she can acquire coping skills and learn to behave in ways that are more successful at home, in school, and in the community (*The Explosive Child*, Greene).

- As an active intervention, the provider along with the parents and child at the time of the visit can identify *one* problem to start working on first and put that plan into place immediately. Often, because the parents are so overwhelmed, the provider will need to elicit the child's input and make the decision as the expert/authority for the first target behavior.

- Brief, simple interventions have an enduring effect on families' abilities to problem-solve.

- The PCP has a major role in preventive mental health strategies; "Early interventions with problem behaviors may eliminate the progression of more serious and persistent mental health concerns" (IOM, 2009).

- Progression from early symptoms to oppositional defiant disorder and conduct disorder frequently follows the path below.

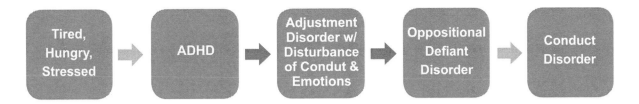

Risk Factors

- Disruptive behaviors can occur in a variety of conditions such as ADHD, anxiety, depressive and psychotic disorders.

- There are complex combinations of risk factors: biological, psychological, and social factors.

- The disruptive, impulse-control, and conduct disorders all tend to be more common in males than in females. These disorders tend to have first onset in childhood or adolescence.

- Biological factors may include family clustering of similar disorders, genetic predisposition, and comorbid conditions, such as ADHD. Disruptive or oppositional behaviors are common in children with language disorders (receptive disorders in particular), cognitive deficits, delays in development with limited problem-solving skills, and other neuropsychological deficits.

- Psychological factors may include temperament, goodness of fit with family, school, and/or neighborhood. Parenting can be a significant factor (e.g., parenting style, parenting inconsistency).

- Social factors may include stress related to the parent-child relationship, child care experiences, and acute stressors in the family or environment, history of abuse, and exposure to parental discord or family violence.

- It is helpful to consider the particular child's risk/protective factor ratio.

Common Presenting Complaints

- Parents, appearing weary from their child's irritable, angry, externalizing behaviors, may present to the primary care or pediatric office with instructions from the school (or child care provider) to "Get my child evaluated and treated for his problem behaviors or he cannot continue to attend here!"

- Parents may describe previous good functioning, but now the child is irritable, does not seem to listen, storms around angrily, and seems preoccupied with his or her own thoughts.

- The child may arrive at the appointment with downcast eyes and a tense, if not angry countenance. He or she may avoid eye contact, refuse to speak, or speak with a defiant, uncooperative attitude.

- The child may talk back to the provider, and present as "the boss" in interactions with family and healthcare team. He/she may be verbally oppositional and argumentative.

- The parent may say, "I can't do anything with him now." "He won't do anything I tell him to do." "He is always throwing temper fits."

- The child's behaviors may be so loud and disruptive in the waiting and exam rooms that it is clear why the referral for evaluation has been made.

- The oppositional defiant (ODD) child is often overly sensitive to authority and the slightest perception of provocation will fuel his or her avoidant, defiant, or oppositional behavior. The pediatric clinician will need to be straightforward with a caring, concerned, matter-of-fact approach, aware that the goal for the clinician is "To not give in, and not give up" (The Psychiatric Interview of Children & Adolescents, Cepeda).

Screening

Two common screening tools found in most pediatric offices, the Vanderbilt and Conner's Assessment/ Rating Scales for ADD, also include items that screen for Oppositional/Defiant Disorder. There are teacher rating scales as well as parent rating scales. These scales are presented in the section on Attention Deficit/Hyperactivity Disorder along with the online links to obtain them. The KySS Worries Questionnaire (also in this manual) can be very helpful in identifying that child's stressors.

Assessment

When addressing problematic or disruptive behaviors, the differential starts with the child's history and physical exam, and interview of the child and parents. The teacher's and parent's completed screening tools (Vanderbilt or Conner's) also provide valuable information for the clinician as the assessment proceeds.

A good beginning assessment/diagnostic guide for the child with aggression is from the T-May – toolkit. (Available online at TMAY.org). Parents and teachers can keep a journal of this information.

The Use of "**BOLDER**" is helpful in the assessment:

B – Behavior: In what ways does the child exhibit aggression?

O – Onset: When does it happen? What triggers it, and why?

L – Location: Where do the symptoms occur – home/school?

D – Duration: How long does it last?

E – Exacerbating factors: What makes it worse?

R – Relief: What makes it better?

**RISK ASSESSMENT: Whenever a young person is seen who has extreme impulsive anger, a risk assessment needs to be conducted. Often we ask parents, "Do you feel safe with this young person?" and we ask the youth, "Do you feel you can keep yourself safe from hurting yourself or hurting others?"

A psychiatry consult or evaluation in the emergency department by a mental health crisis team can always be arranged if the PCP assesses the situation to be acute and requiring immediate psychiatric evaluation and treatment.

Questions to assess RISK from the Reach Institute, Action Signs for Helping Kids program:

Do you have:
> Involvement in many fights, using a weapon, or wanting to badly hurt others?
> Severe out-of-control behavior that can hurt yourself or others?

It is always good to ask the family about a crisis plan. What would they do if the situation became unsafe? Who would they call? Where would they go for immediate help? Having a crisis plan well thought out allows them to react quickly in the event of a crisis.

Used with permission: The REACH Institute and T-MAY Steering Committee,
http://www.thereachinstitute.org/tmay-static.html

DSM-5™ Diagnoses for Disruptive Behaviors

The diagnoses related to disruptive disorders fall on a continuum from ADHD (which needs to be ruled out first) to Adjustment Disorders. If those criteria are not, then consider the behaviors as symptoms of Oppositional Defiant Disorder and Disruptive Disorder NOS or the more serious Conduct Disorder. This section will focus on Adjustment Disorders, Oppositional Defiant Disorder, and Disruptive Disorder NOS. ADHD is covered in a previous section, and Conduct disorders will be covered in the next section.

> In DSM-5™, **Adjustment Disorders with disturbance of conduct and emotions** are found in the section on **Trauma and Stressor-Related Disorders.**

> In DSM-5™, **Oppositional Defiant Disorder and Disruptive Disorder NOS** are found in the section on **Disruptive, Impulse Control and Conduct Disorders**. Specific diagnostic criteria for each disorder will be presented as each is discussed.

Adjustment Disorders

Always consider Adjustment Disorder – (a Trauma – and Stressor-Related Disorder) first while the work-up is in progress. You can always add that a diagnosis is "provisional."

Children's behaviors often represent distress in their home or environment.

When bad things happen, most people get upset. Adjustment disorder is diagnosed when the magnitude of the distress (e.g., alterations in mood, anxiety, conduct) exceeds what would normally be expected. Whenever there is a significant stress, children and teens can respond with externalizing symptoms – anger, impulsivity, and disruptive conduct.

Adjustment disorder is in the trauma and stress section of the DSM-5™, and so are acute stress disorder and PTSD. All three of these disorders involve emotional and behavioral symptoms in response to identifiable stressors. Stressors may be single events, recurrent or continuous. Stressors may affect a single person, an entire family, or a larger group or community (as with disasters). Some stressors accompany specific developmental events (such as starting middle school). Individuals from disadvantaged life circumstances experience a high rate of stressors and may be at increased risk for adjustment disorders. In adjustment disorder the stressor can be of any severity rather than the severity and type required of Acute Stress Disorder and PTSD. There are timing and symptom differences between Adjustment Disorder and Acute Stress Disorder and PTSD. Adjustment disorders can be diagnosed immediately and persist up to 6 months after exposure to the traumatic event. Acute Stress Disorder and PTSD are covered in Section 3 - the anxiety disorders section of this guide.

The prevalence of Adjustment Disorder has been reported to be between 2% and 8% in community samples of children and adolescents. Boys and girls are equally likely to receive this diagnosis.

DSM-5™ Diagnostic Criteria for Adjustment Disorders

A. The development of emotional or behavioral symptoms in response to an identifiable stressor(s) occurring within 3 months of the onset of the stressor(s).

B. These symptoms or behaviors are clinically significant, as evidenced by one or both of the following:

1. Marked distress that is out of proportion to the severity or intensity of the stressor, taking into account the external context and the cultural factors that might influence symptom severity and presentation.

2. Significant impairment in social, occupational, or other important areas of functioning.

C. The stress-related disturbance does not meet the criteria for another mental disorder and is not merely an exacerbation of a preexisting mental disorder.

D. The symptoms do not represent normal bereavement.

E. Once the stressor or its consequences have terminated, the symptoms do not persist for more than an additional 6 months.

Specify whether:

309.0 (F43.21) With depressed mood: Low mood, tearfulness, or feelings of hopelessness are predominant.

309. 24 (F43.22) With anxiety: Nervousness, worry, jitteriness, or separation anxiety is predominant.

309.28 (F43.23) With mixed anxiety and depressed mood: A combination of depression and anxiety is predominant.

309.3 (F43.24) With disturbance of conduct: Disturbance of conduct is predominant.

309.4 (F43.25) With mixed disturbance of emotions and conduct: Both emotional symptoms (e.g., depression, anxiety) and a disturbance of conduct are predominant.

309.9 (F43.20) Unspecified: For maladaptive reactions that are not classifiable as one of the specific subtypes of adjustment disorder.

If the person has had an exposure to actual or threatened death, serious injury, or sexual violation by directly experiencing the traumatic event, witnessing the event, or learning that a traumatic event occurred to a close family member or close friend, then he or she may meet criteria for Acute Stress Disorder for 3 days to a month after trauma exposure.

If a young person has some symptoms of a trauma, or stressor related disorder but does not fully meet DSM 5 criteria for a specific Diagnosis, "Other Specified Trauma and Stressor- Related Disorder": may be used. "Unspecified Trauma and Stressor-Related Disorder" can be used when there is insufficient information to make a specific diagnosis

If the child behaviors cannot be accounted for as: Adjustment Disorder with Mixed Disturbance of Emotion and Conduct, or Adjustment Disorder with Disturbance of Conduct, then the next differential diagnosis to be considered will be: Oppositional Defiant Disorder from the DSM-5™ section Disruptive, Impulse-Control, and Conduct Disorders.

In the DSM-5™, Disruptive, Impulse-Control, and Conduct Disorders are the conditions involving problems in the self-control of emotions (anger and irritation) and behaviors (argumentativeness and defiance). Intermittent Explosive Disorder is also in this section, as is Conduct Disorder, which will be discussed in another section of this guide.

The disruptive, impulse-control, and conduct disorders all tend to be more common in males than in females. These disorders tend to have first onset in childhood or adolescence. Conduct disorder (which now has a childhood onset or adolescent onset clarifier) or intermittent explosive disorder represent patterns of serious disruptive behaviors over time and generally clinicians hold off on assigning these diagnoses in younger patients. Intermittent explosive disorder can include verbal aggression as well as non-destructive, non-injurious behaviors. This must occur after the age of 6 years. The aggressive outbursts are impulsive and anger based.

There is a developmental relationship between ODD and conduct disorder in that most cases of conduct disorder previously would have met criteria for ODD, at least in cases in which conduct disorder emerges prior to adolescence. However, most children with ODD do not eventually develop conduct disorder. Furthermore, children with ODD are at risk for eventually developing other problems besides conduct disorder, including anxiety and depressive disorders (DSM-5™).

Oppositional Defiant Disorder

Children with ODD show extreme levels of argumentativeness, disobedience, stubbornness, negativity, and provocation of others. While such behavior can be true of most children at some point in their lives, this diagnosis is warranted only for the few children (3%-4%) whose symptoms persist over months or years, occur across many situations, and result in pronounced impairment in their functioning in home, school, and peer settings.(theReachinstitute.org/). ODD is a milder form, and sometimes a precursor to conduct disorder. In contrast to children with conduct disorder, the behavior of children with ODD does not involve serious violations of others' rights. It does, however, impair the child's family, academic and social functioning (thereachinstitute.org/).

DSM-5™ Diagnostic Criteria for Oppositional Defiant Disorder

A. A pattern of angry/irritable mood, argumentative/defiant behavior, or vindictiveness lasting at least 6 months as evidenced by at least four symptoms from any of the following categories, and exhibited during interaction with at least one individual who si not a sibling.

Angry/Irritable Mood

1. Often loses temper.

2. Is often touchy or easily annoyed.

3. Is often angry and resentful.

Argumentative/Defiant Behavior

4. Often argues with authority figures or, for children and adolescents, with adults.

5. Often actively defies or refuses to comply with requests from authority figures or with rules.

6. Often deliberately annoys others.

7. Often blames others for his or her mistakes or misbehavior.

Vindictiveness

8. Has been spiteful or vindictive at least twice within the past 6 months.
   Note: The persistence and frequency of these behaviors should be used to distinguish a behavior that is within normal limits from behavior that is symptomatic. For children younger than 5 years, the behavior should occur on most days for a period of at least 6 months unless otherwise noted (Criterion A8). For individuals 5 years or older, the behavior should occur at least once per week for at least 6 months, unless otherwise noted (Criterion A8). While these frequency criteria provide guidance on a minimal level of frequency to define symptoms, other factors should also be considered, such as whether the frequency and intensity of the behaviors are outside a range that is normative for the individual's developmental level, gender, and culture.

B. The disturbance in behavior is associated with distress in the individual or others in his or her immediate social context (e.g., family, peer group, work colleagues), or it impacts negatively on social, educational, occupational, or other important areas of functioning.

C. The behaviors do not occur exclusively during the course of a psychotic, substance use, depressive, or bipolar disorder. Also, the criteria are not met for disruptive mood dysregulation disorder.

Specify current severity:

Mild: Symptoms are confined to only one setting (e.g., at home, at school, at work, with peers).

Moderate: Some symptoms are present in at least two settings.

Severe: Some symptoms are present in three or more settings.

(With the DSM-5™, the same ODD behaviors are included as in DSM-IV, but they are placed in three categories to distinguish emotional and behavioral symptoms)

Presentations in which symptoms characteristic of a Disruptive, Impulse- Control, and Conduct disorder that cause clinically significant distress or impairment in social, occupational, or other important areas of functioning predominate but do not meet fill criteria for any of the specific disorders in the **Disruptive, Impulse-Control, and Conduct Disorder**, in DSM-5TM may be Other Specified **Disruptive, Impulse-Control,** and **Conduct Disorder** and **Unspecified Disruptive, Impulse-Control, and Conduct Disorder**.

Evidence-Based Management

Initial treatment and management planning include:

- Referral to specialty psychiatry services is always considered as an option, depending on patient presentation and availability of such specialists in the community, but in this guide we offer ways to start active intervention with the families – capitalizing on the trusting relationship the family has with the PCP.

  From T-May:

  PRESTO plan:

  P – Partner with the family

  R – Assess risk, identify professional reinforcements, and refer if need be

  E – Educate the family on evidence-based practices and expectations of treatment

  S – Ascertain support in the community

  T – Track signs and symptoms with tools

  O – Objectives and action plans are established with the family.

- In obtaining information for both assessment and subsequent treatment, the success will require building a therapeutic alliance with the parents and the child separately. Engagement with the child is often best achieved by empathizing with the child's anger and unhappiness. Focus on the problem at hand, and let the child know you are aware that he or she is hurting. Engage the child in problem-solving. Most youth realize their behavior is out of line.

- When the child exhibits problems with behavior, the plan of care will routinely include the parents, the child, and the school (or child care provider setting). Parents may need to be informed that, in children, involving the teacher, parent, and healthcare providers is the best evidence-based care. The team approach – multimodal – is most effective and parents and the child need not feel embarrassed – it is standard best practice.

- Initially, with signed consent of the parent or guardian, the PCP will want collateral information from the school regarding the child's behaviors there, and a coordination of care can begin – always keeping the parents and child informed and central to the communications back and forth.

- If the parents request, the PCP can write out a note that the child is being evaluated and followed by that provider. School officials likely will grant an extension for a deadline final decision about the child's continued attendance and this will relieve some of the immediate family pressure.

- Sometimes it takes finesse for the PCP to be the leader/coordinator of the parent/ child/ teacher/ healthcare provider/specialty psychiatry (if involved) team – and keep everyone reminded that the "battle" is against the "problem behaviors" (not blame for each other) and all are on the same team – moving forward, fighting that battle together.

- Identify the child's strengths (and the family's) and praise the child's steps toward solving the problem.

- Pediatric healthcare providers have long recognized the important role of providing guidance to parents. PCPs already provide behavioral interventions in their practice. They have coached many parents through the steps of setting up a reward chart with stickers for a child with an identified problem behavior/habit.

- Most pediatric clinicians have an assortment of favorite behavioral strategies that they use in counseling parents about behavior management (Checklists/monitoring, Reward charts, Special times, Planned ignoring, Time-outs, Logical consequences, Goal setting/ Target behaviors, Positive and negative reinforcements).

- Parents are also reminded that the problem behaviors may escalate at first, as the child "tests" the new parenting approaches.

- Referral to family therapy is often recommended, as well as linking the family to community agencies that provide classes, support, and connections with families struggling with similar challenges.

According to the American Academy of Child and Adolescent Psychiatry, in the Practice Parameter for the assessment and treatment of Children and Adolescents with Oppositional Defiant Disorder, the "treatment of ODD may be particularly problematic and often requires multimodal treatment, including psychosocial interventions and occasionally medication therapy" (2007).

Psychosocial Interventions

The two types of evidence-based treatments for youth with ODD are:

Individual approaches in the form of problem-solving skills training; individual approaches should be specific to problems encountered, behaviorally based, and as much as possible oriented to the development of problem-solving skills.

Examples of problem-solving skills-building programs are:

Collaborative Problem Solving - **www.ccps.info/** and **www.livesinthebalance.org/.**

Child Protective Services (CPS) views the child's disruptive, explosive behavior as the child's inadequate and inappropriate attempt to solve a problem in his world. The child's particular means of "solving his problem" may not be satisfactory to the parent or teacher, but it is the only solution he can figure out at this point. In collaborative problem-solving therapy, the parent's or teacher's role is to "figure out" what problem the child is struggling with, such as having a consistently short fuse, a need to be in control of what seems to be an unpredictable environment, and an inability to understand adults' requests. Once the parents understand the child's problem, their next role is to help the child find a solution, given the problem, and to "scaffold" (assist) the child to a next step in developing new skills and behaviors that help the child solve the problem. (Greene)

Creating Opportunities for Personal Empowerment (COPE) for Children and Adolescents by Dr. Bernadette Melnyk is a seven-session, evidence-based, manualized cognitive behavioral skills building program, presented at length in the Depressive Disorders and Brief Interventions sections of this manual. In the COPE program, there is a major emphasis on teaching the child self-regulation (i.e., how to positively control emotions). The young person learns strategies and skills to positively influence their thoughts, emotions, and behaviors. The homework in COPE provides opportunities for practice of these self-control skills in their home, school, and social environment.

Family interventions in the form of parent management training. The best family interventions encompass training in effective disciplining and age-appropriate supervision. The main principles of evidence-based family interventions are:

Reduce positive reinforcement of disruptive behavior.

Increase reinforcement of prosocial and compliant behavior. Positive reinforcements can vary, but parental attention is the priority. Punishment usually consists of time out and loss of rewards/privileges.

> Apply consequences and/or punishment for disruptive behavior.

> Make parental response predictable, contingent, and immediate.

> The clinician may know of good parenting programs in their community.

Examples of recommended Parent Management Training programs are:

Triple P   http:// **www.triplep.net/**

Incredible Years   **http://www.incredibleyears.com/**

Parent empowerment program   **http://www.thereachinstitute.org/pep.html**

*Practice Parameter for the Assessment and Treatment of Children and Adolescents with Oppositional Defiant Disorder is available at **www.aacap.org.**

Medication
Many primary care/pediatric healthcare providers will consult with child psychiatric clinicians in initiating medication as an adjunct to psychosocial interventions.

According to the AACAP, medications may be helpful as adjuncts to psychosocial treatment for symptomatic treatment and to treat comorbid conditions. Medication should not be the sole intervention in ODD. The following are recommendations from AACAP Practice Parameters for children and teens with ODD.*

- Prescribing medications without enlisting the child's support or assent is unlikely to be successful, especially with adolescents.

- Pharmacological agents for ODD are not well studied, but several agents have received support in double-blind placebo-controlled studies of disruptive behavior.

- Medications such as stimulants and atomoxetine, used to treat ODD in the context of ADHD, may result in improvement of the oppositional behavior.

- Promise has been shown for mood stabilizers such as divalproex sodium and lithium carbonate, anti-psychotics, and stimulants for the target behavior aggression.

- Regardless of diagnosis, atypical antipsychotics seem to be the most commonly prescribed medications for the treatment of acute and chronic maladaptive aggression.

- Typical and atypical antipsychotics are helpful in treating aggression after appropriate psychosocial interventions have been applied in the context of mental retardation and pervasive developmental disorders.

If comorbid conditions are present, then medication should be targeted to those specific symptoms as much as possible.

Consider adding an antipsychotic taking into account the latest available evidence on efficacy and safety if severe aggression persists after an adequate trial of treatments for the underlying disorder.

Start low! Go slow! And stop slowly. Avoid abruptly stopping and/or switching to reduce risk of rebound. Slow switch using cross titration is the preferred method.

Use a recommended titration schedule and deliver an adequate medication trial before changing or adding medication.

Non-responsiveness to a specific compound should lead to a trial of another class of medication instead of adding on medications (to avoid further clouding the case). If a trial of an atypical antipsychotic is not effective, then a trial of another atypical or switch to a mood stabilizer is recommended. Atypical antipsychotics should be prescribed in consultation and collaboration with a mental healthcare provider.

Avoid using more than two psychotropic medications simultaneously.
SSRIs are not considered first-line agents unless MDD or anxiety is diagnosed along with ODD.

Conduct side effect (AIMS) and metabolic assessments and laboratory tests that are clinically relevant, comprehensive, and based on established guidelines.

Provide accessible information to parents and families about identifying and managing side effects. Promote healthy lifestyle changes that may reduce the risk of physical adverse events and medication consequences.

See the T-May Pocket Guide at **www.TheReachInstitute.org/TMAY.html.**

For comorbid ADHD and aggression/ODD, see
http:www.guideline.gov/content.aspx?id=15628&search=antipsychotics+in+primary+care

From the T-May Pocket Guide **www.TheReachInstitute.org/TMAY.html.**

The Reach Institute, Rutgers CERTSs Reference Guide for Primary Care Clinicians and Mental Health Specialist for medication guidelines: "Psychotropic agents, particularly second- generation antipsychotics and mood stabilizers, are increasingly given to youth on an outpatient basis for treatment for overt aggression ….despite troubling side effects and a lack of supportive empirical evidence of their effects on adolescents and children."

Medications are nicely presented in the T-May Reference Guide in a very clear chart (Anticonvulsants, and the atypical antipsychotics – dosages, indications, side effects).

T-MAY Medication Guide for Maladaptive Aggressive Behaviors
(Used with Permission: T-may.org 2010)

TYPICAL MEDICATION DOSING AND TITRATION INTERVALS OF ANTIPSYCHOTICS *

ANTIPSYCHOTIC	DOSE RANGE (mg)	DOSE STRENGTH (mg)	MEDICATION FORMULATIONS (available for use)	STARTING DOSE (mg)	HALF LIFE (hrs)	TIME TO PEAK (hrs)	TITRATION INTERVALS (days)	PRINCIPAL LIVER ENZYME	LIVER ENZYME INDUCER	LIVER ENZYME INHIBITOR
FIRST GENERATION ANTIPSYCHOTICS (FGA)										
HALOPERIDOL (HAL)	1 to 6	0.5, 1, 2, 5, 10, 20 tablets, 2; 10 mg/mL liquid, 5 im	po, im short im long	0.25-1 Chlorpromazine Dose » 2 mg	3 - 6 po 10-20 im	2-6 po .05 im	increase dose by 0.5 kg intervals of 5-7 days	3A4	3A4	3A4
MOLINDONE (MOL)	20 to 140	5, 10, 25, 50	po	0.5-1 mg/kg/d divided in 3-4 doses Chlorpromazine Dose ≈ 10 mg	1.5	1.5	N/A	2D6	2D6	2D6
PERPHENAZINE (PER)	8 to 32	2, 4, 8, 16	po	TBD; no data available Chlorpromazine Dose ≈ 10 mg	8 to 12	1 to 3	TBD; no data available	2D6	2D6	2D6

Modified from: Correll 2008 (Correll CU). Antipsychotics + Adjunctive Medications. Textbook of a Child + Adolescent Psychiatry. M Dulcan (ed.), American Psychiatric Publishing, Inc. New York.

USUAL MEDICATION DOSING AND TITRATION INTERVALS OF ANTIPSYCHOTICS (APs) *

ANTIPSYCHOTIC	DOSE RANGE (mg)	DOSE STRENGTH (mg)	MEDICATION FORMULATIONS (available for use)	STARTING DOSE (mg)	HALF LIFE (hrs)	TIME TO PEAK (hrs)	TITRATION INTERVALS (days)	PRINCIPAL LIVER ENZYME	LIVER ENZYME INDUCER	LIVER ENZYME INHIBITOR
SECOND GENERATION ANTIPSYCHOTICS (SGA)										
ARIPIPRAZOLE (ARI)	Child: 2.5 - 15 Adol: 5 to 15	2, 5, 10, 15, 20, 30 tbl; 10, 15 diss, liquid 1 (30 mg = 25 mL)	po, im short, diss., liquid	2 to 5 / Chlorpromazine Dose ≈ 7.5mg	50 to 72	3 to 5	when starting at 2mg, may increase dose every 3rd day; after steady state, increase dose every 7-14 days	2D6 > 3A4	3A4	2D6 3A4
CLOZAPINE (CLO)	Child: 150 - 300 Adol: 200 - 600	25; 100	po	12.5 / Chlorpromazine Dose ≈ 50 mg	12	1 to 4	25 mg daily or, every other day	1A2>2C19 2C19>3A4 3A4 > 2C9 2C9 > 2D6	1A2 2C19 3A4	1A2 2C19 3A4 2C9
OLANZAPINE (OLA)	N/A	.5, 5, 7.5, 10, 15, 20 tb 5, 10, 15, 20 diss; 10im	po, im short, diss.	5 to 10 Chlorpromazine Dose ≈ 5 mg	30	6	increase at intervals > 5 days	1A2 2D6 3A4	1A2 2D6 3A4	1A2 2D6 3A4
PALIPERIDONE (PAL)	3 to 12	3, 6, 9	po, ER	3 Chlorpromazine Dose ≈ 3 mg	21 to 30	24	increase at intervals > 5 days	<10% Hepatic Clearance	N/A	N/A
QUETIAPINE (QUE)	150 to 750	25, 100, 200	po, XR	50-100 IR 200-300 XR Chlorpromazine Dose ≈ 75 mg	6 to 7	2	100 mg per day	3A4	3A4	3A4
RISPERIDONE (RIS)	Child: 1.5 - 2 Adol: 2 to 4	0.5, 1, 2, 3, 4 tablets; 0.5, 1, 2 diss; liquid 1mg/mL 30ml bottl	po, im long, diss., liquid	0.5 to 1 Chlorpromazine Dose ≈ 2 mg	3	1 to 2	increase at intervals of 0.5-1 per day or > 5 days	2D6 > 3A4	2D6 3A4	2D6 3A4
ZIPRASIDONE (ZIP)	80 to 160	20, 40, 60, 80 tablets	po im short	20 to 40 Chlorpromazine Dose ≈ 60 mg	7	5	increase at 20-40 per day	Aldehyde Oxidase > 3A4	3A4	3A4

Modified from: Correll 2008 (Correll CU). Antipsychotics and Adjunctive Medications. In: Textbook of a Child and Adolescent Psychiatry. M Dulcan (ed.), American Psychiatric Publishing, Inc. New York.
Modified from: 2004 .TRAAY - A Pocket Reference Guide. New York State Office of Mental Health, Research Foundation for Mental Hygiene, Inc. and the Trustees of Columbia University.

USUAL MEDICATION DOSING AND TITRATION INTERVALS OF MOOD STABILIZERS *

MOOD STABILIZER	DOSE RANGE (mg)	DOSE STRENGTH (mg)	MEDICATION FORMULATIONS (available for use)	STARTING DOSE (mg)	HALF LIFE (hrs)	TIME TO PEAK (hrs)	TITRATION INTERVALS (days)	PRINCIPAL LIVER ENZYME	LIVER ENZYME INDUCER	LIVER ENZYME INHIBITOR
CARBAMAZEPINE	100 - 800	100, 200, 100 mg/5mL	po	100 mg B.I.D. (tbl), 1/2 tsp QID (susp) for 6-12 years	Initial 25 - 65 Later 12 to 17	4 to 5	Add < 100 mg/day at weekly intervals, t.i.d or q.i.d. (tbl) til optimal reponse	3A4>2D6 2D6.1A2 Auto-Inducer	3A4 2D6 1A2	3A4 2D6 1A2
CARBAMAZEPINE ER	100 - 800	100, 200, 400	po	100 mg for 6-12 years B.I.D. or T.I.D.	Initial 25 - 65 Later 12 to 17	3 to 12	Add 100 mg/day at weekly intervals b.i.d until optimal response	3A4>2D6 2D6.1A2 Auto-Inducer	3A4 2D6 1A2	3A4 2D6 1A2
DIVALPROEX	500 - 2000	125, 250, 500	po	10 - 15 mg/kg/d B.I.D. or T.I.D.	9 to 16	3 to 4	Add 5-10 mg/kg day q 7 days; give with food. Increase rapidly to lowest effective dose	CYP450 C29 (weak inhibitor)	Rifampin Seco-barbital	# please see footnote
DIVALPROEX ER	500 - 2000	250, 500	po	10-15 mg/kg/day po	9 to 16	7 to 14	Increase dose by 5 - 10 mg/kg/wk until optimal response; clinical response is at plasma levels of 85-125 μg/mL	CYP450 C29 (weak inhibitor)	Rifampin Seco-barbital	# please see footnote
LAMOTRIGINE	50 - 200	25, 100, 150, 200	po	only 25mg < 16 yo, or on DVP	24 - 34	1.4 - 4.8	Keep starting dose stable for 2 wks, increase by 12.5 - 25 mg; but if < 16 yo, or on DVP, increase by 12.5 mg	Glucu-ronidation	N/A	N/A
LITHIUM	600 - 1800	8mEq/5mL	po	15 - 20 mg/kg/d B.I.D or T.I.D.	20 - 24	1 to 3	Dose wkly based on plasma Li+ levels	Renal Elimination Only	Renal Elimination Only	Renal Elimination Only
LITHIUM CR	1800 mg/d, serum level 1-1.5mEq/L adults	300, 450	po	150 - 300 mg B.I.D.	24	4	Dose according to need	Renal Elimination Only	Renal Elimination Only	Renal Elimination Only

Modified from: Correll and Schenck. Correll CU and Schenck EM. Assessing and Treating Pediatric Bipolar Disorder. Oxford American Psychiatry Library. In preparation.

Resources for Providers

American Academy of Child and Adolescent Psychiatry. (2007). Practice Parameters for the Assessment and Treatment of Children and Adolescents with Oppositional Defiant Disorder. *Journal of the American Academy of Child & Adolescent Psychiatry*, 46(1), 107-125.

American Psychiatric Association. (2013). *Diagnostic and Statistical Manual of Mental Disorders, Fifth Edition*, **www.dsm5.org.**

Cepeda, C. (2010) Clinical Manual for the Psychiatric Interview of Children and Adolescents, Arlington, VA: American Psychiatric Publishing, Inc.

Greene, R. W. (2010). The explosive child: A new approach for understanding and parenting easily frustrated, "chronically inflexible" children (Revised 4th edition). New York: HarperCollins.

Parent Empowerment Training - **http://www.thereachinstitute.org/pep.html**

The Reach Institute **www.thereachinstitute.org/** behavior therapy, **http://www.thereachinstitute.org/behavioral-therapy.html**

R.W. Greene's Website with resources for his collaborative problem solving **http://www.livesinthebalance.org/;** this Website has an extensive Q&A section for parents, and audio lectures by Dr. Greene. It is factual and positive.

T-May *(Treatment of Maladaptive Aggression in Youth) Rutgers CERTs Pocket Reference Guide for Primary Care Clinicians and Mental Health Specialists.* (2010). Center for Education and Research on Mental Health Therapeutics (CERTs) Rutgers University , The REACH Institute, University Texas at Austin College of Pharmacy, New York State Office of Mental Health, California Department of Mental Health).

Another Website with information on Collaborative Problem Solving is **http://www.thereachinstitute.org/cps.html.**

Resources for Families

AACAP *(American Academy of Child and Adolescent Psychiatry Campaign for America's Kids* website - information pages: Facts for Families. Children with ODD, "Facts for Families," No. 72 (3/11). **http://www.aacap.org/cs/root/facts_for_families/facts_for_families_numerical_list**

COPE – Creating Opportunities for Personal Empowerment, a manualized, seven-session, evidence-based, cognitive-behavioral skills building program for children, adolescents, and young adults by Bernadette Melnyk. To obtain the COPE program, contact **cope.melnyk@gmail.com.**

Greene **http://www.explosivechild.com** and **http://www.livesinthebalance.org/** This Website has very useful information and links for parents and healthcare providers. These sites focus on the collaborative problem-solving approach.

Incredible Years Program: **http://www.incredibleyears.com**

Oppositional Defiant Disorder Resource Center link: **www.aacap.org/cs/ODD.Resource_Center**

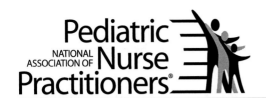

Information for Parents About Behavior Problems in Children and Teens

- Pediatric healthcare providers recognize how difficult your role as a parent is with this challenging child. You still may want to remind us about how exhausting it is to have a child with behavior issues.

- Please write down and tell us about every positive step that is being made as you parent your child.

- Always build on your child's particular positives; give your child praise and positive reinforcement when he shows flexibility or cooperation.

- Your child's problems are "loud" problems – they stand out for all to notice (as opposed to anxiety, which is more of a private child problem). You may be bombarded by others in your community telling you about your child's behaviors.

- The journey of working with a child who has problem or disruptive behaviors can be frustrating, draining, and isolating. This Website connects you to a vast array of resources and links that can help you better understand challenging children: http://www.livesinthebalance.org/.

- We want you to be well informed so you can teach others what you know. Your child's behaviors get "louder" and more obvious to others when he or she doesn't have the skills to deal with the demands being placed on him or her.

- Your child's difficulties are complicated, and may have come with the child. Maybe it is in their hard wiring – their brain anatomy and connections. Maybe it is in subtle temperament qualities; maybe it is compounded with traumatic experience. Maybe your style of parenting is perfect for one type of child but not such a "good fit" with this child's strong personality traits. Another significant factor is family stress, and family distress, including socioeconomic status.

- Whatever the combination of factors, there is no blame, rather there is assurance that your child can learn to be more flexible, and can learn problem-solving skills, and can get better at tolerating frustration.

- Recognize that, as Dr. Greene writes in the "Explosive Child," **"children do well if they can."**

- Your child longs for your approval, so provide it when your child does something positive.

- Because your child has some very real challenges with his or her "wiring" and temperament, possibly genetics and early developmental stress, it is very likely that your child has trouble with 1) flexibility, 2) frustration tolerance, and 3) problem solving (From The Explosive Child, by Ross W. Greene, 2010), just as other children lag behind in acquiring academic or athletic skills.

- Some of the skills that children similar to yours (with problem behaviors) have trouble with include:**

    Difficulty handling transitions – shifting from one mind-set task to another

    Difficulty reflecting on multiple thoughts or ideas simultaneously (disorganized)

    Difficulty considering a range of solutions to a problem

    Difficulty considering the likely outcomes or consequences of actions (impulsive)

    Difficulty expressing concerns, needs, or thoughts in words

    Difficulty managing emotional response to frustration in order to think rationally

    Chronic irritability and/or anxiety, which significantly impede capacity for problem solving

- One of the biggest favors you can do for an explosive child is to identify the lagging skills that are setting the stage for his challenging behavior so that you and others understand what is getting in his way. Also, identify what problems may be causing explosive episodes and what helps to calm your child down. You and the teacher can keep a journal of these observations.

- Build in some extra minutes for the child to comply with your request. Your child may have trouble "switching gears" and moving to the new activity. Don't add time for their time-out for every minute they stall on the way. That is the way they are wired -- they are slower to process a change in activity.

- Take a break or time-out if you are about to make the conflict with your child worse. This is good modeling for the child for using self-control strategies.

- The best parenting style is a warm and involved guiding approach – providing discipline. Being consistent and firm, yet loving, is the best approach.

- Build on the positives of your individual child (an example would be the COPE exercise in the Child Handout – where you and your child list three positive things particular to your child, and you display those prominently and bring those up regularly and add to them).

- Dr. Greene writes, "Good parenting means being responsive to the hand you were dealt."

- Your child likely had developmental "lags" or challenges in these areas:

  Difficulty seeing the "grays": concrete, literal, black and white thinking

  Difficulty deviating from rules or routine

  Difficulty handling unpredictability, ambiguity, uncertainty, or novelty

  Difficulty shifting from original idea or solution

  Difficulty taking into account situational factors that would suggest the need to adjust a plan

- Pick your battles. Prioritize the tasks you want the child to do, or habits you want to develop.

- Avoid power struggles. The child with ODD has trouble avoiding power struggles so you may have to go the "extra mile" to avoid getting into the battle of wills.

- Set up reasonable, age-appropriate limits with consequences that can be enforced consistently. Review these with an expert you trust, such as your pediatrician or nurse practitioner. Once these are set, feel confident they are what are best for the child, and stick consistently with your limits and consequences.

- All "adults" that are authorities in your child's life should also know your rules and also consistently enforce them. If the other parent disagrees, then there must be a plan made that all of the important adults in that child's life can consistently enforce.

- Your child has difficulty sorting out what to do if rules are not black and white.

  Because of this difficulty – the adults caring for and parenting this child will have to be SUPER CONSISTENT in consistently enforcing the rules.

- Sticking to your expectations is very important. If you eventually give up your resolve and give in, the child will learn to persist until you give in.

- Remember that the problem behaviors may escalate, get worse at first, as the child "tests" the new parenting approaches.

- Parents will need to make special efforts to care for themselves. The strong-willed, explosive child consumes so much of the parent's time and energy; it is easy to become exhausted physically and mentally. Maintain interests other than your child and ODD.

- Parents can seek out support from other parents who are raising challenging children. When you receive regular calls from the school or child care setting with complaints about your child's behavior, you need sounding boards. You need people around you who support your heroic efforts in parenting this child.

- Remember, much of the intense effort you are putting into your child is directly focused on making sure that other people will want to be around them. You have a good parenting goal.

- Please know that your healthcare provider knows and applauds how much time and energy you are investing – to make the tiny steps that seem undetectable but, in fact, are the necessary steps for your child's march toward success.

The *Explosive Child* book by Dr. Greene promotes a collaborative problem-solving approach. That approach has been incorporated into this resource page for parents. There is an excellent Website for you to check out this approach to see if it fits with your family values/preferences.

Resources

Fact Sheet: Children with Oppositional Defiant Disorder
http://www.aacap.org/cs/root/facts_for_families/children_with_odd

Lives in the Balance: a nonprofit organization to advocate on behalf of behaviorally challenging children and their parents, teachers, and caregivers. Free Web-based resources are available at http://www.livesinthebalance.org/.

The research evidence to support "collaborative problem solving "can be found on this Website: http://www.explosivechild.com

Handouts for Children to Help Them Cope and Behave in Positive Ways

Your doctor/nurse practitioner, parents/guardians, and you are all on the same team, helping you to deal with things that you find hard to do. As a team, we want to help you deal with things and behaviors at home and school that tend to get you in trouble. We are on your side. The other team is the problem behaviors. We know what behaviors will help you to be accepted by others at school and other places you go, and we are going to work with you so that you can learn behaviors that are positive. We may have to all take tiny steps, but with one step at a time, we will get there to watch you succeed.

Here are two handouts that will help you to feel more positive about yourself and deal with things that you find hard. It is a good idea to work on these with your parents, teacher, doctor, or nurse practitioner.

Positive Things about Me

(From: *COPE For Children* by Bernadette Melnyk, ©)

Positive self-talk helps you to fill your mind with positive thoughts. Thinking positive thoughts will help you to feel better and behave in positive ways.

Here are some examples:

- **I am a good friend.**

- **I am really good with my dog.**

- **I am good at running.**

- **I really like to go to the park with my family.**

- **I can keep in control of my anger when my little brother bothers me.**

Let's write out your own positive self-talk statements.

List 3 positive things about you.

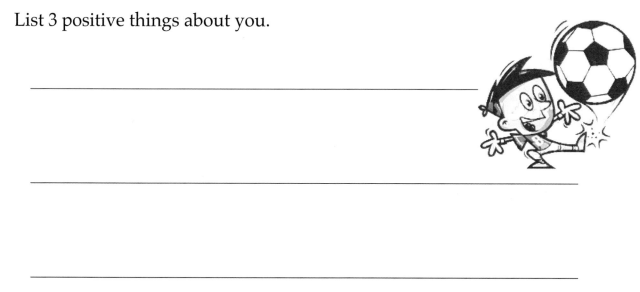

Place this paper where you can see it, and say these positive things about you out loud at least 10 times every morning and every night. Keep adding to the list as you and your parents notice more positive things about you.

Strong Feelings – Anger, Hurt, Fear, Sadness

(From: *COPE For Children* by Bernadette Melnyk, ©)

Children, like adults, have times when they feel hurt, sad, fear or anger. These are all normal feelings. All people feel angry, sad or afraid sometimes.

These can be very strong feelings, but we can control how we COPE with these feelings in positive ways.

Our bodies might signal strong feelings by:

A hot face

Tense muscles

A fast heartbeat

Fast or loud breathing,

Feeling like exploding with my hands, feet or mouth

Sweating

Restlessness (feeling like you have to keep moving)

Headaches

Stomachaches

Trouble thinking clearly

Sometimes when young people feel afraid or hurt, or sad or angry, they act in unhealthy ways that might hurt them or others.

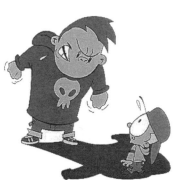

- Fighting with parents or friends
- Hitting, kicking, screaming, or using mean words
- Getting bad grades or not doing homework
- Tearing up things, or hitting walls
- Not showering or taking care of your body
- Staying alone in your room too much

Name things you do when you have strong feelings (Fear, sadness or anger).

_____

_____

Taking Control of your Anger (Strong Feelings)

(From: *COPE For Children* by Bernadette Melnyk, ©)

Let's list some positive things you can do when you are feeling angry, sad or afraid, that don't hurt you and don't hurt other people.

Here are some ways children COPE and take control of their strong feelings in a positive way

- Talking about how you feel
- Exercise/playing outside
- Going to family or friends for help
- Counting to 10 or saying the ABCs
- Walking away and deep breathing
- Thinking of a time when you did something great
- Writing your thoughts and feelings down
- Using positive self-talk (saying your positive self-statements)
- Doing something that you enjoy (like reading or drawing)

Which of these do you do?

_____

_____

Which sound like new ideas you can practice doing to deal with your feelings in positive ways?

_____

_____

Draw a picture of a time when you had strong feelings – were sad hurt, afraid or angry.

You can decide to make healthy choices about your feelings—it is under your control. At first, it may be hard to make good choices. But, with practice, it will get easier over time. (It will feel good to be in control!)

Let's write down a plan. When I feel angry, sad or afraid,

I will:

_____

_____

_____

I can talk to:

_____

_____

_____

(Adapted with permission from COPE for Children by Bernadette Melnyk, ©)
For the entire COPE for Children Program, contact cope.melnyk@gmail.com)

Some books that you might like to read

Cook, J. (2011) *I Just Don't Like the Sound of No! My Story about Accepting No for an Answer and Disagreeing the Right Way! (Best Me I Can Be)* Boys Town, NE: Boys Town Press.

Meiners, C. (2010) *Cool Down and Work Through Anger: Learning to Get Along.*
Minneapolis, MN: Free Spirit Publishing.

REFERENCES

American Academy of Child and Adolescent Psychiatry: Facts for Families - *www.aacap.org/cs/root/facts_for_families/facts_for_families* and *www.aacap.org/cs/root/facts_for_families/children_with_odd*

American Academy of Child and Adolescent Psychiatry. (2007). Practice Parameters for the Assessment and Treatment of Children and Adolescents with Oppositional Defiant Disorder. *Journal of the American Academy of Child & Adolescent Psychiatry*, 46(1), 107-125.

Cepeda, C. (2010) Clinical Manual for the Psychiatric Interview of Children and Adolescents, Arlington, VA: American Psychiatric Publishing, Inc.

Child and Adolescent Mental Health Division. (2007). 2007 Biennial Report: Effective psychosocial interventions for youth with behavioral and emotional needs. Retrieved from *http://oregon.gov/DHS/mental health/ebp/reports/biennial07effective-hawaii.pdf*

Greene, R. W. (2010). The Explosive Child: A new approach for understanding and parenting easily frustrated, "chronically inflexible" children (Revised 4th edition). New York, NY: HarperCollins.

Knapp, P., Chait, A., Pappadopulos, S., Crystal, S., Jensen, P., &T-May Steering Group. (2012). Treatment of maladaptive aggression in youth: CERT guidelines. Pediatrics. 129(6), e1562.

Melnyk, B.M. (2003) COPE – Creating Opportunities for Personal Empowerment for children, adolescents and young adults. Powell, Ohio: COPE2Thrive.

The Reach Institute *www.thereachinstitute.org/*

T-May *(Treatment of Maladaptive Aggression in Youth) Rutgers CERTs Pocket Reference Guide for Primary Care Clinicians and Mental Health Specialists. (2010)* Center for Education and Research on Mental Health Therapeutics (CERTs) Rutgers University , The REACH Institute, University Texas at Austin College of Pharmacy, New York State Office of Mental Health, California Department of Mental Health).

Yearwood, E., Pearson, G., & Newland, J. (2012). Child and Adolescent Behavioral Health: A Resource for Advanced Practice Psychiatric and Primary Care Practitioners in Nursing, West Sussex, And UK: John Wiley & Sons, Inc.

SECTION 8
Richard Kreipe

Eating Disorders

Fast Facts

- Currently, more than 10 million people are afflicted with eating disorders and, of those, 87% are children and teens under the age of 20 years.

- Approximately 7% of adolescent males and 13% of adolescent females struggle with eating disorders.

- Eating disorders tend to occur in early to mid-adolescence, ranging from 13 years to 18 years of age, in response to body image disturbance; however, they are now occurring in younger children. Overindulgent eating patterns emerge earlier as well.

- Correlates of eating disorders include overweight status, low self-esteem, anxiety, depression, suicidal ideation, obsessive-compulsive traits, and substance use.

Disordered Eating Patterns Include

- Anorexia nervosa

- Bulimia nervosa

- Binge/compulsive eating disorder

- Eating disorder not specified

- Antecedents of bulimia nervosa and anorexia nervosa include perfectionism, conflict avoidance, and negative self-evaluation.

Bulimia Nervosa has been found to be influenced by

- Parental obesity

- Childhood obesity

- Critical comments by family (especially by males) about body shape, weight, or eating

- Early menarche

- Parental psychiatric disorder

- Certain parental problems (e.g., low contact and high expectations, and alcohol use)

Screening Questions for Eating Disorders

Questions for Parents

- Are you concerned about your child's weight?
- Does your son or daughter make negative comments about his or her weight or shape?

Questions for Children and Teens

- Are you concerned about your weight or shape?
- Do you eat breakfast every day?

Guidelines for Adolescent Preventative Services (GAPS) (AMA, 1994) (contained in Section 1).

Questions for the Younger Adolescent

- Do you spend a lot of time thinking about ways to be skinny or lose weight?
- Do you do things to lose weight (e.g., skip meals, take pills, starve yourself, or vomit)?
- Do you work, play, or exercise to make yourself sweat or breathe hard at least 3 times a week?

Questions for the Middle to Older Adolescent

- Are you satisfied with your eating habits?
- Do you ever eat in secret?
- Do you spend a lot of time thinking about ways to be thin?
- In the past year, have you tried to lose weight or control your weight by vomiting, taking diet pills or laxatives, or starving yourself?
- Do you exercise or participate in sports activities that make you sweat and breathe hard for 20 minutes or more at a time at least 3 times during the week?

A Thorough Mental Health Evaluation Is Necessary

Teens with eating disorders often have comorbid mental health disorders (e.g., anxiety, depression) that also must be ruled out.

The Following Laboratory Tests Should Be Considered

- Serum electrolytes
- Renal function tests
- Complete blood count
- Liver function tests
- Electrocardiogram

DSM-5™ Diagnostic Criteria for Anorexia Nervosa

Diagnostic Features

There are three essential features of anorexia nervosa: persistent energy intake restriction; intense fear of gaining weight or of becoming fat, or persistent behavior that interferes with weight gain; and a disturbance in self-perceived weight or shape.

A. Restrictions of energy intake relative to requirements, leading to a significantly low body weight in the context of age, sex, developmental trajectory, and physical health. Significantly low weight is defined as a weight that is less than minimally normal or, for children and adolescents, less than that minimally expected.

B. Intense fear of gaining weight or of becoming fat, or persistent behavior that interferes with weight gain, even though at a significantly low weight.

C. Disturbance in the way in which one's body weight or shape is experienced, undue influence of body weight or shape on self-evaluation, or persistent lack of recognition of the seriousness of the current low body weight.

Coding note: The ICD-9-CM code for anorexia nervosa is 307.1, which is assigned regardless of the subtype. The ICD-10-CM code depends on the subtype (see below).

Specify whether:

(F50.01) Restricting type: During the last 3 months, the individual has not engaged in recurrent episodes of binge eating or purging behavior (i.e., self-induced vomiting or the misuse of laxatives, diuretics, or enemas). This subtype describes presentations in which weight loss is accomplished primarily through dieting, fasting, and/or excessive exercise.

(F50.02) Binge-eating/purging type: During the last 3 months, the individual has engaged in recurrent episodes of binge eating or purging behavior (i.e., self-induced vomiting or the misuse of laxatives, diuretics, or enemas).

Specify if:

In partial remission: After full criteria for anorexia nervosa were previously met, Criterion A (low body weight) has not been met for a sustained period, but either Criterion B (intense fear of gaining weight or becoming fat or behavior that interferes with weight gain) or Criterion C (disturbances in self-perception of weight and shape) is still met.

In full remission: After full criteria for anorexia nervosa were previously met, none of the criteria have been met for a sustained period of time.

Specify current severity:

The minimum level of severity is based, for adults, on current body mass index (BMI) (see below) or, for children and adolescents, on BMI percentile. The ranges below are derived from World Health Organization categories for thinness in adults; for children and adolescents, corresponding BMI percentiles should be used. The level of severity may be increased to reflect clinical symptoms, the degree of functional disability, and the need for supervision.

Mild: BMI ≥ 17 kg/m²
Moderate: BMI 16-16.99 kg/m²
Severe: BMI 15-15.99 kg/m²
Extreme: BMI ≤ 15 kg/m²

Prevalence: Rates of 0.5 to 1% among females in late adolescence and early adulthood.

Course: The mean age of onset for anorexia nervosa is 16 years, with some suggesting bimodal peaks at ages 14 and 18 years. The onset is often associated with a stressful or traumatic life event, such transitioning to middle school, high school, or college, or having difficulty in peer relationships. The course and outcome are highly variable. Some individuals recover fully after a single episode, while others relapse and experience a chronic debilitating course of the illness over many years.

DSM-5™ Diagnostic Criteria for the Diagnosis of Bulimia Nervosa

Diagnostic Features

There are three essential features of bulimia nervosa: recurrent episodes of binge eating (Criterion A), recurrent inappropriate compensatory behaviors to prevent weight gain (Criterion B), and self-evaluation that is unduly influenced by body shape and weight (Criterion D). To qualify for the diagnosis, the binge eating and inappropriate compensatory behaviors must occur, on average, at least once per week for 3 months (Criterion C). An "episode of binge eating" is defined as eating, in a discrete period of time, an amount of food that is definitely larger than most individuals would eat in a similar period of time under similar circumstances.

A. Recurrent episodes of binge eating. An episode of binge eating is characterized by both of the following:

1. Eating, in a discrete period of time (e.g., within any 2-hour period), an amount of food that is definitely larger than what most individuals would eat in a similar period of time under similar circumstances.

2. A sense of lack of control over eating during the episode (e.g., a feeling that one cannot stop eating or control what or how much one is eating).

B. Recurrent inappropriate compensatory behaviors in order to prevent weight gain, such as self-induced vomiting; misuse of laxatives, diuretics, or other medications; fasting; or excessive exercise.

C. The binge eating and inappropriate compensatory behaviors both occur, on average, at least once a week for 3 months.

D. Self-evaluation is unduly influenced by body shape and weight.

E. The disturbance does not occur exclusively during episodes of anorexia nervosa.

Specify if:

In partial remission: After full criteria for bulimia nervosa were previously met, some, but not all, of the criteria have been met for a sustained period of time.

In full remission: After full criteria for bulimia nervosa were previously met, none of the criteria have been met for a sustained period of time.

Specify current severity:

The minimum level of severity is based on the frequency of inappropriate compensatory behaviors (see below). The level of severity may be increased to reflect other symptoms and the degree of functional disability.

Mild: An average of 1-3 episodes of inappropriate compensatory behaviors per week.

Moderate: An average of 4-7 episodes of inappropriate compensatory behaviors per week.

Severe: An average of 8-13 episodes of inappropriate compensatory behaviors per week.

Extreme: An average of 14 or more episodes of inappropriate compensatory behaviors per week.

Prevalence: Approximately 1 to 5% among adolescent and young adult females. Approximately 1 male for every 10 females experiences from bulimia nervosa.

Course: Bulimia nervosa usually begins in adolescence or young adulthood. The binge-eating frequently begins during or after an episode of dieting. Disturbed eating behavior persists for at least several years in a high percentage of clinic samples. The long-term outcome is variable, often associated with substance abuse and personality disorder traits. The mortality rate is higher than that of anorexia nervosa, due to an increased suicide risk.

Reprinted with permission from the Diagnostic and Statistical Manual of Mental Disorders, Fifth Edition, (Copyright ©2013). American Psychiatric Association. All Rights Reserved.

Management of Anorexia Nervosa

- Treatment for anorexia nervosa requires the reestablishment of nutritional intake to restore physical health upon which mental health treatment can succeed.

- Parents have a central role in family-based treatment models, which have been shown to be the most effective in resulting in recovery from anorexia nervosa.

- Medications, such as antidepressants or anti-anxiety medications, may be used along with intensive counseling, but food remains the most important "medicine' in the initial phase of treatment.

- Nutritional counseling by a trained specialist is often helpful.

- Adolescents with anorexia nervosa who have fasted for long periods often will not be able to eat normal amounts of food and will need to begin eating small amounts of food more often.

- Some patients with anorexia nervosa will require hospitalization if their weight loss is so extreme that health is poor (e.g., if heart rate or blood pressure becomes too low), or the pattern of inadequate nutritional intake cannot be interrupted in intensive outpatient therapy.

Management of Bulimia Nervosa

- Restoring nutritional balance and maintaining structured nutritional intake is central to the success of counseling by a trained mental health provider/counselor.

- Counseling is often directed toward the person's distorted self-image, uncontrollable and excessive eating, profound guilt, and embarrassment.

- Treatment usually includes the use of antidepressants (especially selective serotonin reuptake inhibitors) and/or other medications to help the obsessive thinking and uncontrollable compulsive behaviors.

- Occasionally, some adolescents need to be admitted to the hospital if their fluid loss is extreme and/or health is threatened (e.g., if heart rate becomes too irregular or if blood pressure becomes too low).

- Sometimes intermediately intensive partial hospitalization programs are required to interrupt the harmful dieting-binge eating-purging cycle that affects individuals.

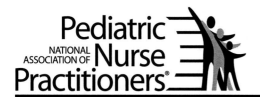

What Is Anorexia Nervosa?

Anorexia nervosa is the most common eating disorder among girls entering puberty, although there is an increasing trend of adolescent boys developing this disorder; it is more common among younger than older boys, but only about 50% of patients are males. Anorexia nervosa is an eating disorder that makes eating very distressing. People who struggle with this disorder become very anxious or obsessed with maintaining or reducing their body weight through rigid control and restriction of their caloric intake, and/or intensive exercise. These people have intense drive to lose weight and feel that their self-worth is directly affected by their body weight or shape.

What Are Common Signs and Symptoms of Anorexia Nervosa?

- Weight loss
- Food rituals
- Frequent weighing
- Loss of menstrual periods
- Feeling cold much of the time

- Dietary restriction
- Avoiding public eating
- Excessive focus on exercise or dieting
- Hair loss or growth of baby-fine hair on face or body

How Can Anorexia Nervosa Affect Someone's Health?

It can cause:

- Low blood pressure
- An inability to concentrate
- Irritability
- Loss of menstrual periods/sterility
- Brittle bones

- Low heart rate
- Fatigue/muscle weakness
- Constipation
- Dehydration
- Kidney damage

What Causes Anorexia Nervosa?

Eating disorders have been called "brain circuit disorders" because there is emerging evidence that the way in which the brains of affected individuals respond to food, eating and body image is different, so that what is positive for most people is either threatening or overly rewarding for those with an eating disorder. Previously held beliefs that parents cause eating disorders have been definitively debunked. Eating disorders occur when several biological, psychological and social factors interact in a vulnerable individual. For many individuals, simple dieting may be the trigger to weight control becoming out-of-control. For those with anorexia nervosa, the desire to be thinner and to restrict their eating habits is constantly on their mind. Anorexia literally means to lose one's appetite; however, people with anorexia nervosa do not truly lose their appetite. Instead, the fear of weight gain causes them to go on strict diets that may result in the inability to eat normally. People who struggle with anorexia nervosa feel driven to lose weight, and their desire to control their weight is tied to their self-worth. They often feel that eating is a sign of a lack of self-control.

Some people who develop anorexia nervosa may have emotional needs that are not being met in their lives. They may have difficulty in social relationships or have problems making friends. The development of anorexia nervosa is sometimes a physical way for adolescents to deal with overwhelming and emotional issues that can occur during the transition to adulthood. Still others develop anorexia nervosa in the face of puberty and the emergence of emotional tensions with family or peers. This may be related to concerns about their own normal body changes that occur with puberty, or an unpleasant social experience.

It is very common for teens with anorexia nervosa to be high achievers and perfectionists; however, they feel that they are underachievers. Frequently, people with anorexia nervosa set unrealistically high standards for themselves that are impossible to achieve or sustain. As a result, they are left with feelings of failure and inadequacy.

What Are the Treatments for Anorexia Nervosa?

Treatment for anorexia nervosa requires the restoration of nutritional intake to establish physical health upon which mental health treatment can succeed. Parents have a central role in family-based treatment models, which have been shown to be the most effective in resulting in recovery from anorexia nervosa. Medications, such as antidepressants or anti-anxiety medications, may be used along with intensive counseling, but food remains the most important "medicine' in the initial phase of treatment. Nutritional counseling by a trained specialist is often helpful. Adolescents with anorexia nervosa who have fasted for long periods often will not be able to eat normal amounts of food and will need to begin eating small amounts of food more often. The digestive tract of someone who has dieted extremely may have difficulty digesting certain foods until their system becomes used to eating more food. Some patients with anorexia nervosa require hospital admission if their weight loss is so extreme that the person's health is poor (e.g., if their heart rate or blood pressure becomes too low), or the pattern of inadequate nutritional intake cannot be interrupted in intensive outpatient therapy.

What Can You Do If You Think You Have Anorexia Nervosa?

If you believe that you may have anorexia nervosa, you should seek professional help from your doctor or nurse practitioner right away. The longer that you have fixed patterns and attitudes toward eating, the more difficult it will be to begin to change those habits. It may feel very upsetting and scary for you to think of changing these habits.

Specialists will be able to offer you many suggestions, even if you are uncertain you would like to change things. Below are some suggestions that other people have said have been helpful to them:

- Find ways to pamper yourself that have nothing to do with food (perhaps something that you used to enjoy).

- Put your energy into different channels. Find activities that you are good at or that give you satisfaction, or do something to make someone else happy.

- Try to do what you want to do, not just what other people want you to do (or what you think other people would like you to do), at least some of the time.

- Focus on finding ways to like yourself that do not involve a "target weight" or anything to do with eating.

- Believe that you can overcome this problem and get the help you need to do it NOW!

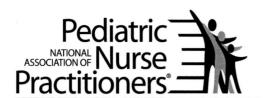

What Is Bulimia Nervosa?

Bulimia nervosa is an eating disorder that commonly occurs in adolescent girls and rarely occurs in males. It is defined by episodes of "binge" eating or eating large quantities of food in a short time. This behavior may be severe with very large quantities of food being eaten, often containing carbohydrates or fat. People who struggle with bulimia try to prevent weight gain that would normally occur after bingeing by following the binge-eating with periods of food restriction, vomiting, laxative abuse, and/or excessive exercising (otherwise known as "purging"). In severe cases, when vomiting is used, the binge episodes may become more common with the cycles repeating over several hours. Without treatment, the severity of this eating disorder increases and the teen's life becomes more chaotic and focused on purging behavior. The drive to eat is so strong that the teen may steal food in order to satisfy his or her compulsion. Teens with this disorder are usually ashamed of their behavior, so they often keep their bingeing secret because of the guilt associated with eating and weight control.

Who Has Bulimia Nervosa?

Many people don't know when a family member or friend has bulimia because the binge-eating and purging (ridding the body of calories by laxative use, vomiting, or excessive exercise) occurs in private and there may not be noticeable weight loss or weight gain.

What Are Common Signs or Symptoms of Bulimia Nervosa?

- Dental cavities
- Enlarged parotid glands, which are by the back portion of the face below the jaws
- Puffy cheeks
- Uncontrollable gastro-esophageal reflux
- Abdominal pain and bloating
- Constipation
- Secret eating or large amounts of food disappearing
- Excessive exercise
- Preoccupation with food
- Going to the bathroom directly following meals
- Using laxatives and vomiting to control weight
- Intestinal problems from frequent laxative use
- Kidney problems from use of "water" pills (diuretics)
- Irregular heartbeat
- Muscle weakness or fatigue

What Causes Bulimia Nervosa?

Eating disorders have been called "brain circuit disorders" because there is emerging evidence that the way in which the brains of affected individuals respond to food, eating and body image is different, so that what is positive for most people is either threatening or overly rewarding for those with an eating disorder. Worry, stress, or feeling angry, lonely or abandoned are common triggers to binge eating. Dieting and missing meals as a form of weight control may trigger food cravings and overeating. Sometimes bulimia can develop as a complication of some emotional trauma or upsetting event, such as family breakdown, death of a friend or relative, or abuse. Other risk factors for the development of bulimia include poor self-esteem, extreme anxiety, and a highly sensitive nature, or a family history of substance abuse.

What Are the Treatments for Bulimia Nervosa?

As with anorexia nervosa, restoring nutritional balance and maintaining structured nutritional intake is central to the success of counseling by a trained mental health provider/counselor is one of the primary treatments used for people with this disorder. This therapy should help the person to understand the complex emotions that trigger bingeing and purging behaviors. The counseling is often directed toward the person's distorted self-image, uncontrollable and excessive eating, profound guilt, and embarrassment. Treatment usually includes the use of antidepressants (especially selective serotonin reuptake inhibitors) and/or other medications to help the obsessive thinking and uncontrollable compulsive behaviors. Occasionally, some teens need to be admitted to the hospital if their fluid loss is extreme and/or health is threatened (e.g., if heart rate becomes too irregular or if blood pressure becomes too low). Sometimes intermediately intensive partial hospitalization programs are required to interrupt the harmful dieting-binge eating-purging cycle that can trap individuals.

What Can I Do to Help?

- Strongly suggest that the teen get help
- Be positive and supportive
- Be empathetic to the teen's feelings
- Go to a support group
- Don't blame the teen
- Give written information that encourages the teen to get help early

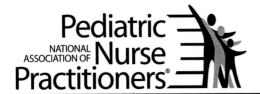

Information about Bulimia Nervosa for Teens

What Is Bulimia Nervosa?

Bulimia nervosa is an eating disorder that most commonly occurs in adolescent girls, but can occur in males. It is defined by episodes of "binge" eating or eating large quantities of food in a short time. This behavior may be severe with very large amounts of food being consumed, often containing carbohydrates and fat. Teens who struggle with bulimia try to prevent weight gain that would normally occur after binge-eating by not eating for a period of time, vomiting, using laxatives and/or excessive exercising (otherwise known as "purging"). In severe cases when vomiting is used, the bingeing may become more frequent. Without treatment, this disorder can become severe. The drive to eat can become so strong that people with this disorder may even steal food to satisfy their compulsive eating. Teens are often ashamed of their behavior, so they often binge in secret.

Who Has Bulimia Nervosa?

Many people don't know when a family member or friend has bulimia because the binge-eating and purging (ridding the body of calories by laxative use, vomiting, or excessive exercise) often occurs in private, and there may not be visible weight loss or weight gain.

What Are Common Signs or Symptoms of Bulimia Nervosa?

- Dental cavities
- Enlarged parotid glands, which are in the back portion of the face, below the jaws
- Puffy cheeks
- Uncontrollable stomach acid that comes up in the throat
- Abdominal pain and bloating
- Constipation
- Secret eating or large amounts of food inexplicably disappearing
- Excessive exercise
- Preoccupation with food
- Going to the bathroom directly following meals
- Using laxatives and vomiting to control weight
- Intestinal problems from frequent laxative use
- Kidney problems from use of "water" pills (diuretics)
- Irregular heartbeat
- Muscle weakness or fatigue

What Causes Bulimia Nervosa?

Eating disorders are caused by many things, but a common feature of bulimia is changes in the reward system of the brain, which drives much of the behaviors. Worry, stress, or feeling angry or lonely may trigger binge eating. Dieting and missing meals as a form of weight control may also trigger food cravings and overeating. Sometimes bulimia can develop after an emotional trauma or upsetting event (e.g., family breakdown, death of a friend or relative, abuse). Other risk factors for the development of bulimia include poor self-esteem, extreme anxiety, and a highly sensitive nature (anxious).

What Are the Treatments for Bulimia Nervosa?

Counseling by a trained mental healthcare provider/counselor is one of the primary treatments used for teens with this disorder. But effective therapy requires a well-nourished body and brain, meaning that focusing on eating and weight control patterns is also important. This therapy should help these teens to understand the complex emotions that trigger these bingeing and purging behaviors. Counseling is often directed toward the teen's distorted self-image as well as the excessive eating and guilt. Treatment often includes the use of antidepressants and/or other medications to help the obsessive thinking and compulsive behaviors. Some teens need to be admitted to a partial hospital program to break the cycle of binge eating and purging while receiving intensive mental health treatment, or to the hospital if their fluid loss is extreme and/or their health is threatened (e.g., if the heart rate becomes too irregular or if their blood pressure becomes too low).

What Can I Do?

If you think that you or a friend has this eating disorder, talk to your doctor/nurse practitioner, parent, or trusted adult about it right away. The earlier that treatment is started, the better. You won't be helping yourself or your friend by keeping it a secret.

Internet Resources

Academy for Eating Disorders
www.aedweb.org//AM/Template.cfm?Section=Home

A global professional association committed to leadership in eating disorders research, education, treatment and prevention. This Website contains a lot of practical information for both professionals and the lay public.

American Academy of Child and Adolescent Psychiatry
www.aacap.org

This Website is an excellent source of information on the assessment and treatment of child and adolescent mental health disorders. Handouts for use with families (*i.e., Facts for Families*) are available on a multitude of problems, including eating disorders.

American Academy of Pediatrics
www.aap.org

This Website contains information for both healthcare providers and parents, including excellent clinical practice guidelines and handouts.

Bright Futures in Practice: for Nutrition, Physical Activity, and Mental Health
www.brightfutures.org

This Website contains outstanding materials for healthcare professionals on a variety of topics that can be easily implemented in practice.

Centers for Disease Control and Prevention
www.cdc.gov

The CDC Website contains outstanding materials for healthcare professionals and the public on a variety of topics, including the latest information on overweight and obesity.

National Eating Disorders Association (NEDA)
www.nationaleatingdisorders.org/

NEDA is the largest not-for-profit organization in the United States that works to prevent eating disorders and provide treatment referrals to those suffering from anorexia, bulimia, and binge-eating disorder and to those concerned with body image and weight issues. NEDA is dedicated to expanding public understanding of eating disorders and promoting access to quality treatment for those affected along with support for their families through education, advocacy, and research. The organization develops prevention programs for a wide range of audiences, publishes and distributes educational materials, and operates the nation's first toll-free eating disorders information and referral helpline.

REFERENCES

American Psychiatric Association. (2013). *Diagnostic and Statistical Manual of Mental Disorders, Fifth Edition* (DSM-5). Washington, DC: APA.

Kaye, D.L., Montgomery, M.E., & Munson, S. (2002). *Child and Adolescent Mental Health.* Philadelphia, PA: Lippincott.

Jellinek, M., Patel, B.P., & Froehle, M. (2002). *Bright Futures in Practice: Mental Health- Vol I. Practice Guide.* Arlington, VA: National Center for Education in Maternal and Child Health.

Jellinek, M., Patel, B.P., & Froehle, M. (2002). *Bright Futures in Practice: Mental Health- Vol II. Tool Kit.* Arlington, VA: National Center for Education in Maternal and Child Health.

Melnyk, B.M., Brown, H., Jones, D.C., Kreipe, R., & Novak, J. (2003). Improving the mental/psychosocial health of U.S. children and adolescents. Outcomes and implementation strategies from the national KySS summit. *Journal of Pediatric Healthcare*, 17(6 Suppl 1), S1- S24.

SECTION 9
Deborah A. Napolitano and Holly E. Brown

Autism and Pervasive Developmental Disorders

Autism Spectrum Disorder

Fast Facts

- The diagnostic category of Autism Spectrum Disorder (ASD) refers to a group of symptoms characterized by delays in the development of socialization and communication skills.

- Parents may note symptoms as early as infancy, although the typical age of onset is before 3 years of age.

- Symptoms may include problems with using and understanding language; difficulty relating to people, objects, and events; unusual play with toys and other objects; difficulty with changes in routine or familiar surroundings, and repetitive body movements or behavior patterns.

- Prior to the publication of the DSM-5™, Autism was one of several categories under the Pervasive Developmental Disorder (PDD) "umbrella." Autism (a developmental brain disorder) characterized by impaired social interaction and communication skills, and a limited range of activities and interests) was the most characteristic and best studied of the three. Other types of ASD include Asperger's Syndrome, Pervasive Developmental Disorder – Not Otherwise Specified, Childhood Disintegrative Disorder, and Rett's Syndrome. Children with ASD vary widely in abilities, intelligence, and behaviors.

- The new diagnostic criteria support and allow for some characterization of these associated symptoms (e.g., ASD with or without accompanying intellectual impairment).

- Some children do not speak at all, others speak in limited phrases or conversations, and some have relatively normal language development. Repetitive play skills and limited social skills are generally evident.

- Unusual responses to sensory information, such as loud noises and lights, are also common.

- Information about autism has become readily available in mainstream and social media, making it easily accessible to the general population. This has the impact of raising parent anxiety about whether their child might have an ASD. It is quite common for parents and parents-to-be to ask the question, "Does (or will) my child have autism?"

- Primary care providers play an integral role in screening for an ASD and, therefore, are the first line of defense in detecting symptoms associated with ASDs.

- The earlier an accurate diagnosis can be made, the earlier treatment can begin.

- The PCP is often the medical professional most trusted by the parents. Their opinion and information may be held with a great deal of trust and respect, so it is incumbent upon those individuals to have accurate and sufficient information to help guide the parents towards the next steps on what will likely be a life-long journey. Therefore, questions being asked by parents are important and are not to be dismissed or overlooked by PCPs. That said, this is a topic that also can strike fear in a parent who has begun to imagine their child's future almost as soon as they know they will be parents. This is a sensitive topic and should be carefully addressed with accurate and reliable information about autism.

- Even more importantly, it is critical to also provide families with anticipatory guidance about what to expect in terms of further evaluation, treatment, and resources once an autism diagnosis is suspected.

- Information about ASD has become quite easy to obtain. Unfortunately, for many reasons, there is a great deal of information out there that would not meet a best practice or "evidence-based litmus test." Controversies abound and are often promulgated by parents trying to find the next best treatment, practitioners who think they have hit upon the next best thing, or in some cases people who are looking to make a lot of money.

- The best place to quickly find information is the Internet. Unfortunately, it is also the best place to quickly find misinformation or become connected to groups who promote treatments that may sound great, but are ineffective at best and harmful at worst.

Some Key Points to Consider:

- ASD is a neurodevelopmental disorder.

- The prevalence of Autism Spectrum Disorder (ASD), including the previous diagnostic categories of Pervasive-Developmental Disorders-NOS and Asperger's disorder, is currently reported as 1:88 children (CDC).

- ASD is 5 times more common among boys (1:54) than among girls (1:252) (CDC).

- The etiology of ASD is not well understood but there is clearly a genetic link as evidenced by occurrence among siblings, and the research is increasingly demonstrating gene-related mutations and structural variations (Abrahams & Geschwind, 2008; Ronald and Hoekstra, 2011).

Descriptions of the disorders and categories previously diagnosed under the PDD "umbrella" are based on descriptions provided by Healthy Children.org: http://www.healthychildren.org/English/health-issues/conditions/developmental-disabilities/Pages/Asperger-Syndrome.aspx.

Autistic Disorder

Autistic disorder is characterized by language and communication problems, problems with social relationships, and repetitive or rigid behaviors. Children with an ASD may have intellectual disabilities or challenges that make testing intelligence and development difficult. Others with an ASD may score well on standardized testing but struggle with abstract concepts, subtle social cues and concepts, and language variations (e.g., slang).

Pervasive Developmental Disorder-Not Otherwise Specified (PDD-NOS)

A diagnosis of PDD-NOS is given when a child meets some of the criteria for an ASD, but may not exhibit all of the symptoms or to the degree that would meet the criteria for ASD under the DSM-IV. Additionally, individuals with PDD-NOS may not be diagnosed until later. Some of the signs of PDD-NOS, similar to those of autistic disorder, include impaired social skills, difficulty with communication, and repetitive behavior or rigid thinking and behaving. Although symptoms for a child with PDD-NOS may be milder than for those with autism or Asperger syndrome, children with this diagnosis are faced with many of the same challenges.

Asperger Syndrome

Asperger syndrome is named for Hans Asperger. Traits observed in persons with Asperger are similar to those observed in persons with ASDs. These include social difficulties such as concerns in social situations, with social reciprocity, social skills and interactions (e.g., how to initiate a conversation), and difficulty with eye contact. Although individuals with Asperger do not have delayed language skills, they may struggle with understanding complexities of language such as humor, slang, or figures of speech. Other common features of persons with Asperger are repetitive motor movements, fixation or preoccupation with one topic or object, and the need for routine or sameness.

Typical language development -- and even early language development and/or reading skills -- is a primary difference between Asperger syndrome and other ASDs. Another difference is that individuals with Asperger syndrome do not have cognitive delays.

Associated Disorders

From the National Institute for Mental Health (NIMH) Parent Guide to Autism Spectrum Disorders (http://www.nimh.nih.gov/health/publications/a-parents-guide-to-autism-spectrum-disorder/what-are-the-symptoms-of-asd.shtml):

- Rett syndrome is a rare PDD/ASD that is characterized by a regression in development. Unlike other PDDs, Rett syndrome is almost exclusively seen in girls. Regression is typically seen between 6 and 18 months after typical development. Children who are suspected of having Rett syndrome or for whom regression was seen in skills at an early stage of development should be offered genetic testing (HealthyChild.org).

- Childhood disintegrative disorder (CDD) also is a rare (more rare than Rett syndrome) form of ASD. Onset typically occurs between the ages of 3 and 4 and also is characterized by regression in normal development of communication and social skills. CDD, unlike Rett syndrome, is most often seen in boys.

- Due to the rare nature of Rett syndrome and CDD, the focus of this section will be on the three primary PDD diagnostic categories of autistic disorder, PDD-NOS, and Asperger syndrome.

Screening for Autism

It is recommended by the American Academy of Pediatrics that screening for autism be conducted at regular intervals. The American Academy of Pediatrics (AAP) recommends that all children be screened for developmental delays and disabilities during regular well-child doctor visits at 9, 18, and 24-30 months with specific screenings for ASD at 18 and 24 months. Additional considerations for screening should occur if there are risk factors present for developmental problems (e.g., low birth weight or a sibling diagnosed with autism).

There are specific screening tools that may be used in addition to some critical history-taking questions. The questions include:

a. Does your child make eye contact?

b. Does your child look to you to share his or her toys and activities?

c. Does your child share his/her enjoyment with you?

d. Does your child point to things he or she wants to show you?

e. Does your child respond to his/her name or other attempts to get his/her attention?

f. Does your child repeat words or phrases over and over?

g. Does your child have any repetitive movements or behaviors that makes him/her different from other same-age children?

h. Does your child have very specific interests (e.g., lining up toys, schedules, pre-occupation with wheels on a car)?

You will want to collect a basic medical history as outlined in Table 9.1.

Table 9.1. Medical History

Birth History	Any known risk factors for ASD such as: a. Parental age b. Drug or alchohol use c. Method of pregnancy
Developmental History	Has the child developed typically and met his or her milestones (e.g., sitting and babbling at 6 months), beginning word use at 1 year, following two-step commands, or using two-to-three phrases by 24 months).
Behavioral or Medical History	May include sleep difficulties, gastrointestinal problems, intellectual disability, or neurological problems such as seizures.
Family History	Research has demonstrated that autism is a genetic, neurological disorder. This is due to the number of twims diganosed with the disorder and family members with associated dianoses. Some questions to consider asking are: a. Is there a twin or sibling with an autism diagnosis? b. Is there a family history of autism, intellectual disabilities, known syndromes (e.g., fragile X syndrome), metabolic disorders, or epilepsy? c. Do any family members appear socially awkward

Source: Adapted from Mazefsky, C. A., Filipink, R., Lindsey, J., & Lubetsky, M. (2011). Medical Evaluation and Comorbid Psychiatric Disorders. In Lubetsky, M. J., Handen, B. L., & McGonigle, J. J. (Eds.), Autism Spectrum Disorders: Pittsburgh Pocket Psychiatry New York, NY: Oxford Press, p. 44.

Medical Conditions With Neurologic Symptoms That Overlap With Those of ASD

McFadden, Minshew, and Scherf (2011) describe syndromes with specific genetic markers associated with syndromic ASD. These include Fragile X, tuberous sclerosis, Smith-Magenis syndrome, and Rett syndromes. These are often associated with higher rates of both dysmorphic features (e.g., intellectual disability) and chromosomal abnormalities. Up to 20% of persons with previously diagnosed ASD PDD may have one of these genetic markers or genetic lesions, making genetic testing an important recommendation for any child who receives a diagnosis on the autism spectrum.

Behavioral characteristics of all the associated syndromes are similar to those in non-syndromic ASD. Some key concerns with each syndrome include:

a. Fragile X. Individuals with Fragile X may have facial (e.g., protruding ears) and other physical differences (e.g., large hands). They also may have joint hyperextension, mitral valve prolapse, and 20% may have epilepsy (Mazefsky et al., 2011).

b. Tuberous Sclerosis Complex (TSC) is most often characterized by intellectual disabilities (ID) and benign tumors throughout the body (e.g., brain, heart, lungs, eyes). Additionally, up to 80% of individuals with TSC have a seizure disorder (Mazefsky et al., 2011).

c. Smith-Magenis syndrome. Individuals with Smith-Magenis often have intellectual disabilities. As with individuals with Fragile X, they also have some craniofacial abnormalities. These individuals may also have hearing loss and other sensory-related difficulties (e.g., ear infections, eye abnormalities) (Elsea & Girirajan, 2008).

DSM-5™ Diagnostic Criteria for Autism Spectrum Disorder

A. Persistent deficits in social communication and social interaction across multiple contexts as manifested by the following, currently or by history (examples are illustrative, not exhaustive; see text):

1. Deficits in social-emotional reciprocity, ranging, for example, from abnormal social approach and failure of normal back-and-forth conversation; to reduced sharing of interests, emotions, or affect; to failure to initiate or respond to social interactions.

2. Deficits in nonverbal communicative behaviors used for social interaction, ranging, for example, from poorly integrated verbal and nonverbal communication; to abnormalities in eye contact and body language or deficits in understanding and use of gestures; to a total lack of facial expressions and nonverbal communication.

3. Deficits in developing, maintaining, and understanding relationships, ranging, for example, from difficulties adjusting behavior to suit various social contexts; to difficulties in sharing imaginative play or in making friends; to absence of interest in peers.:

Specify current severity:

Severity is based on social communication impairments and restricted, repetitive patterns of behavior (see Table 2*).

B. Restricted, repetitive patterns of behavior, interests, or activities, as manifested by at least two of the following, currently or by history (examples are illustrative, not exhaustive, see text):

1. Stereotyped or repetitive motor movements, use of objects, or speech (e.g., simple motor stereotypes, lining up toys or flipping objects, echolalia, idiosyncratic phrases).

2. Insistence on sameness, inflexible adherence to routines, or ritualized patterns of verbal or nonverbal behavior (e.g., extreme distress at small changes, difficulties with transitions, rigid thinking patterns, greeting rituals, need to take same route or eat same food every day).

3. Highly restricted, fixated interests that are abnormal in intensity or focus (e.g., strong attachment to or preoccupation with unusual objects, excessively circumscribed or perseverative interests).

4. Hyper- or hyporeactivity to sensory input or unusual interest in sensory aspects of the environment (e.g., apparent indifference to pain/temperature, adverse response to specific sounds or textures, excessive smelling or touching of objects, visual fascination with lights or movement).

Specify current severity:

Severity is based on social communication impairments and restricted, repetitive patterns of behavior (see Table 2*).

C. Symptoms must be present in the early developmental period (but may not become fully manifest until social demands exceed limited capacities, or may be masked by learned strategies in later life).

D. Symptoms cause clinically significant impairment in social, occupational, or other important areas of current functioning.

E. These disturbances are not better explained by intellectual disability (intellectual developmental disorder) or global developmental delay. Intellectual disability and autism spectrum disorder frequently co-occur; to make comorbid diagnoses of autism spectrum disorder and intellectual disability, social communication should be below that expected for general developmental level.

Note: Individuals with a well-established DSM-IV diagnosis of autistic disorder, Asperger's disorder, or pervasive developmental disorder not otherwise specified should be given the diagnosis of autism spectrum disorder. Individuals who have marked deficits in social communication, but whose symptoms do not otherwise meet criteria for autism spectrum disorder, should be evaluated for social (pragmatic) communication disorder.

Specify if:

With or without accompanying intellectual impairment

With or without accompanying language impairment

Associated with a known medical or genetic condition or environmental factor (Coding note: Use additional code to identify the associated medical or genetic condition.)

Associated with another neurodevelopmental, mental, or behavioral disorder (Coding note: Use additional code[s] to identify the associated neurodevelopmental, mental, or behavioral disorder[s].)

With catatonia (refer to the criteria for catatonia associated with another mental disorder, pp.119-120, for definition) (**Coding note:** Use additional code 293.89 [F06.1] catatonia associated with autism spectrum disorder to indicate the presence of the comorbid catatonia.)

*See Table 2 on page 52 of the DSM-5™ for a description of severity levels: 3) requiring very substantial support; 2) requiring substantial support; and 1) requiring support.

Screening Tools for Autism

There are a variety of screening tools and checklists for the primary care professional to use in identifying whether further evaluation for an autism disorder (previously pervasive developmental disorder/PDD) is warranted. These tools have varying evidence of sensitivity and treatment validity (Livanis & Mouzakitis, 2010); however, they all provide some information that helps the front-line professional identify whether additional screening and evaluation are necessary. This is critical as early intervention is the key to an effective treatment plan. Samtani et al. (2011) provide a nice review of these tools. Below is a description of the most commonly used checklists, screening tools, and diagnostic instruments.

Table 9.2. Screening Tools for Autism

Name	Description	Ordering and Additional Information
Checklists		
Modified Checklist of Autism in Toddlers (M-CHAT™)	M-CHAT is a copyrighted instrument, and use of the M-CHAT must follow these guidelines. No modifications can be made to items or instructions without permission from the authors. The M-CHAT must be used in its entirety. Parties interested in reproducing the M-CHAT in print (e.g., a book or journal article) or electronically (e.g., as part of digital medical records or software packages to be distributed to others) must contact Diana Robins to request permission. There are many Websites where a practitioner or parent can go to download or take the M-CHAT.	http://www.autismspeaks.org/what-autism/diagnosis/screen-your-child http://www.firstsigns.org http://www2.gsu.edu/~wwwpsy/faculty/robins.htm
Screening for Autism in Two-Year Olds (STAT)	The STAT is an interactive measure designed for use with children aged 24-35 months. It is a screening tool to be administered by community providers who have experience with ASD. There are 12 activities in which early social and communication behaviors are observed.	http://kc.vanderbilt.edu/triad/training/page.aspx?id=821
Social Communication Questionnaire (SCQ; previously called Autism Screening Questionnaire [ASQ])	SCQ was developed by Michael Rutter, MD, FRS, Anthony Bailey, MD, and Catherine Lord, PhD. It is a brief instrument completed by a parent or primary caregiver. The SCQ evaluates communication skills and social functioning in children aged 4 years or older who may have autism or autism spectrum disorders. The SCQ is available in English and Spanish.	http://portal.wp-spublish.com/portal/page?_pageid=53,70432&_dad=portal&_schema=PORTAL
Communication and Symbolic Behavior Scales (CSBS)	The CSBS Developmental Profile Infant/Toddler Checklist is designed to measure the seven language predictors, including emotion/eye gaze, communication, gestures, sounds, words, understanding of words, and object use. It can be used as part of a routine developmental screening/well-child visit for children as young as 6 months, through 24 months. The CSBS is to be completed by a parent or other familiar caregiver.	http://firstwords.fsu.edu/pdf/Checklist_Scoring_Cutoffs.pdf http://products.brookespublishing.com/CSBS-DP-Manual-P273.aspx

Rating Scales		
Childhood Autism Rating Scale 2 (CARS2):	The CARS2 has been in use for many years. Based on direct observation, it yields a composite score to help differentiate autism from developmental disabilities. The tool can be used by clinicians, parents and teachers. The CARS2 includes a rating scale to identify individuals with high-functioning autism.	SAGE Publications. 2455 Teller Road, Thousand Oaks, CA 91320. Tel: 800-818-7243; Tel: 805-499-9774; Fax: 800-583-2665; e-mail: journals@sagepub.com. http://sagepub.com
Guilliam Autism Rating Scale-2 (GARS-2):	The GARS-2 is a norm-referenced instrument that assists teachers, parents, and clinicians in identifying and diagnosing autism in individuals ages 3 through 22. Items were developed based on the DSM-IV-TR.	http://www.proedinc.com/customer/ProductView.aspx?ID=3754&sSearchWord=gilliam
Diagnostic Assessments		
Autism Diagnostic Interview – Revised (ADI-R)	The ADI-R is a structured interview used for diagnosing autism, planning treatment, and distinguishing autism from other developmental disorders. To administer the ADI-R the clinician must be trained. Levels of training are determined by the purpose of the assessment (diagnosis or research).	Purchase: http://portal.wpspublish.com/portal/page?_pageid=53,70436&_dad=portal&_schema=PORTAL Training: http://www.cornellpsychiatry.org/education/adi-r.html
Autism Diagnostic Observation Schedule (ADOS) and Autism Diagnostic Observation Schedule 2 (ADOS-2)	The ADOS allows for accurate assessment and diagnosis of autism and PDD in toddlers, children, teens, and adults. This is a standardized observational measure that requires specific training to implement. The ADOS-2 offers revised algorithms and a new Comparison Score for Modules 1 through 3, a new Toddler Module, and updated protocols with clearer administration and coding guidelines for all modules.	ADOS: http://portal.wpspublish.com/portal/page?_pageid=53,288971&_dad=portal&_schema=PORTAL ADOS-2 : http://portal.wpspublish.com/portal/page?_pageid=53,288914&_dad=portal&_schema=PORTAL

Medical Conditions Associated With PDDs

Obsessive Compulsive Disorder (OCD) is the disorder most often associated with an ASD. This is due to an overlap in symptoms as well as a relationship between parents with OCD and children with an ASD. A diagnosis of OCD in an individual with an ASD can be difficult. Because of the overlap in symptoms (i.e., repetitive behaviors), it is very important to rule OCD out as the primary condition. In a study where children with ASD and children with OCD were compared, children diagnosed with ASD and those with OCD were reported to display similar levels of sameness behavior and repetitive movements. While both groups were reported to have more compulsions than a typical population, children with OCD were more likely than those with ASD to display compulsions. One important distinction between the groups may be in the types of routines, compulsions, and other repetitive-like behaviors displayed. Persons with OCD tended to display more sophisticated or complex sets of behaviors than those with ASD.

Additional Associated Conditions Include:

a. *Endocrine diseases*, such as hypothyroidism, tend to occur in individuals with PDDs more frequently than in a typically developing population. In the case of endocrine diseases, the estimated prevalence of two or more forms of autism was 0.7%, approximately 7 times greater than in the general population.

b. *Metabolic diseases*, such as homocysteinuria, have been associated with ASDs. This indicates that metabolic testing should be considered when clinical symptoms are present, such as lethargy, seizures, and dysmorphic features (Manzi et al., 2008).

Comorbidities Important for Consideration When Assessing PDDs

There are many physical and psychiatric symptoms associated with PDDs that may in fact be symptoms of other disabilities or disorders. In all cases it is important to determine the primary presenting problems in assessing for an ASD, a disorder or disability with similar features, or co-occurring disorders and disabilities. Some that may warrant particular attention (and some which have been taken into consideration in the recent edition of the DSM-5 include:

a. Intellectual disabilities

b. Learning disabilities

c. Development language disorders

d. Developmental delay

e. Reactive attachment disorder

f. Anxiety spectrum disorders (e.g., OCD)

g. ADHD

h. Mood dysregulation

i. Childhood onset schizophrenia

Psychiatric comorbidities are of particular interest when evaluating individuals with PDDs as evidence has indicated that comorbidity between ASD and psychiatric diagnoses may be quite common. While there is debate about diagnosing comorbid disorders with overlapping symptoms to an ASD, research has demonstrated a high rate of psychiatric disorders present in individuals with an ASD. For example, in a recent study, deBruin et al. (2007) identified at least one comorbid disorder in 81% of a sample of 94 children between the ages of 6 and 12 diagnosed with PDD-NOS. Of the 81%, almost 62% met the criteria for a disruptive behavior disorder such as ADHD or ODD and 55% met the criteria for anxiety disorders. Furthermore, 13.8% of the participants met the diagnostic criteria for mood disorders. These results are similar to those reported in a study by Simonoff et al. (2008). The authors found that for 112 individuals diagnosed with ASD, ranging in age from 10-14, 70% had at least one comorbid disorder; however, anxiety was scored most often (29%), with ADHD and ODD both at 28%. It is unclear whether the differences in comorbid disorders are due to the differing diagnoses or the differing ages of the participants; however, these studies and others confirm the high prevalence of comorbid symptoms.

Identifying a comorbid psychiatric diagnosis is particularly difficult due to the lack of measures specifically designed to detect these disorders in a population with an ASD. Because persons with PDDs present with behavioral symptoms that may mimic symptoms of other disorders (e.g., difficulty with change, difficulty in social situations), it is important to consider the person's baseline presentation when determining a diagnosis of a psychiatric disorder for a person with a PDD. A change or increase in impairment is important when considering a diagnosis in addition to a PDD.

Persons with ASD and comorbid psychiatric diagnoses often have greater difficulty with behavioral symptoms. To a varying degree, this may impact all core features of the disorder. Common assessment measures for assessment of behavioral and emotional concerns in children with a PDD include:

Table 9.3 Assessments for Children with PDD

Instrument	Brief Description	Age Range	Assessment Type	Number of Items
Aberrrant Behavior Checklist (ABC; Aman & Singh)	Usually completed by an adult who knows the child well. It has five subscales, including irritability, lethargy/social withdrawal, stereotypy, hyperactivity, and inappropriate speech.	6-54 years	Rating scale	58 items
Behavior Assessment System for Children (BASC-2)	To be completed by teachers, parents, and the child. There also is a structured observation and history taking, to help the assessor understand the behaviors and emotions.	2-5, 6-11, 12-21 years	Rating scale	134-160 items
Behavior Problem Inventory (BPI-01; Rojhan et al., 2001)	Filled out by a respondent who knows the child well. It measures self-injurious, stereotypic, and aggressive destructive behavior.	14 and up (adolescents and adults)	Rating scale	52 items
Child Behavior Checklist (CBCL)	Completed by a parent or caregiver. They rate the child on a variety of areas, including aggressive behavior, anxiety or depression, attention problems, rule-breaking, social problems, somatic complaints, thought problems, and withdrawal.	1.5-5 years, 6-18 years	Rating scale	99 items, 112 items
Developmental Behavior Checklist (DBC)	A questionnaire completed by parents or other primary caregivers or teachers to assess behavior or emotional problems	4-18 years	Rating scale	96 items
Repetitive Behavior Scale – Revised (RBS-R)	Completed by caregiver. Measures ritualistic and sameness, stereotypic, self-injurious, compulsive, behavior, and restricted interests.	2-18 years	Rating scale	43 items

Signs of the most common comorbid disorders (Mazefsky et al., 2011):

Signs of ADHD

ADHD symptoms in individuals with PDDs include inattention, hyperactivity, and impulsivity. When considering a diagnosis of ADHD in an individual with a PDD it is important to consider:

*The child's mental age as related to the degree to which behavior is atypical

*The differences between inattention and skill deficits or hearing impairments

*Distractibility versus over-focus or preoccupation with irrelevant stimuli (e.g., motor movements or lights)

Signs of an anxiety disorder

It is not uncommon for individuals with an ASD to be more likely to experience fears due to their difficulty with change, social situations, and other situations related to the core features of ASD. This is the reason why anxiety disorders are not typically diagnosed separate from an ASD diagnosis. When specific treatment is warranted for anxiety, however, it may be warranted to do so. Specific anxiety symptoms and classifications may include:

*Separation anxiety

*Panic disorder

*Generalized anxiety disorder

*Social phobias

*Obsessive-compulsive symptoms

Depressive and Anxiety disorders

Depressive and anxiety disorders may be prevalent in individuals with ASD due to a genetic risk and/or due to environmental stressors. As with all comorbid disorders with ASD, consideration of the severity of symptoms as they relate to ASD versus a mood disorder is important. For this reason, historical information is critically important. For example, measures on the Aberrant Behavior Checklist of social withdrawal are often high for individuals with ASD due to impairments in social functioning. For individuals without an ASD, this may indicate a concern about a mood disorder; however, this is typical for individuals with ASD. Some key considerations are: are there changes in affect (which may already be impaired), increased isolation, increased emotional dysregulation (e.g., frequent crying) that was not present previously?

Associated Behavioral and Cognitive Features

Severe or serious challenging behaviors are often associated with the disorder. The most common behaviors observed are aggression, tantrums, property destruction, and self-injury (Horner et al., 2002). Additional behavioral concerns that can have life-threatening implications are elopement (wandering away) and pica (eating inedible objects). All of the behaviors can significantly affect an individual's quality of life and place the person in danger. If children are exhibiting these behaviors it is important that they are referred to a board-certified behavior analyst (BCBA) and a qualified medical professional with expertise in assessing and treating these behaviors.

Additional behavioral challenges that may be encountered include:

a. Feeding challenges

b. Sleep challenges

c. Toileting difficulties

Each of these may impact the progress that an individual with an ASD can make in the typical environment. Feeding challenges also may impact an individual's health as he or she may not eat a full range of nutritious foods. Sleep challenges may have an impact on the functioning of the individual and of the family. Toileting difficulties may particularly impede an individual from fully participating in their school and community.

Treatment

It is critical that treatment and intervention for ASD is initiated as early as possible. Early intervention is particularly critical with this disorder. Referral to a specialist in diagnosis of an ASD is the first step. You may be asked to assist in providing information about professionals in your community who provide treatment. This is where it is important to understand the evidence currently available for the treatment of ASD. Best practice would dictate a well-functioning, multidisciplinary team to evaluate and assess the presence of the disorder, treat and psychiatric and mental health needs, provide training and support for the family, and specific, evidence-based treatment of the child with ASD. There are several resources describing the evidence for treatment of ASD. These include the CDC (http://www.cdc.gov/ncbddd/autism/treatment.html) and the American Academy of Pediatrics (http://pediatrics.aappublications.org/content/early/2011/04/04/peds.2011-0426.abstract).

The review of the literature conducted by Warren and his colleagues (2011) states that interventions based on Applied Behavior Analysis (ABA) and the Denver Early Start Model have the most evidence for efficacy to date. Additional sources, such as the National Standards Project completed by the National Autism Center (http://www.nationalautismcenter.org/nsp/) categorize treatments as "established," "emerging," and "unestablished." The National Autism Center lists the following interventions, all based on ABA, as established:

a. Antecedent Package

b. Behavioral Package

c. Comprehensive Behavioral Treatment for Young Children

d. Joint Attention Intervention

e. Modeling

f. Naturalistic Teaching Strategies

g. Peer Training Package

h. Pivotal Response Treatment

i. Schedules

j. Self-management

k. Story-based Intervention Package

l. All other interventions were either considered emerging or unestablished at the time of their report (2011).

Best practice in treatment for ASD is far from a resolved issue. There are a number of schools of thought on the best treatment approach and there are a number of well-circulated myths or unproven treatments widely used and widely available. Sifting through the evidence can often be time consuming, overwhelming, and difficult for the most sophisticated parent and practitioner. Additionally, new treatments are often developed and advertised without much evidence of their efficacy. There are some tools to help the practitioner in evaluating treatment claims. The Association for Science in Autism Treatment (ASAT) recommends reading the article, "Sense About Science" (http://www.senseaboutscience.org/pages/peer-review.html), which discusses the peer-review process. On its Website, ASAT provides a description of autism treatments and the research studies supporting those (http://www.asatonline.org/treatment/autismtreatments) and some warning signs of pseudoscientific therapies (http://www.asatonline.org/treatment/articles/evaluate.htm).

Medication Guide for ASD

Although the evidence is still emerging for most medications, medication may play an important role in the treatment of associated symptoms of ASD and comorbid disorders. Psychopharmacological interventions applied to ASD are somewhat of a double-edged sword. Specifically, there is no evidence to support the use of these agents to treat the core symptoms of ASD (e.g.,. social reciprocity, language/communication, and restricted repetitive behaviors/interests); however, they have been used widely to treat features associated with the disorder (e.g. irritability, aggression, self-injury [SIB], inattention, hyperactivity, repetitive behaviors, anxiety and depression) (Kaplan & McCracken, 2012; Westphal & Pelphrey, 2011).

Symptom-based approaches to management using psychopharmacological interventions have afforded youth diagnosed with ASD the opportunity to enjoy improved functioning and quality of life. For example, the FDA approved the prescription of risperidone in 2006 and aripiprazole in 2009, to treat irritability (e.g., moderate to severe tantrums, aggression, and SIB) in youth diagnosed with ASD ages 5-16 and 6-17 years of age, respectively. When prescribed these agents, youth diagnosed with ASD seem to be afforded improved functioning, such as reduction in challenging behaviors. What is not well understood is whether these agents impact the core social abilities of youth versus a reduction in irritability that enables better compliance with routines, demand activities, and improved functional communication (Williams et al., 2006).

This symptom-based approach has several limitations. Outside of the agents mentioned above, there are few randomized controlled trials that have evaluated the effects of psychopharmacological agents in populations diagnosed with ASDs. In essence, providers need to rely on evidence conducted in typically developing populations and extrapolate to individuals diagnosed with ASD. In addition, in some instances these agents can exacerbate core symptoms of ASD (i.e., use of stimulants to treat inattention may result in excessive focus on a different and socially inappropriate target). This point is made to simply underscore the importance of careful monitoring of youth diagnosed with ASDs and the importance of an interprofessional team to optimize outcomes.

Prior to initiating a psychopharmacological intervention, it is important that individuals have a complete clinical assessment and evaluation that identifies strengths and opportunities in adaptive functioning as well as associated target symptoms. A comprehensive evaluation should include assessments of: 1) developmental psychiatric functioning; 2) medical history; 3) medication history with a focus on the child's response to these interventions (positive and adverse), including dosages, length of trial and reasons for discontinuation. (Given the popular use of supplements, vitamins, and complementary and alternative medicine interventions, review of these agents should also be conducted and assessed for potential drug-drug interactions.); 3) history of current and past educational, psychosocial, and behavioral interventions; and finally, 4) inclusion of behavioral observations and results of rating scales (described above) (AACAP, 1999).

Additionally, a functional behavior assessment (FBA) to determine environmental variables contributing to the challenging behavior is considered best practice. Additional assessments, such as physical exam, neurological assessment, imaging studies, audiology and vision evaluation, routine laboratory studies (including lead levels), and EKG should also be included in a comprehensive evaluation. Further, psychological assessment (IQ testing, adaptive skills), speech-language-communication assessments (vocabulary, language skills, articulation and oral-motor skills, pragmatic skills), and occupational and physical therapy assessments will likely also be included in a comprehensive assessment of youth diagnosed with an ASD (AACAP, 1999). Each of these evaluations will provide vital information for decisions about psychopharmacological interventions. They will also serve as important points of contrast to evaluate response to treatment.

As mentioned previously, there are no current psychopharmacological interventions available to treat the symptoms of ASD. Educational systems are required to provide functional behavioral assessments and behavioral treatment plans, and to evaluate their outcome when associated behaviors impact the learning environment. Psychopharmacological intervention may be considered when the following criteria are met: 1) the behavioral symptoms persist and continue to interfere with the individual's overall functioning after a behavioral plan is implemented; 2) the behavior or symptoms continue to occur at a significant frequency, duration, and/or intensity; and 3) the behavior or symptoms are impacting the safety of the individual or others. If these items are deemed significant, in spite of behavioral interventions, a targeted medication trial should be considered.

Target symptoms that may be responsive to psychopharmacological intervention may include: hyperactivity, impulsivity, distractibility, inattention, anxiety, obsessions, perseverations, compulsions, irritability, agitation, depression, aggression, self-injury, repetitive or stereotypic behaviors.

Evidence for psychopharmacological interventions for the listed target symptoms include:

1) Psychostimulants (RUPP Autism Network, 2005):

- **Agent:** Methylphenidate

- **Target symptom and/or behavior:** hyperactivity

- **Adverse events:** irritability, anorexia, sleep disturbance, emotional outbursts

2) Alpha-adrenergic Agents (Posey & McDougle, 2007)
- **Agent:** Guanfacine (Tenex, Intuniv) and clonidine (Catapress, Kapvay)
- **Target symptom and/or behavior:** hyperactivity
- **Adverse events:** hypotension, sedation, fatigue, irritability

3) Norepinephrine Reuptake Inhibitors (Arnold et. al., 2006)
- **Agent:** Atomoxetine (Strattera)
- **Target symptom and/or behavior:** ADHD symptoms
- **Adverse events:** irritability, GI upset, nausea/vomiting, fatigue, tachycardia

4) Selective Serotonin Reuptake Inhibitors (McDougle et al., 2000; Hollander et al., 2005; King et al., 2009)
**Please review literature as results for SSRIs are quite mixed despite frequency of use.

- **Agent:** Fluvoxamine (Luvox), fluoxetine (Prozac), citalopram (Celexa)
- **Target symptom and/or behavior:** repetitive thoughts and/or behaviors
- **Adverse events:** activation syndrome (increased activity and/or energy, mood changes, insomnia, agitation), aggression, nausea, sedation, impulsiveness. **Carefully consider Black Box Warning: increased suicidal thinking**

5) A typical Antipsychotics (Marcus et al., 2009; Owen et al., 2009; RUPP, 2002; RUPP Autism Network, 2005)

- **Agent:** Aripiprazole (Abilify) and risperidone (Risperdal)
- **Target symptom and/or behavior:** Irritability, mood instability, hyperactivity, stereotypies, social withdrawal, inappropriate speech, severe tantrums, aggression, and self-injury
- **Adverse events:** weight gain, increased appetite, vomiting, somnolence, drowsiness, drooling, tremor, fatigue, and dizziness

6) Mood Stabilizers (Hellings et al., 2005; Hollander et al., 2005; Belsito et al., 2001)

- **Agent:** valproic acid (Depakote) and lamotrigine (Lamictal)
- **Target symptom and/or behavior:** irritability, aggression
- **Adverse events:** insomnia, hyperactivity, irritability, aggression, increased appetite, skin rash

Considerations for Office Visits

Being prepared to support an individual with an ASD and the family when they come for office visits is an important part of primary care. Individuals with an ASD may have difficulty with office visits for a variety of reasons. First, the visit is not part of their typical routine which may make them anxious. Social situations can be hard for some persons with an ASD, making a visit to a crowded office even more difficult. While waiting can be hard for many children, waiting can be highly problematic for an individual with an ASD. All of these may combine to increase the likelihood the visit will not go smoothly. Some suggestions for easing these concerns might be:

a. Provide the family with pictures of the office, the people in the office, and a description (e.g., story) of what they child can expect.

b. Suggest that the caregivers show the individual the pictures and review the "story" before they come to the office to help the individual prepare.

c. Try to schedule the visit for a time when there are likely to be few people in the office and for a time when the wait is likely to be short (e.g., the first appointment in the morning).

d. Be sure to have objects that might be dangerous or that can be thrown both in the exam and waiting rooms out of reach if the individual has a history of displaying challenging behavior.

e. Speak with the person with ASD, not just with the caregiver.

f. Use language that matches the individual's level of comprehension (take your cues from the caregiver).

g. Use visuals to describe what you are doing as often as possible. For example, you might show a picture of a person listening to a child's heart, then say, "Now this is what I am going to do."

h. Make the visit with the individual with ASD as short as possible. Consider having some toys or play objects in the room to engage the individual with ASD while you speak with the caregiver after the exam.

Individuals with ASD often have impairments in their ability to communicate. This can make your ability to identify symptoms and medical concerns very difficult. Some considerations to help in this process are provided by Mazefsky et al. (2011). These include:

a. A child with an ASD may not look ill, but may display challenging behavior as the only outward symptom.

b. Challenging behavior may reflect pain that the child is not able to communicate. Understanding whether the behavior displayed is part of his or her typical repertoire or whether it has changed will be critical in detecting whether the behavior is communicating a change in pain.

c. The child with ASD may be in need of care for injuries that are self-inflicted or as a result of a lack of understanding of danger (e.g., ran into the woods).

d. Be aware of the child's history and provide adequate space during an exam if the child has a history of displaying challenging behavior.

e. Consider obtaining information for the appointment in advance via phone call with the caregiver (e.g., history, concerns, changes).

f. Ask the parent for advice on how to make optimal use of the visit (e.g., reinforcers for the child, communication modalities, whether a second adult would be beneficial).

g. For children who cannot tolerate blood draws, consider prescribing an anesthetic cream in advance for the parent to apply.

Information for Parents About ASD in Children

There are many resources for parents who are either concerned their child might have autism or whose child has been diagnosed with an ASD.

- Autism Speaks (http://www.autismspeaks.org/), in particular, has a wealth of information and kits to help parents navigate the often overwhelming dearth of information available on the assessment and treatment of children with ASD. Some resources available on their Website include tool kits (http://www.autismspeaks.org/family-services/tool-kits) such as the 100-day kit that helps parents navigate the first 100 days after their child's diagnosis and a variety of others to help families (e.g., Tips for Successful Hair Cuts).

- The National Institute of Mental Health has a parent's guide to autism spectrum disorders (http://www.nimh.nih.gov/health/publications/a-parents-guide-to-autism-spectrum-disorder/parent-guide-to-autism.pdf), and the National Autism Center has a Parent's Guide to Evidence-Based Practice (http://www.nationalautismcenter.org/pdf/nac_parent_manual.pdf).

- The American Academy of Pediatrics also has a book for purchase, Autism Spectrum Disorders: What Every Parent Needs to Know, edited by Alan I. Rosenblatt, MD, FAAP, and Paul S. Carbone, MD, FAAP (http://www.healthychildren.org/English/bookstore/Pages/Autism-Spectrum-Disorders-What-Every-Parent-Needs-to-Know.aspx).

Additional Internet Resources

- American Academy of Child and Adolescent Psychiatry (AACAP) - AACAP Practice Parameter: Autism

- American Academy of Pediatrics AAP Autism Tool Kit 2nd Edition (www.aap.org)

- Association for Science in Autism Treatment

- Autism Speaks (www.autismspeaks.org)

- Caring for Children with Autism Spectrum Disorders: a resource toolkit for clinicians (www.2.aap.org/publiced/autismtoolkit.cfm)

- CDC Act Early Campaign (www.cdc.gov/ncbddd/actearly/autism/html)

- CDC Autism Case Training (www.cdc.gov/ncbddd/actearly/autism/index.html)

- International Rett Syndrome Foundation (http://www.rettsyndrome.org/)

- National Institute of Mental Health: A Parent's Guide to Autism Spectrum Disorders (http://www.nimh.nih.gov/health/publications/a-parents-guide-to-autism-spectrum- disorder/index.shtml)

- National Institute of Neurological Disorders and Stroke (http://www.ninds.nih.gov/disorders/pdd/pdd.htm)

REFERENCES

Abrahams, B. S. & Geschwind, D. H. (2008). Advances in autism genetics: on the threshold of new neurobiology. *Nature Reviews, Genetics*, 9(5), 344.

Chen, C-Y, Chen, K-H, Liu, C-Y, Huang, S-L, Lin, K-M, (2009). Increased risks of congenital, neurologic, and endocrine disorders associated with autism in preschool children: Cognitive ability differences. *The Journal of Pediatrics*, 154(3), 345-350.

deBruin, E. I., Ferdinand, R. F., Meester, S., de Nijs, P. F. A., & Verheij, F. (2007). High rates of psychiatric co-morbidity in PDD-NOS. *Journal of Autism and Developmental Disorders*, 37(5), 877-886.

Diagnostic tests for Autism Spectrum Disorders (ASD) in preschool children (Protocol). *Cochrane Database of Systematic Reviews*, 3. Retrieved from http://onlinelibrary.wiley.com/doi/10.1002/14651858.CD009044/full

Elsea, S. H. & Girirajan, S. (2008). Smith-Magenis syndrome. *European Journal of Hman Genetics*, 16(4), 412–421.

Horner, R. H., Carr, E. G., Strain, P. S., Todd, A. W., & Reed, H. K. (2002). Problem behavior interventions for young children with autism: A research synthesis. *Journal of Autism and Developmental Disorders*, 32(5), 423-446.

Livanis, A. & Mouzakitis A. (2010). Treatment validity of autism screening instruments. *Assessment for Effective Intervention*, 35(4), 206-217.

Manzi, B., Loizzo, A. L., Giana, G., & Curatolo, P. (2008). Autism and metabolic diseases. *Journal of Child Neurology*, 23(3), 307-314.

Mazefsky, C. A., Filipink, R., Lindsey, J., & Lubetsky, M. J. (2011). Medical evaluation and co-morbid psychiatric disorder. In: Lubestky, M. J., Handen, B. L., & McGonigle, J. J. (Eds.). *Autism Spectrum Disorder: Pittsburgh Pocket Psychiatry* New York, NY: Oxford Press.

Samtani A, Sterling-Levis K, Scholten RJPM, Woolfenden S, Hooft L, Williams K. (2011). Diagnostic tests for Autism Spectrum Disorders (ASD) in preschool children (Protocol). Cochrane Database of Systematic Reviews 2011, Issue 3. Art. No.: CD009044. DOI: 10.1002/14651858.CD009044.

Simonoff, E., Pickles, A., Charman, T, Chandler, S., Loucas, T., & Baird, G. (2008). Psychiatric disorders in children with autism spectrum disorders: prevalence, comorbidity, and associated factors in a population derived sample. *Journal of the American Academy of Child & Adolescent Psychiatry*, 47(8), 921-929.

Warren, Z, McPheeter, M. L., Sathe, N., Foss-Feig, M. A., Glasser, A., & Veenstra-Vanderweele, J. (2011). A systematic review of early intensive intervention for autism spectrum disorder. *Pediatrics*, 127(5), e1303-e1311.

Zandt, F., Prior, M., & Kyrios, M. (2007). Repetitive behaviour in children with high functioning autism and obsessive compulsive disorder. *Journal of Autism and Developmental Disorders*, 37(2), 251-259.

SECTION 10
Patrice Rancour

Helping Children Deal With Death, Loss, and Grief

Fast Facts

- These three things are true: we live in a death-phobic society, children do grieve, and while it can be extremely painful, grief is a normal healing response to all loss.

- An estimated 3.5% - 4-5% of children in this country (or 1.2-2.5 million children) will lose a parent before the age of 18.

- While the vast majority of grieving children receive the support they need in order to grow into healthy adulthood, it is estimated that 40% of children bereaved by sudden parental death may require preventive intervention in order to avoid complications later in adulthood (Melhem et al., 2008; Melhem et al., 2011).

- Normal grief requires facilitation, while complicated grief requires intervention.

- Common comorbid conditions of complicated grief, such as depression and PTSD, require treatment.

- Not all loss and grief are about the death of a parent, or even death in general. Grief responses are associated with many other kinds of changes (e.g., moving homes, foster placement, changes in health status, separation, divorce or incarceration of parents, and moving to a new school).

- A 2011-2012 New York Life Foundation/National Alliance for Grieving Children poll identified that 68% of the polled children reported that the death was the worst thing that had ever happened to them, 45% reported they acted in ways they know aren't healthy and that they can't concentrate on school work, and 39% have trouble sleeping. (National Alliance for Grieving Children, 2012).

- Helping children come to terms with loss and grief becomes a teachable moment in learning to adapt to the vagaries of change over the course of a lifetime.

Table 10.1 Age-Related Responses to Loss and Grief

Age Stage	Concept	Presentation	Assistance
Infants-Toddlers (0-2)	No understanding of death; no language; recognizes changes in family	Separation anxiety, anxious, crying, problems with appetite or sleep, fearfulness, needy, irritable	Provide parental warmth and physical closeness, meet needs, maintain routine, include in family rituals as much as possible, provide verbal love and reassurance.
Preschool (3-5)	Believes death is temporary, magical thinking, fantasies	Crying, anxious, irritable, regressed behavior, temper tantrums, problems eating or sleeping, separation anxiety, acting out	Provide parental warmth and physical closeness, maintain routines, include in family rituals as much as possible, be honest in responses to questions, listen to and accept children's need to express themselves, make time for play.
School-age (6-9)	Now understands that death is permanent; starts to wonder what happens after death	Asking questions, problems with sleeping/appetite, withdrawn, anxious, guilty, nightmares, problems in school, acting out, crying, angry	Provide parental warmth and closeness, be honest, answer questions, accept feelings, encourage use of play and art to express self, maintain routines, work with school, encourage inclusion in family mourning rituals.
Pre-teen (10-12)	Understands finality of death, magical thinking, understands that life will go on without the loved one	Confusion, denial, shock, lonely, angry, anxious, fearful, problems with sleep/appetite, acting out, problems in school, may self-isolate, guilty, physical problems, questioning existential issues	Provide opportunities to tell his/her story, include in family rituals, provide parental warmth, encourage expressive arts, be honest, work with school, provide information.
Teenager (13-18)	Understands the universality and finality of death, magical thinking, understands that life will go on without the loved one, spiritual concepts evolving	Confusion, denial, shock, sadness, lonely, angry, self-conscious, guilty, anxious, fearful, acts out, problems with sleep-appetite, problems in school, self-isolation, other physical problems	Provide parental warmth, be honest, opportunities for expressive arts, peer group support, anticipate risky behaviors, include in family mourning rituals, work with school, be honest.

Adapted from Children's Grief Education Association, 2004

Facilitating Normal Grief in Children

- The goals of helping children grieve include helping them redefine their relationship with their lost loved one or object, hold onto meaningful memories in order to continue the relationship, and maintain an inner connection with the deceased as they continue to grow and develop (Haine et al., 2008; Mitchell, Wesner, Brownson, Gale, Garand, & Havill, 2006; Wesner, Garand, Gale, Havill & Brownson, 2007).

- According to the transitional events model, Haines and colleagues (2008) propose that "the primary goal of interventions should be to decrease children's exposure to stressful changes following the death and to strengthen child and family resources for dealing with those stressors."

In general, small children respond to loss and grief after a death with several common questions:

- "Can I catch this too?" (fear of contagion)

- "Who will take care of me now?" (fear of abandonment) (Schoenfelder et al., 2011)

- "I told Daddy to drop dead last week. Did I cause this?" (magical thinking) (Schoenfelder et al., 2011)

These become opportunities to teach about the inevitability of loss and how we die. Generally speaking, make sure children are reassured that they can't "catch" what the dead person had, and that they are surrounded by adults who will take care of them. Ensuring that children understand that they are not so powerful as to have had thoughts that could actually kill another person is reassuring. In general, teenagers are often catapulted into taking on more responsibility before they are ready, and so tend to be angrier about less disposable time and money for themselves. It is important to remember that 13-year-old Tom is indeed not the new man of the house.

Guidelines for Management

- In order to help others, become more comfortable with *facing your own mortality* so that death is a discussable subject.

- The best way to ensure healthy grieving in children is to ensure that the surviving parent remains supported and healthy in his/her own grief work. Complicated grief on the part of the parent is a predictor of complicated grief in the child. (Haine et al., 2008; Cohen, & Mannarino, 2010).

- Screening caregivers who display complicated grief, mood disorders, substance abuse, and PTSD ensures that they receive proper treatment in order to care for their children.

- Be watchful for evidence of child abuse in parents who are not coping well with loss. Support demonstrations of parental warmth with one-on-one time (Melhem et al., 2011; Haine et al., 2008; Schoenfelder et al., 2011).

- Counsel parents not to lie to children. Tell the truth in brief, age-appropriate conversations in a safe place and at a pace that affords them the opportunity to ask questions. Use the correct language.

- Do not say the person "passed away" or "went to sleep." Use the word "died," otherwise children may be afraid that they themselves might die in their sleep or that perhaps the lost one will "pass back." It is not the talking about death that triggers the hurt; the hurt is already there. It is about choosing between being sad together or being sad separately (Goldman, 2001).

- Provide information about the grief process to children and their adults. Remind parents that misbehaving and regressing are often how children communicate their grief (Haine et al., 2008).

- Counsel parents not be afraid to express their feelings openly and normalize them. However, they should not overwhelm children with parental grief that needs to be handled by other adults. Crying is a normal human emotion and sharing it with children lets them know that the parent can handle sadness. Ensure that children understand they are not responsible for fixing parental distress, and that the family's situation will improve over time.

- Include 'Family Fun Time' as a weekly way to break from grief (Haine et al., 2008).

- Counsel parents to include children in the family life of grief and mourning as much as possible. This means encouraging them to attend funerals and other rites of mourning where they see their family members coming together for support. Packing a bag of drawing materials, paper, small toys, and books will help occupy young children as they watch adults cry, tell stories, and basically reduce a sense of isolation. Many adults who were prevented from attending funerals of deceased friends and relatives as children report feeling resentment later that they were excluded. They also did not develop life skills related to loss and grief as a result. Children tend to fantasize the worst when left to their own devices. Letting children know what the ground rules are during these rituals will prepare them to participate. Let children know that if they feel overwhelmed by their experiences, they can take breaks and that their adults will debrief them about their experience later (Goldman, 2001).

- Creating farewell ceremonies, such as writing a message and sending it off on a balloon, can help the child find ways to create his/her own ritual (Goldman, 2001; Swank & Robinson, 2009).

- Use the death of pets as intentional teachable moments about coping with loss.

- Become familiar with the family's cultural and spiritual beliefs as to what happens when people die, their customs surrounding mourning, any special rituals, prayers and devotionals that are important to them. Ask them to educate you about their beliefs in order to avoid inadvertently offending their sensibilities.

- Referral for family therapy may be in order if the loss exacerbates pre-existing dysfunction.

- Play therapy utilizes therapeutic story-telling, drama, role play, puppets and masks, dance and movement, and sand and clay trays to help children work through feelings for which they often do not have vocabulary (Swank & Robinson, 2009).

- Support groups are particularly effective for teenagers whose need for peer support steadily increases as they work towards self-acceptance and acceptance by their peers. In particular, group work helps normalize their feelings during a time when they feel self-conscious or when they believe that expressing vulnerable emotions makes them look weak (Mitchell et al., 2007).

- Social networking blogs, chat rooms and other Web-based communication portals can reduce a sense of social isolation and promote a feeling of protected anonymity; however, teens need to be counseled that there is no such thing as confidentiality once it goes out on the Internet (Wagneret al., 2006).

- Animal-assisted therapy is an intervention whereby children can to relate to non-threatening contact with specially trained service dogs, horses, etc. in helping them cope with loss. Interaction with therapy animals and their own pets often helps children reduce stress levels.

- Cognitive-behavioral therapy may be useful for children whose language skills have developed to a level whereby their myths about death can be challenged, and more healthy thought substitutions can help them transform maladaptive coping with healthier grief work (Haine et al., 2008; Cohen & Mannarino, 2010; Swank & Robinson, 2009).

- Expressive arts like music, journaling, and painting give children and teenagers a creative outlet that can release emotional material in non-threatening ways. For example, giving sentence-completion exercises such as answering questions like "The day my dog died…." or "The thing that I am most afraid of now that my mother has died is…" Asking children to paint pictures of their family before the loss occurred and then afterward can act as a springboard for discussion (Haine et al., 2008; Goldman, 2001; Swank & Robinson, 2009).

- Creative visualization/relaxation training can maximize the innate tendency of children to use their imaginations by helping them induce a relaxation response prior to taking them to a safe space. Remember that children will not have learned to censor unusual sensory experiences that adults have censored. They will report auditory, visual, olfactory, tactile, and other sensory stimulation that adults might feel uncomfortable with and identify as hallucinatory. Unless there are other disturbing symptoms, accept these experiences that children report as normal. Children can also be guided into having conversations with their lost loved one in order to speak with them, especially if they did not have a chance to say good-bye prior to the death.

- Therapeutic letter writing can also be used as a vehicle to write to the lost person to explain what it has been like since the lost person died.

- Use memory boxes, collages, scrap books, photos, souvenirs, and other related memoirs to build a concrete reminder of positive memories of time spent together.

- Bibliotherapy and movies provide a non-threatening introduction of how other children and teenagers respond to loss and grief. Debriefing the book or movie with questions that then bring up the child's own experiences feels natural. It can also be a prelude to the child or teen writing his/her own personal story to work through their experiences (Haine et al., 2008; Swank & Robinson, 2009).

- Holidays and anniversary dates present special challenges for incorporating the lost person into the life of the family. Lighting candles, decorating graves with flowers on special dates of remembrances, and other tender rituals can help keep the memories of deceased family members alive so that family members can feel connected to the one who has been lost (Haine et al., 2008; Wesner et al., 2006; Mitchell et al., 2007).

The DSM-5™ and the Newly-Emerging Criteria for Persistent Complex Bereavement-Related Grief Disorder (CG)

Complicated grief research is a work in progress. There has been a great deal of controversy over whether or not there is sufficient evidence to include it as a new diagnostic category for complicated grief. At this time, this condition is being recommended for further study in Section III of the DSM-5™ in order for further research to clarify evidence for its inclusion. This decision should provide opportunities to collect ongoing data to determine if there indeed are sufficient clinical differences between normal grief, and persistent complicated grief, which require different interventions. It also is hypothesized that PTSD and depression can be comorbid with persistent complex Bereavement-Related Grief Disorders (Shear et al., 2011; Shear et al., 2005; Prigerson, et al., 2009; American Psychiatric Association, 2010).

Table 10.2 Differences Between Normal Grief, Complicated Grief, Depression, PTSD, and Anxiety Disorder

Normal Grief	Complicated Grief (CG)	Depression	PTSD	General Anxiety Disorder
Sadness	Yearning	Sadness	Numbness	Anxiety
Improves over time	Overwhelmed by the loss	Does not improve over time	Disconnection	Does not improve over time
Childhood attachment issues may or may not be an issue	*Childhood attachment issues create vulnerability	No evidence of childhood attachment issues	No evidence of childhood attachment issues	No evidence of childhood attachment issues
No significant functional impairment	Significant functional impairment	Functional impairment	Functional impairment	Functional impairment
Vivid dreaming may be present	Changes in EEG sleep physiology	No changes in EEG sleep physiology	No changes in EEG sleep physiology	No changes in EEG sleep physiology
No reward-related neural activity	Reward-related neural activity in nucleus accumbens in response to reminders of the deceased	No reward-related neural activity	No reward-related neural activity	No reward-related neural activity
Suicidal ideation not prominent	Elevated rates of suicidal ideation and attempts, cancer, immunological dysfunction, hypertension, cardiac events, functional impairments, hospitalizations, adverse health behaviors, reduced quality of life	Rates are not as high as CG	Rates are not as high as CG	Rates are not as high as CG
Absenteeism rates are not as high as for CG	Increased absence from home and work	Absenteeism rates are not as high as CG	Absenteeism rates are not as high as CG	Absenteeism rates are not as high as CG
Treatment not necessary	Treatment: tricyclics alone and interpersonal psychotherapy are ineffective. Focused complicated grief therapy is efficacious	Tricyclics and SSRIs, psychotherapy efficacious	Tricyclics and SSRIs, psychotherapy efficacious	Tricyclics and SSRIs, psychotherapy efficacious

Adapted from Shear et al., 2011; Prigerson et al., 2009; Treating Post-traumatic Stress, 2008

*Childhood attachment issues refer to history of childhood separation anxiety, controlling parents, parental abuse or death, close kinship relationship to deceased, insecure attachment, marital supportiveness and dependency, lack of preparation for the death.

Persistent Complex Bereavement-Related Grief Disorder in Children

Why screen for complicated grief in children? Depending on the source, 10% of all grieving people (an estimated 1 million people annually) develop complicated grief, which is often under-identified and, therefore, under-treated. The inherent risk is to either pathologize a normal grief reaction or to miss treating a pathological one (Shear et al., 2005).

Loss during childhood is normal; however, not receiving support for it is what creates complications. The goal of early identification and treatment is prevention of morbidity *and* premature mortality by promoting adaptive coping, promoting a healthy lifestyle and managing the stress response, treating complicated grief, comorbid depression, and PTSD early in **both** parent and child (Melhem et al., 2008; Shear et al., 2011).

It is important to note that complicated grief is reported across all cultures, so that while it is universal, its manifestation is also affected by the cultural mores and spiritual beliefs of the families who experience it (Haine et al., 2008).

Children most at risk for complicated grief include those:

- Who already suffer from a mood disorder
- Whose caregivers suffer from mood disorders, substance abuse, or PTSD
- Whose loved ones died traumatically
- Who might have suffered multiple losses
- Whose losses involve social stigma (e.g., HIV/AIDS, suicide, incarceration of a parent)
- Whose past relationship with the deceased might have involved abuse, abandonment, or neglect
- Who experience low perceived social support
- Whose surviving caregiver or parent is so disabled by his/her own grief process that s/he is not able to attend to the needs of the grieving child.
- Who have been victims of community violence or war (Developmental Trauma Disorder) (Melhem et al., 2008; Haine et al., 2008; Shear et al., 2011;Cohen & Mannarino, 2010; Felitti, 2002; Kersting, 2004)

Left untreated, complicated grief in children can lead to:

- Poor academic performance
- PTSD
- Depression (risk is 3x higher in bereaved youth)
- Sleep disorders
- Impairment in relationships due to problems with attachment
- Chronic illnesses later in life due to poor coping/lifestyle choice
- Self-medication with drugs and/or food
- Legal issues including misbehavior, aggression, incarceration, delinquency
- Increased cortisol responses to stress
- Increased family adversity
- Suicide (Melhem et al., 2008; Schoenfelder et al., 2011; Prigerson et al., 2009; Brent, 2012)

Symptoms

A. For children, the death must have occurred at least 6 months ago.

B. At least one of the following symptoms must be present more days than not and must result in functional impairment:

a. Persistent yearning which may be expressed in play and behavior, including separation-reunion behavior with caregivers

b. Intense pain

c. Preoccupation with deceased

d. Preoccupation with the circumstances of the death, such that it may be expressed through play and behavior, and worry about the possible death of others close to them

C. At least six of the following symptoms must be present more days than not and must result in functional impairment:

a. Depending on the child's capacity to understand, difficulty accepting the death

b. Feeling shocked, stunned, or numb

c. Difficulty with positive reminiscing about the deceased

d. Anger about the loss

e. Maladaptive self-appraisals in relation to the death

f. Avoidance of thoughts and feelings regarding the deceased

g. A desire to join the deceased by death

h. Difficulty trusting others

i. Detachment from other relationships

j. Feeling life cannot be lived without the deceased

k. Diminished self-identity

l. Inability to look forward to the future

D. If the death occurred under traumatic circumstances, persistent flashbacks and magical thinking regarding the death (Shear et al., 2011; Prigerson et al., 2009; Grohol, 2005)

Screening Tools for Persistent Complex Bereavement-Related Grief Disorder in Children

1. *Inventory for Complicated Grief-Revised for Children* (ICG-RC)
   See tool on next page.

2. *Complicated Grief Assessment Interview (Child Version)-Short Form, revised (parent form also available)*
   This is a 23-item questionnaire which can be administered to children. It evaluates yearning, level of denial, trust, hopelessness and relationships since the death. It can be obtained from the author, Dr. Holly Prigerson at measures@twosuns.org.

3. *Prolonged Grief Disorder (PG-13)*
   This is a 13-item questionnaire which can be administered to children as above. It evaluates similar responses as the above questionnaire, and can also be obtained from the author, Dr. Holly Prigerson at holly_prigerson@dfci.harvard.edu.

Inventory for Complicated Grief-Revised (ICG-RC) for Children

Each of the 28 items is scored on a 5-point Likert scale with an overall score ranging from 28 to 140:

1 = Almost never (less than once a month)

2 = Rarely (monthly)

3 = Sometimes (weekly)

4 = Often (daily)

5 = Always (several times a day)

INVENTORY OF COMPLICATED GRIEF–REVISED (ICG-RC) FOR CHILDREN					
Item	Almost never (< than once/ month) 1	Rarely (monthly) 2	Sometimes (weekly) 3	Often (daily) 4	Always (several times a day) 5
1) The death feels upsetting, overwhelming or devastating	☐	☐	☐	☐	☐
2) I think about....[a] so much that it can be hard for me to do the things I normally do	☐	☐	☐	☐	☐
3) Memories of.... upset me	☐	☐	☐	☐	☐
4) I feel that I cannot accept the death[b]	☐	☐	☐	☐	☐
5) I very much miss....[b]	☐	☐	☐	☐	☐
6) I feel angry about the death	☐	☐	☐	☐	☐
7) I feel that I cannot believe the death[b]	☐	☐	☐	☐	☐
8) I feel shocked over the death[b]	☐	☐	☐	☐	☐
9) Ever since the death, it is hard for me to trust people	☐	☐	☐	☐	☐
10) Ever since the death, I feel like I don't care about other people as much and I don't feel as close to people I care about as I used to	☐	☐	☐	☐	☐
11) I avoid reminders of....	☐	☐	☐	☐	☐
12) I avoid reminders that he/she is dead	☐	☐	☐	☐	☐
13) Sometimes people who lose a loved one feel that they cannot go back to normal life and be able to make new friends and do new activities. Do you feel that making new friends or doing new activities would be difficult for you?	☐	☐	☐	☐	☐
14) I feel that life is empty or has no meaning without....	☐	☐	☐	☐	☐

15) I hear the voice of….speak to me	☐	☐	☐	☐	☐
16) I feel like I have become numb (or has no feelings) since the death	☐	☐	☐	☐	☐
17) I feel that it is unfair that I should live when he/she died	☐	☐	☐	☐	☐
18) I am bitter (or angry) over the death	☐	☐	☐	☐	☐
19) I feel jealous of others who have not lost someone close	☐	☐	☐	☐	☐
20) I feel like the future has no meaning or purpose without….	☐	☐	☐	☐	☐
21) I feel lonely ever since the death [b]	☐	☐	☐	☐	☐
22) It is difficult for me to imagine life being satisfying without….	☐	☐	☐	☐	☐
23) I feel that a part of myself died with….	☐	☐	☐	☐	☐
24) I feel that the death made me see the world differently [b]	☐	☐	☐	☐	☐
25) I don't feel safe since the death	☐	☐	☐	☐	☐
26) I feel that I don't have control over things since the death	☐	☐	☐	☐	☐
27) I am jumpy or easily startled since the death	☐	☐	☐	☐	☐
28) Since the death, my sleep has been disturbed	☐	☐	☐	☐	☐

[a]"My parent" or the relationship lost.

[b]Items constitute the ICG-RC screen.

Reprinted from the Journal of the American Academy of Child & Adolescent Psychiatry, 52(6), *Melhem, N. M., Porta, G., Walker Payne, M., & Brent, D. A. Identifying Prolonged Grief Reactions in Children: Dimensional and Diagnostic Approaches, 599-607.e7,* Copyright (2013), with permission from Elsevier.

Complicated Grief Therapy (CGT)

In addition to those aids designed to help facilitate normal grief in children, CGT represents an emerging compendium of new treatment tools when normal grief in interrupted. While many of these are in development for adults, one can see their utility in adapting them for age-appropriate use with children and teenagers. The goal of therapy is not so much helping the individual let go and say good-bye to the lost person as it is to "construct a continuing bond with the deceased, remembering good times, using guided conversations, and revisiting techniques that help the individual imagine what the lost loved one's response to present day situations might be" (Haine, et al., 2008; Kersting, 2004).

Potential Interventions for Children Experiencing Complicated Grief

- Screen for parental/caregiver complicated grief. The primary predictor of complicated grief in children is the incapacitation of the caregiver to make him/herself available to support the child's normal grieving process (Haine et al., 2008; Cohen & Mannarino, 2010).

- Support positive parenting and the provision of warmth. Watch for signs of parental distress, such as evidence of self-medication or child abuse due to the unusual nature of the stress.

- Psycho-education: normalize grief by teaching parents and children about it.

- Offer cognitive-behavioral therapy (Wagner, Knaevelsrud & Maercker, 2006) (see information about the adolescent coping with depression course and the COPE CBT-based skills building program in the Brief Interventions Section)

- Antidepressants and other medications may be indicated for comorbid conditions of depression, PTSD, or anxiety.

- Relaxation training and thought/stopping therapy.

- Telling the story of the death or "revisiting" it. With older children and teenagers, taping their narration and encouraging them to listen to it might have the effect of desensitization (Shear et al., 2005; Kersting, 2004; Grohol, 2005; Silberner, 2005).*

- Guided conversations with the deceased individual help the child connect with the memory of the lost loved one and assist the child to give voice to those thoughts and feelings which were never shared (Shear et al., 2005; Kersting, 2004; Grohol, 2005; Silberner, 2005). *

- Healthy coping skills designed to improve self-care with emphasis on stress management, healthy nutrition and fitness can help prevent cortisol reactivity which can lead to chronic illnesses later in life (Felitti, 2002).

- Reintroduce fun activities whether the child thinks s/he will have fun or not.

- Reintroduce avoided activities (e.g., going to the park if that is where the lost loved one took the child, etc.)

- Encourage reminiscence through story-telling.

- Encourage reengagement with significant others.

- Bibliotherapy (Swank & Robinson, 2009)

- Visualizing hurt, especially for children who do not have access to emotional vocabulary (e.g., "If your tears could talk, what would they say?")

- Creating a time loss line to help the child understand the basis for the grief (Goldman, 2001)

- Creating a loss genogram to assist the child to understand the extent of loss across close generations within his/her family. This is especially relevant in situations involving community violence or war (Goldman, 2001).

- Play therapy and/or play groups (Swank & Robinson, 2009)

- Narrative therapy, such as writing letters to the lost person

- Art therapy

- Creating commemoration works such as scrapbooks, CDs, journals and memory books.

- Creating rituals or ceremonies (Goldman, 2001; Swank & Robinson, 2009).

- Therapy groups with the goal of resuming normal childhood development (Mitchel et al., 2007)

- Challenging cognitive distortions and correcting dysfunctional automatic thoughts (e.g,. "The grown-ups in my family will not abandon me," or "I did not cause this.") (Haine et al., 2008)

- Refer to a child mental health therapist for more intense treatment

*These interventions are specific to complicated grief.

Special Considerations

Suicide

Annually, between 7,000 and 10,000 children lose a parent to suicide. Due to the social stigma, shame, abandonment and anger issues that suicide brings up in youthful survivors, they can grow up to replicate their parents' choice. They represent a portion of the 40% of children bereaved by sudden parental death who will require some sort of preventive intervention (Melhem et al., 2008; Melhem et al., 2011; *JAMA* and Archives *Journals* , 2011)

When the child is orphaned by a suicide:

1. Define suicide as when 'someone chooses to make his/her body stop working. Remember to tell the child that the person who committed suicide was sick (i.e., depressed).

2. Give age-appropriate facts and explanations. Tell the truth, answering questions as they come up. It is not necessary to share every detail. If the truth is not shared, and the child finds out later from outside of the family, the child can often feel betrayed and resentful.

3. Dispel myths of suicide.

4. Re-tell good memories to help balance the weight of the trauma.

5. Model feelings and thoughts for children that normalize grief.

6. Emphasize that suicide is a mistake because there is 'always another way out.' (Haine et al., 2008; Wesner, S., et al., 2006; Mitchell, A. M., et al., 2007)

Military Deployment or Death in the Line of Duty

Children of military families face special needs related to prolonged absences of the military parent. During deployment, it is important to have regularly scheduled time to communicate with the absent parent.

When death in the line of duty happens (military, police, fire, etc.), many children will be told that they should be proud of their dead parents for their service. This leaves the child in an untenable position in which to grieve the very real loss of the parent. For children of military parents, the death is only one of many major losses that happen quite immediate to the death, and which can include moving away from military support and housing, relocating to a new school (again non-military) so that the customary family supports are stripped away at a time when they are most needed. These children often respond well to the interventions listed above. (Swank & Robinson, H. M., 2009).

When the Initial Presentation Is Misbehavior or Delinquency

Anger, fighting, irritability and misbehavior are normal responses to loss due to death. Incarceration and foster care placement also may yield this type of response. Grief can be hidden because of the social stigma associated with the loss (e.g., HIV/AIDS, substance abuse). Therefore, it is very important to ask troubled children about loss. Punishing these children without attending to their grief needs is unfair.

Summary

Experiencing loss as a child is inevitable. Learning how to cope with grief through the support of loving adults is what helps the vast majority of children weather its vagaries and grow into healthy adults. However, there is indeed a subset of adults and their children who are at risk for complicated grief for whom early identification and intervention are critical in preventing serious complications later in life. Screening for complicated grief and referring for specialty care can prevent a sad experience from turning into a bad one.

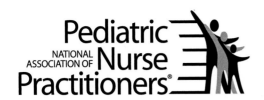

How Parents Can Help Children/Teens to Cope with Loss and Grief

What is Grief
Grief is a term used for the many feelings and behaviors we experience when we are faced with loss. The loss may be from the death of a significant other, relocation, or divorce. Grief is a normal reaction to loss and change. Children do experience grief as they have feelings and are aware of losses. However, children grieve differently based upon age and personality.

What Are Some of the Feelings Children Might Have
Children may have one more of these feelings: abandonment of the feelings of being left alone, anxiety, confusion, anger, guilt, fear, body distress, rejection, sadness, and panic. It is important to help children identify, label, and label about these different feelings.

What Is the Effect of Age on Children Who Are Grieving
Children's development and age will have an impact on how they think about deal and the loss.

Age	Reaction
Infants and young Children (0 - 2 years)	React the way they see their caretakers react. They may resist change and separation from caretakers.
Preschool aged children (3 - 5 years)	Do not accept death as permanent. They will often ask when the deceased person will return. They may react primarily to separation.
Young school-aged children (5 - 9 years)	Accept that death is permanent, but not universal. Question about why their loved one had to die and not someone else is common.
Older school-aged children (9 - 12 years)	See death as permanent and universal. They take death personally and understand they also will die someday. They are interested in concrete details about death, such as funeral and burial.
Older children (12 years and older)	Have started to reach an adult understanding of death. They spend a significant amount of time thinking about death and trying to understand what happens after death. They have very intense emotions during this time.

As children go through the different developmental stages, they re-grieve the loss and try to understand their loss in new ways. This can be confusing and difficult for adults.

What are Some of the Behaviors You May See in Your Child Who Is Grieving

Children will normally act out some of their feelings. In a supportive way, let children know what behavior you see that has changed. Continue to expect that the child will function. It is important to se limits on destructive behavior should disappear.

Temper outbursts, panic attacks, regression or less mature behavior, disinterest in usual activities, increased dependency on adults, stomachaches and headaches, silence, model child behaviors or trying to be "the perfect child", withdrawal, adult role behaviors or taking on adult responsibilities, over-activity.

What Is The Difference Between Grief and Mourning

Grief can be though of as the internal experience about a loss. Mourning and bereavement are words that people use about the outward signs of grief. The goal of dealing with children who are grieving is to help them talk about how they feel.

What is the Difference Between Grief and Depression

The symptoms of depression and grief are similar. If you have any concerns about how your child is adjusting to the loss or whether your child has slipped into depression... TALK TO SOMEONE! People that can help you are nurses, doctors, nurse practitioners, school counselors, and psychologists.

How do Children Grieve Differently than Adults

Adults often feels sad over an extended period of time, whereas children's grief tends to come and go. Children's expression of grief may flare up and then be over relatively quickly as they move on to the next activity. This "volcano"-like mourning, though different from that experienced by adults and possibly uncomfortable for adults, is a normal grief pattern for children.

Section 10 - Helping Children Deal With Death, Loss, and Grief

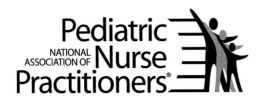

How Can I Help My Child Deal With Loss and Grief?

The following tasks help the child in adjusting to a loss. Each child will complete these tasks in his or her own way and on his/her own time schedule. The below suggestions may help you.

Task	Activites to Assist Child
Understanding: facing the reality of death	• Offer the child time to talk about death and loss as he/she experiences it in everyday life. Allow the child to tell his or her "story" of death of the loved one. • Be there to listen, including long after you think the child should be moving on, as he or she will revisit this grief throughout his/her life. • Answer questions about death and loss as honestly as possible.
Identifying and expressing feelings	• Show the child how you talk about feelings and help the child identify and express feelings. • Tell the child that his/her feelings are normal and that others feel the same way. • Offer age-appropriate expressions of feelings such as: writing about feelings; talking to someone about feelings; crying; laughing; snuggling; singing; arts and crafts; walking or other physical activity like dance and martial arts.
Commemorating/ honoring the person who died	• Assist your child with creating an ongoing list and put it on the refrigerator."Things I remember about _____" and have family members contribute to it when they want • Help your child write a story, poem, prayer, or song for the loved one. • Assist your child in creating a memory book or box with photographs and/or other items. • Take your child to the cemetery. Take flowers or a balloon. • Plant a tree or some flowers with your child in honor of the loved one.
Going on - not "getting over"	• Create a ritual good-bye to the loved one. • Ask your child to create a collage of the things that make him/her happy to be alive. • Express and validate the child's mixed feelings about "going on." • Develop rituals around anniversary dates for remembering the loved ones.

Adapted from: Nussbaum, K. (1998). Preparing the Children: Information and Ideas for Families Facing Terminal Illness and Death. Burnsville, North Carolina: *Compassion Books.*

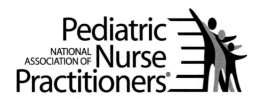

Information For Teens About Coping with Loss and Grief

What is Grief
Grief is the term used for many feelings and behaviors we experience when we are faced with loss. The loss may be from the death of a significant other, relocation, or divorce. Grief is a natural and normal reaction to loss and change. Teens do experience grief as they have feelings and are aware of losses. However, everyone experiences grief differently.

What Are Some of the Feelings I May Have
You many have 1 or more of these feelings: abandonment or feeling of being left alone, anxiety, confusing, anger, guilt, fear body, distress, rejection, sadness, and panic. It is important to try to identify, name, and talk about these different feelings with your parent, a health professional, or counselor.

Some Teens Who Are Grieving May Notice Some of These Behaviors
Temper outbursts, panic attacks, regression or less mature behavior, disinterest in usual activities, increased dependency on adults, stomachaches and headaches, silence, trying to be "the perfect child", withdrawal, taking on adult activities, over-activity. If you notice any of these changes in your behavior, again share this with your parent, a health professional, or counselor.

What Is the Difference between Grief and Depression
The symptoms of depression and grief are similar. If you have any concerns about how you are adjusting to your loss or wondering if you depressed........ TALK TO SOMEONE! People that can help you are nurses, doctors, nurse practitioners, school counselors, and psychologists.

How do Teens Grieve Differently than Adults
Adults often feel sad over an extended period of time, whereas a teen's grief tends to come and go. Your expression of grief may flare up and then be over quickly as you move on to the next activity. This "rollercoaster" feeling, though different from that experiences by adults and possibly uncomfortable for adults, is a normal grief pattern for teens.

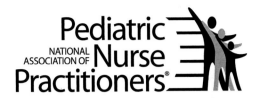

What Can I Do To Help Myself Deal with Loss and Grief?

There are certain tasks that help people adjust to a loss. Every person will complete these tasks in his or her own time and in his/her own way. The below suggestions may help you.

Understanding: facing the reality of death

1. Take the time to talk about death and loss as you experience it in everyday life. Tell your "story" of the death of your loved one.

2. Find someone who will listen -- a parent, a trusted adult, a health professional, or counselor.

3. Find someone who will listen long after you think you should be moving on, as you will revisit this grief in some way throughout your life.

4. Ask questions about death and loss.

Identifying and expressing feelings

1. Notice how other people talk about feelings.

2. Trying to identify and express your feelings.

3. Try one of these activities:
   - ♥ writing about feelings
   - ♥ talking to someone about feelings
   - ♥ snuggling
   - ♥ arts and crafts
   - ♥ physical activity like dance, martial arts.
   - ♥ crying
   - ♥ laughing
   - ♥ singing
   - ♥ walking

Commemorating/honoring the person who died

1. Create an ongoing list and put it on the refrigerator: "Things I remember about _____" and have family members contribute to it when they want.

2. Write a story, poem, prayer, or song for the loved one.

3. Create a memory book or box with photographs and/or items.

4. Plan a visit to the cemetery with your family. Take flowers or a balloon.

Going on - not "getting over.

1. Create a ritual to say good-bye to the loved one.

2. Create a collage of the feelings that make you happy to be alive.

3. Express your mixed feelings about "going on".

4. Develop rituals around anniversary dates for remembering the loved one.

Adapted from: Nussbaum, K. (1998). Preparing the Children: Information and Ideas for Families Facing Terminal Illness and Death. Burnsville, North Carolina: *Compassion Books.*

REFERENCES

American Psychiatric Association. (2010). *A Statement on the proposal to eliminate the grief exclusion criterion from major depression.* Arlington: Kenneth S. Kendler, M.D.

Brent, D. (2012). *Resilience in the face of loss; promoting healthy development in parentally bereaved youth* [PowerPoint slides]. Retrieved from STAR-Center, Services for Teens at Risk Website: www.starcenter.pitt.edu.

Children's Grief Education Association (2004). *Navigating children's grief: How to help following a death.* Mary M. Lyles, MSW, LCSW.

Cohen, J. A. & Mannarino, A. P. (2010). Psychotherapeutic options for traumatized children. *Current Opinion in Pediatrics,* 22(5), 605-609. Retrieved Oct. 25, 2012, from http://dx.doi.org/10.1097/MOP.0b013e32833e14a2

Felitti, V.J. (2002). The relation between adverse childhood experiences and adult health: Turning gold into lead. *The Permanente Journal,* 6(1), 44-47. Retrieved Oct. 25, 2012, from http://xnet.kp.org/permanentejournal/winter02/goldtolead.pdf.

Goldman, L. (2001). *Breaking the silence: A guide to help children with complicated grief—suicide, homicide, aids, violence, and abuse.* New York, NY: Brunner-Routledge.

Grohol, J. M. (2005). New complicated grief treatment holds promise for millions, Pitt researchers report. *Psych Central - Trusted mental health, depression, bipolar, ADHD and psychology information.* Retrieved Oct. 25, 2012, from http://psychcentral.com/news/archives/2005-05/uopm-ncg052505.html

Haine, R. A., Ayers, T. S., Sandler, I. N., & Wolchik, S. A. (2008). Evidence-based practices for parentally bereaved children and their families. *Professional Psychology: Research and Practice, 39*(2), 113-121. Retrieved Sept. 18, 2012, from http://dx.doi.org/10.1037/0735-7028.39.2.113

JAMA and Archives Journals (2011). Grief reactions subside in most children and teens whose parent dies suddenly, but may persist or increase in some cases. *ScienceDaily.* Retrieved Oct. 25, 2012, from http://www.sciencedaily.com/releases/2011/09/110906183111.htm

Johns Hopkins Medical Institutions (2010). Children who lose a parent to suicide more likely to die the same way, study finds. *ScienceDaily.* Retrieved Oct. 25, 2012, from http://www.sciencedaily.com /releases/2010/04/100421160013.htm

Kersting, K. (2004). A new approach to complicated grief. *American Psychological Association,* 35(10), 51. Retrieved Sept. 18, 2012, from http://www.apa.org/monitor/nov04/grief.aspx

Mayo Clinic Staff (2011). Complicated grief: Treatments and drugs. *Mayo Clinic.* Retrieved Oct. 25, 2012, from http://www.mayoclinic.com/health/complicated-grief/DS01023/DSECTION=treatments-and-drugs

Melhem N. M., Porta G., Shamseddeen W., Walker Payne M., Brent D. A. (2011). Grief in children and adolescents bereaved by sudden parental death. *Archives of General Psychiatry. 68*(9):911-919. doi:10.1001/archgenpsychiatry.2011.101.

Melhem N. M., Walker M., Moritz G., Brent D. A. (2008). Antecedents and sequelae of sudden parental death in offspring and surviving caregivers. *Archives of Pediatric and Adolescent Medicine.* 162(5):403-410. doi:10.1001/archpedi.162.5.403.

Mitchell, A. M., Wesner, S., Brownson, L., Gale, D. D., Garand, L., & Havill, A. (2006). Effective communication with bereaved child survivors of suicide. *Journal of Child and Adolescent Psychiatric Nursing,* 19(3), 130-136. Retrieved Sept. 18, 2012, from http://dx.doi.org/10.1111/j.1744-6171.2006.00060.x

Mitchell, A. M., Wesner, S., Garand, L., Gale, D. D., Havill, A., & Brownson, L. (2007). A support group intervention for children bereaved by parental suicide. *Journal of Child and Adolescent Psychiatric Nursing,* 20(1), 3-13. Retrieved Sept. 18, 2012, from http://dx.doi.org/10.1111/j.1744-6171.2007.00073.x

National Alliance for Grieving Children (2012). *National poll of bereaved children & teenagers.* Stuart, FL: Andy McNiel.

Prigerson, H. G., Horowitz, M. J., Jacobs, S. C., Parkes, C. M., Aslan, M., Goodkin, K., et al. (2009). Prolonged grief disorder: Psychometric validation of criteria proposed for DSM-5™ and ICD-11. *PLoS Medicine,* 6(8). Retrieved Sept. 18, 2012, from http://dx.doi.org/10.1371/journal.pmed.1000121

Ryan's Heart. (2009). *Just for me! Healing activities for grieving children and teens.* Presque Isle: www.ryansheartnpo.org.

Schoenfelder, E. N., Sandler, I., Wolchik, S., & MacKinnon, D. (2011). Quality of social relationships and the development of depression in parentally-bereaved youth. *Journal of Youth and Adolescence,* 40(1), 85-96.

Shear, K., Frank, E., Houck, P., & Reynolds, C. I. (2005). Treatment of complicated grief: A randomized controlled trial. *JAMA: The Journal of the American Medical Association*, 293(21), 2601-2608. Retrieved Oct. 25, 2012, from http://dx.doi.org/10.1001/jama.293.21.2601

Shear, M. K., Simon, N., Wall, M., Zisook, S., Neimeyer, R., Duan, N., et al. (2011). Complicated grief and related bereavement issues for DSM-5. *Depression and Anxiety*, 28(2), 103-117. Retrieved Sept. 18, 2012, from http://www.ncbi.nlm.nih.gov/pmc/articles/PMC3075805/?tool=pmcentrez

Silberner, J. (2005). Research points to new method of treating severe grief. *NPR Radio*. Retrieved Sept. 18, 2012, from www.npr.org/templates/story/story.php?storyId=4674922&ps

Swank, J. M. & Robinson, E. H. M. (2009). *Addressing grief and loss issues with children and adolescents of military families*. Presentation delivered at The American counseling association annual conference and exposition, Charlotte, North Carolina.

University of California - Los Angeles (2008). Addicted to grief? Chronic grief activates pleasure areas of the brain. *ScienceDaily*. Retrieved Sept. 18, 2012, from http://www.sciencedaily.com/releases/2008/06/080620195446.htm?utm_source=feedburner&utm_medium=feed&utm_campaign=Feed%3A+sciencedaily+%28ScienceDaily%3A+Latest+Science+News%29

University of Georgia (2008). Treating post-traumatic stress first helps children overcome grief, study shows. *ScienceDaily*. Retrieved Oct. 25, 2012, from http://www.sciencedaily.com /releases/2008/04/080408160631.htm

Wagner, B., Knaevelsrud, C., & Maercker, A. (2006). Internet-based cognitive-behavioral therapy for complicated grief: A randomized controlled trial. *Death Studies*, 30(5), 429-453. Retrieved July 11, 2013, from http://dx.doi.org/10.1080/07481180600614385

SECTION 11
Bernadette Mazurek Melnyk and Linda J. Alpert-Gillis

Marital Separation and Divorce

Fast Facts

- Divorce affects more than 1 million children every year.

- Over 30 years of research indicates that the outcomes for children and adolescents following divorce are determined by numerous factors that can increase risk or foster resilience.

- The risk of emotional, behavioral, social, and academic problems for children of divorced parents (25%) is more than double than that of children whose parents are continuously married (10%). However, the differences between children of divorced and married families are modest and not universal.

- Externalizing problems (e.g., acting out behaviors, impulsivity) have been consistently identified as the most common problems identified in children after divorce.

- Between 75% and 80% of children of divorce fall within the average range or better on objective measures of adjustment 2-3 years after parental divorce.

- Interparental hostility and lack of cooperation between parents following divorce is the most consistent predictor of poor outcomes among children.

- Risk factors linked to negative outcomes following divorce with robust empirical support include: parental conflict, psychological adjustment of the parents, quality and type of parenting and parent-child relationships, loss of important relationships, parental cohabitation and remarriage, family structure transitions, and economic resources.

- Protective factors linked to resilience in children with strong empirical evidence include: reduced or encapsulated parental conflict, good adjustment of the residential parent, competent parenting of both parents and cooperative or parallel co-parenting styles, higher levels of involvement of the nonresidential parent, limited number of family transitions, and economic stability.

- The child's age at the time of divorce affects outcomes related to the developmental tasks associated with that age.

- No consistent gender differences are attributable to divorce.

Additional Facts About Conflict

- Parents' post-separation conflict levels are not predicted by level of conflict prior to separation.

- 8%-12% of parents exhibit high levels of conflict 2-3 years after divorce.

- Intensity, conflict style, and focus of marital conflict are better predictors of child outcomes than frequency of conflict or legal conflict.

- There are direct and indirect effects of high levels of conflict on children's adjustment. A direct effect is that children often model their parents' aggressive behavior in their own relationships and do not learn age-appropriate social skills for conflict resolution. Indirect effects are mediated through variables such as quality of parenting which impacts emotional security.

- Most deleterious impact of post-divorce conflict occurs when parents involve their children directly in the conflict including using them as messengers as well as when parents talk in a hostile and demeaning manner about the other parent. The degree of legal conflict between parents is not associated with child adjustment.

- Protective factors in families that have high conflict include: warm, competent parenting; not exposing children directly to the conflict; not using children to express anger to the other parent; refraining from making negative comments about the other parent; and positive sibling relationships.

- A good relationship with at least one caregiver or adult mentor and supportive sibling relationships are buffers against the effects of high parental conflict.

Additional Facts About Parents and Parenting

- The adjustment of the parent with primary residential custody is one of the most powerful predictors of children's psychological adjustment following divorce. Parental depression, anxiety, and long-term mental health problems, such as personality disorders, are associated with externalizing, internalizing and academic problems in children. Significant mental health problems interfere with the quality of parenting and the parent-child relationship which is associated with children's adjustment.

- Shortly after separation, some parents experience a "honeymoon" period in which they feel relieved that a stressful marriage has ended, whereas others feel anxiety, anger/guilt, depression, exhaustion, and helplessness.

- Most adults report that their low point is a year after marital separation, with full adjustment taking 2 to 3 years.

- Quality of parenting is a major predictor of adjustment and academic performance at least of equal importance as conflict in determining risk. Positive adjustment is associated with effective parenting, greater father involvement, and close father-child relationships. Children are found to function best when both parents provide adequate and nurturing parenting in each home and have a cooperative or parallel co-parenting relationship.

- Economic difficulties are associated with increased parental conflict and poorer parental functioning, which predict poorer child adjustment.

Additional Facts About Remarriage and Family Transitions

- Remarriage is not a protective factor and does not in itself decrease the risk of adverse outcomes for children.

- Cohabitation is associated with more negative outcomes for children compared to children in remarried families.

- Positive stepfather-child relationships and nonresident father-child relationships are associated with lowered risk for both externalizing and internalizing symptoms.

- Each change in family structure increases the risk of behavioral and social problems, drug use, and poorer academic achievement.

Typical Responses to Marital Separation

Young Children

- Regression
- Irritability and restlessness
- Temper tantrums
- Sleeping difficulties
- Separation problems
- Anger
- Increased whining and crying
- Sadness
- Guilt
- Fear of abandonment
- Excessive clinging
- Withdrawal

School-Aged Children

- Sadness
- Depression
- Longing for parent's return
- Withdrawal
- Denial
- Somatic complaints
- Parentification
- Deterioration in school performance
- Low self-esteem
- Anger
- Preoccupation with parent's departure from home
- Decrease in peer relations
- Shame
- Loyalty conflicts
- Reunification fantasies
- Behavioral problems

Adolescents

- Anger
- Blaming one paren
- Attempts to gain control
- Denial
- Somatic complaints
- Low self-esteem
- Sadness
- Depression
- Loyalty conflicts
- Acting out or immature behaviors
- Parentification
- Increase in sexual activity and drug and alcohol usage
- Withdrawal

Responses to Marital Separation That Require Immediate Assessment and Intervention

- Self-injury, cutting or eating disorders
- Frequent angry/violent outbursts
- Severe depression and/or withdrawal from primary relationships
- Significant academic or social difficulty at school
- Drug or alcohol abuse
- Hopelessness or suicidal ideation

Critical History-Taking Questions When a Divorce or Separation Has Occurred

- Have there been any changes in your family since your last visit? (This is an essential question as parents may not disclose a marital transition unless directly asked.)

- What are the parents' and child's perceptions of the divorce?

- How are the parents and child coping with the divorce and what are their responses? Specifically, how have their emotions and behaviors changed?

- What is the parents' knowledge of the impact of divorce on their children and the typical responses that children have when adjusting to the transition?

- What changes have occurred in parenting practices and daily routines (e.g., limit setting, child care arrangements)?

- What are the family's other major life stressors (e.g., move to a new home, change in job, financial difficulties)?

- How much and what type of conflict between the parents is occurring, and is the child a witness or involved in that conflict?

- What social supports do the parent and child have in place to assist them in coping with the separation and divorce?

- What is the level of involvement of the non-residential parent?

- What is the parents' and child's mood state (e.g., anxiety, depression)?

- Specifically ask, on a scale of 0 to 10, "How stressed/anxious as well as depressed are you (your child) on a daily basis?"

- What is the parents' and child's current level of functioning (e.g., at work and at school)?

- What is worrying the parent and child most at this time?

Early Interventions

- Educate parents about **risk factors** that can lead to child adjustment difficulties: parental conflict, psychological adjustment of the parents, quality and type of parenting and parent-child relationships, loss of important relationships, parental cohabitation and remarriage, family structure transitions, and economic resources.

- Educate parents about **protective factors** linked to resilience in children: low levels of parental conflict or encapsulated parental conflict, good adjustment of the residential parent, competent parenting of both parents and cooperative or parallel co-parenting styles, higher levels of involvement of the nonresidential parent, limited number of family transitions, and economic stability.

- When there are high levels of conflict in the family, it is especially important to share with families the factors that can ameliorate its impact: warm, competent parenting; positive sibling relationships; not exposing children directly to the conflict; not using children to express anger to the other parent; and refraining from making negative comments about the other parent.

- Emphasizing the importance of self-care for the parent and discussing with parents that their own functioning is one of the most powerful predictors of children's psychological adjustment following divorce. Advise the parent to obtain counseling if he or she is having difficulty coping and notice that this is affecting their parenting.

- Inform the parent that it is not helpful to set unrealistic expectations for themselves or their children and that the process of adjustment to this transition may take up to 2 to 3 years.

- Educate the parents about typical age-appropriate responses that children have to separation and divorce.

- Counsel parents about age-appropriate strategies to help their children cope with the transition.

- Provide parents with the handout, "A dozen ways to help your child deal with divorce," available in this guide.

- Advise parents to consistently reinforce to their child that: (a) the divorce is not the child's fault (as children often feel guilty about it); and (b) that they will not abandon him or her (children need this reinforcement). However, it is important to not make promises that you do not have control over such as frequency of contact with the nonresidential parent.

- Encourage parents to help their children openly express their feelings about the divorce (younger children often express their feelings by talking about how their stuffed animal or puppet feels).

- Encourage parents to spend special time with their child every day, even if only for 15 minutes, without interruptions, and to maintain routines.

- Assist the parent with discipline; encourage the importance of setting of limits and reinforcing them consistently. (Although he or she cannot control what happens at the other parent's home, the parent can implement limits at his or her own home.)

- Offer parents the COPE program (Creating Opportunities for Parent Empowerment), an evidence-based user-friendly program designed to assist parents in helping 3 to 7 year old children cope with divorce. The program can be obtained from Bernadette Melnyk at cope.melnyk@gmail.com.

- Provide local resources to help parents and children deal with the divorce (e.g., Parents without Partners).

- Inform the parents to contact you with any concerns or worries about their child.

Screening for Marital Transitions

Because of the major impact that marital transitions (i.e., separation, divorce, remarriage) have on families, it is very important to ask the following questions at each healthcare encounter.

For Parents and Children/Teens:

Have there been any changes in your family in the past year, such as marital separation/divorce or remarriage?

On a scale of 0 to 10, if 0 means "there is no fighting" and 10 means "there is a lot of fighting," how much arguing/fighting goes on between family members?

On a scale of 0 to 10, if 0 means you "have no stress" and 10 means you have "a lot of stress," how much stress is the family situation causing you?

On a scale of 0 to 10, if 0 means "not at all" and 10 means "a lot," how much is the family situation affecting your ability to work (for parents) or to do well in school (for children/teens)?

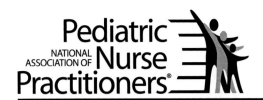

A Dozen Ways to Help your Child Deal with Marital Separation/Divorce

1) Understand the impact of divorce on children	Marital separation involves stressful and difficult transitions for children and parents. It is common for children to show some behavioral changes in response to such transitions. There are parenting strategies that can help you and your children cope effectively with your family situation.
2) Prepare your children for the changes changes involved in a divorce.	Give children information about family in a way they can understand. Tell children in advance about the changes they are about to experience.
3) Accept children's feelings and encourage talking them.	Help your children learn to talk about their about feelings and express feelings in acceptable ways. When children can put their feelings into they are much less likely to act out inappropriately.
4) Reassure your children.	Make sure that your children know that you love them and that you will take care of them. Inform your children that you are divorcing the other parent, not them. Provide assurance that a parent's love for a child is a special kind that does not stop.
5) Allow your children to be children.	Avoid having your child take on too many adult responsibilities. Discussing family finances with them or telling them that they are now the "little man or woman of the house" can be a burden. Instead, encourage them to become involved in school activities, clubs, or hobbies that develop their own strength and abilities.
6) Give children permission to love both parents. Support your children's relationship with their other parent.	Children benefit from a positive relationship with both a consistent schedule of when children will be with each parent is very important. Also, not talking in a negative way about the other parent can allow your children a healthier relationship with both parents.
7) Problem solve together.	Talk with your children about how to make things better or more comfortable for them.
8) Work on your relationship with your children.	Set aside special time to spend with each child, doing things together such are reading, playing a game, or taking a walk.
9) Keep conflict away from your children.	Keep arguments with your former spouse as far away from your children as possible, especially if they involve verbal or physical aggression. Intense conflict between parents is likely to lead to adjustment problems in children. Do not use your children as messengers or as weapons to get back at your former spouse.
10) Maintain as much structure and predictability in your everyday routine as possible.	Children thrive on routine, including regular bedtimes, having meals together and consistent rules. Setting limits on children's inappropriate behavior helps children feel safe and communicate to them that you will provide order and control when they are not able to do so.
11) Listen to children's verbal and nonverbal communication.	Listen to what your children say and watch what they do. Remember children often state things indirectly. For, example, "I hate the woman you're dating" may mean "I am worried that you like her more than me."
12) Take care of yourself.	Reach out to resources such as trusted friends, family members, Support groups, members of the clergy and mental health professionals. Research has emphasized the important link between parents' emotional and physical well-being and children's healthy development.

Reprinted with permission from: Melnyk, B.M. & Alpert-Gillis, L.J. (1997). Coping with marital separation. Smoothing the transition for parents and children. Journal of Pediatric Health Care, 11: 165-174.

Internet Resources

American Academy of Child and Adolescent Psychiatry Facts for Families
www.aacap.org

This Website is an excellent source of information on the assessment and treatment of child and adolescent mental health disorders. The AACAP developed Facts for Families Handouts to provide concise and up-to-date information on issues that affect children, teens, and their families. These handouts are available in English and Spanish and can be duplicated and distributed free of charge as long as AACAP is properly credited and no profit is gained from their use.

HELPGUIDE.org
www.helpguide.org

HELPGUIDE is a non-profit organization that maintains a Website to assist individuals and families with accurate information about a variety of mental health disorders and challenging family issues, such as divorce and remarriage.

KidsHealth
www.kidshealth.org

This is an outstanding Website that contains health information for healthcare providers, parents, teens, and children. Many of the topics relate to emotions and behaviors (e.g., anxiety, fears, and depression) as well as family changes and are developmentally sensitive to specific age groups. Physicians and other healthcare providers review all material before it is posted on this Website.

REFERENCES

Amato, P.R. (2000). The consequences of divorce for adults and children. *Journal of Marriage and Family*, 62(4), 1269-1287.

Emory, R.E. (2004). *The Truth About Children and Divorce: Dealing with the Emotions so You and Your Children Can Thrive*. New York, NY: Viking Penguin.

Jellinek, M., Patel, B.P., & Froehle, M. (2002). *Bright Futures in Practice: Mental Health- Vol 1Practice Guide*. Arlington, VA: National Center for Education in Maternal and Child Health.

Jellinek, M., Patel, B.P., & Froehle, M. (2002). *Bright Futures in Practice: Mental Health- Vol II. Tool Kit*. Arlington, VA: National Center for Education in Maternal and Child Health.

Kelly, J.B. (2012). Risk and protective factors associated with child and adolescent adjustment following separation and divorce: Social science applications. In Kuehnle, K. & Drozd, L. (Eds.) *Parenting Plan Evaluations: Applied Research for the Family Court* (pp.49-84). UK: Oxford University Press.

Leon, K. (2003). Risk and protective factors in young children's adjustment to parental divorce: A review of the research. *Family Relations*, 52(3), 258-270.

SECTION 12
Pamela Herendeen

Child Maltreatment

Fast Facts

- Child maltreatment is defined as the causation of a non-accidental injury. It may be physical or sexual abuse, and includes inflicting a physical or sexual offense against a child or allowing a physical/sexual offense to be inflicted on a child.

- Child neglect is defined as the omission in care of a child's basic needs that may result in harm or potential harm. It is a significant cause of morbidity and mortality in children.

- Psychological maltreatment is a repeated pattern of damaging interactions from a parent to a child.

- About 3 million reports are filed each year on children suspected to have been abused or neglected. Out of these less than1 million are substantiated. Most of child maltreatment falls under neglect.

- Every day, four children in our country die of child maltreatment. Most victims are under 6 years of age.

- Annual costs of child abuse are estimated at $80 billion.

- Most perpetrators are primary caregivers.

- Domestic violence is significantly correlated with child maltreatment. Millions of children witness domestic violence in their lifetime, significantly increasing the risk of child maltreatment

- Girls who are abused as children may be more likely to become victims of violence as adults. Boys abused as children may be more likely to commit acts of violence as adults.

- Child maltreatment tends to be repetitive and frequently will escalate over time. In many cases the abuser does not intend to hurt the child. Rather, abuse is the result of unrealistic caretaker expectations and poor coping mechanisms of the caregiver.

- Although child maltreatment crosses all socioeconomic, racial, and religious boundaries, high-risk socioeconomic factors are associated with an increased risk of abuse and neglect.

Risk Factors

- Young and/or single caregivers

- Unrealistic expectations of caregivers

- Caregivers with a history of being abused

- Unwanted pregnancy

- Economic or social stressors

- Substance abuse/mental illness/developmental delay of the caregiver

- Domestic violence in the home

- Children who have fussy/challenging behavior, are under 3 years old, have chronic medical conditions, developmental disabilities , or in foster care

Common Presenting Complaints

Any one indicator is not definitive – it just raises questions. Many primary care providers (PCPs) are resistant to making Child Protective Service (CPS) reports -- they feel they "know" the family well and want to spare the "nice" family the aggravation of dealing with CPS – but please try to be objective and make referrals to CPS based on the history and indicators.

- Triggers of Abuse
- Excessive crying/fussy
- Acute illness
- Frequent nighttime awakenings
- Toilet training
- Feeding issues
- Oppositional behavior

Behavioral Indicators

- Behavioral extremes and mood swings
- Mental health disorders/suicidal ideation
- Anger issues/harming of others or animals
- Alcohol or substance abuse
- School problems
- Poor social interactions with peers
- Conversion reactions/psychosomatic illnesses
- Sleep/appetite/behavior changes
- Self-injurious behavior

Behavioral Indicators Specific for Sexual Abuse

- Provocative behavior
- Aggressive sexual behavior
- Increased sexual knowledge
- Regression/new fearfulness
- New money or gifts
- Depression/self-mutilation

Physical Indicators of Concern:

- Bruises, burns, fractures not consistent with developmental stage or a delay in care; injuries to mouth (especially in an infant); any bruise/burn/fracture in a non-ambulatory child that lacks a very corroborating history
- Bruising on the face, neck, wrists, ankles, back, genitals, thighs; bruises in the shape of a hand or object
- Bites that are too large to be a child's
- Burns that are patterned, immersion, cigarette shaped

- Any fracture occurring in a child aged 1 year or younger; fractures of the skull, spiral, rib, metaphyseal, spinal, hands/feet, or fractures in multiple stages of healing
- Head trauma with subdural hematomas, retinal hemorrhages
- Neglect issues (e.g., inappropriate clothing, poor weight gain, poor medical compliance, lack of appropriate supervision, poor hygiene)
- Itching, discomfort, lesions, bleeding, discharge in genitals
- Pain with bowel movements/dysuria
- New-onset encopresis/enuresis
- STDs/pregnancy depending on age or situation
- Any injury that does not fit the history

Screening Tools

There are very few screening tools that have been methodically tested to assist in the identification of child abuse. Currently, there are a number of studies that are evaluating the feasibility of using a tool for this purpose. However, there is insufficient evidence that these tools will adequately predict child maltreatment, though some have demonstrated promise. Dubowitz has demonstrated that the SEEK Model of focused questions for the caregiver may identify/prevent child maltreatment. The Edinburgh Postnatal Depression Scale or Beck Post-partum Depression Screening Scale are tools that are currently being utilized in some pediatric practices to screen families. There is evidence to support that a mother who is depressed is at high risk for neglect and abuse of her child. The GAPS (Guidelines for Adolescent Preventive Services) form for adolescents briefly addresses abuse and may provide insight to the provider. Any of the many tools that are currently being utilized for mood/ mental health disorders may be useful in identifying abuse and neglect. Anticipatory guidance regarding child maltreatment and violence should be done at every well child visit. One of the main challenges for healthcare providers is how to add more questions in an already limited time period. Another major concern is how to adequately screen the parent for domestic violence issues with the child in the room, and how to screen the child for abuse issues with the parent in the room. The following brief screening questions may be utilized during a visit to identify abuse and violence in the home.

Questions for Parents

- Because violence is so common, ask about violence in the home.
- Are you in a relationship where you are being hurt physically or emotionally?
- Have you ever been emotionally or physically abused by your partner (e.g., have you ever been hit, kicked, slapped, punched, isolated from your family or someone important to you by your partner?)
- Are you afraid of anyone in your home?
- Do you ever feel so frustrated/overwhelmed that you fear you may hit or hurt your child?
- Have the police come to your home?
- The U.S. Preventive Services Task Force (USPSTF) recommends that clinicians screen women of childbearing age for intimate partner violence (IPV), such as domestic violence, and provide or refer women who screen positive to intervention services. This recommendation applies to women who do not have signs or symptoms of abuse. See http://www.uspreventiveservicestaskforce.org/uspstf12/ipvelder/ipvelderfinalrs.htm#summary

Screening Tools for Intimate Partner Violence (IPV)

Several screening instruments can be used to screen women for IPV. Those with the highest levels of sensitivity and specificity for identifying IPV are:

- Hurt, Insult, Threaten, Scream (HITS) (English and Spanish versions available)
- Ongoing Abuse Screen/Ongoing Violence Assessment Tool (OAS/OVAT)
- Slapped, Threatened, and Throw (STaT)
- Humiliation, Afraid, Rape, Kick (HARK)
- Modified Childhood Trauma Questionnaire–Short Form (CTQ-SF)
- Woman Abuse Screen Tool (WAST)

Questions for Children/Teens

- Are you afraid of anyone in your home?
- Whom could you tell if anyone has touched you in your private area? Has this ever happened to you?
- What happens when your parents are angry with you or you get into trouble?
- Do you ever get hit or spanked? What do they hit you with? Are there ever marks left?
- What happens when adults in your home are angry at each other?
- Have the police been to your home?

Assessment

- Thorough psychosocial assessment including current concerns, history of violence in the home, family constellation, day care arrangements, custody issues, economic stressors, child's behavior, prior involvement with police/child protective services
- Complete medical history including any presenting physical symptoms, behavior – especially recent changes, psychosocial history, current/past medications, allergies, chronic illnesses
- Complete physical exam, including the genital area

  — Carefully examine head to toe for any bruises, burns, bites, abrasions, erythema, swelling, old patterned scars (especially in soft tissue areas)-extra concern for patterned or shaped injuries, limited mobility of an extremity. Note growth pattern. Genitalia examine for erythema, swelling, bruising, tears, friability, fissures, bleeding, discharge, lesions.

  — Any injury (bruising, burns fractures) in a non-ambulatory child deserves a full child abuse work up unless you have a detailed, corroborating history. For other children it would be dependent on the history provided.

  — Medical photography is advised with any physical injuries for documentation.

  —A full child abuse work-up would include a skeletal survey for any child <u>younger than 2 years of age,</u> head imaging and ophthalmology exam for retinal hemorrhages (especially with any facial bruising, head injury, neurological impairment), labs inclusive of bleeding studies and a trauma panel, abdominal imaging if symptomatic or belly bruising, other labs as indicated.

  —Sexual abuse history/disclosure or symptoms very dependent on timing and community protocols. A disclosure of sexual abuse <96 hours often requires an evidence collection kit. Cultures may need to be obtained; prophylactic medications usually not given to pre-pubertal children with the possible exception of HIV meds.

- Many communities now have a child abuse team or child advocacy center staffed with experts to assist you through the process of the assessment and management of child abuse. Please be aware of your community resources and utilize to help you complete an accurate and safe assessment and plan for your patient.

Diagnosis

The identification of child maltreatment is a very complex diagnosis based on psychosocial factors, social history, medical history, and physical findings. It is advisable to consult a child abuse expert to assist you in your diagnosis. Be extraordinarily careful of your documentation, first presenting the history and your objective findings. It is always recommended to consult with an expert unless you are very sure of your diagnosis as you may find yourself in a legal court of law.

Over 90% of known sexual abuse victims have a normal exam. Please refer to the scale developed by Dr. Joyce Adams for child sexual abuse in the reference section.

Management is very specific for the type of child maltreatment that is diagnosed. A child abuse expert should be consulted whenever possible. Foremost, the safe disposition of the child needs to be considered. Use of a child advocacy center is encouraged if there is one located in your region. An interview and/or an exam by a formally trained child abuse specialist is always advised.

Sexual Abuse: A full exam, including genitals with cultures for gonorrhea, chlamydia, with any disclosure is necessary. An evidence collection kit should be considered if the contact was less than 96 hours. Blood work for Hepatitis B & C, HIV, and RPR is recommended. With the exception of HIV (consult Peds ID), no prophylactic treatment of a prepubescent child is recommended. An adolescent needs pregnancy and STD prophylaxis if indicated. Photograph any injuries noted.

Physical Abuse: Very dependent on sustained injuries. Must consider a skeletal survey if <u>child is younger than 2</u> years of age, head imaging, trauma labs, ophthalmology exam, abdominal imaging – this is all very individualized. The history must be correlated with the injuries before you can determine a diagnosis. It is recommended that the skeletal survey be repeated in two weeks to ascertain the healing of possible injuries.

Neglect: Often CPS and other agencies need to intervene to ensure that appropriate resources are implemented. These children all need a full physical, including genitals, and further work ups as indicated.

Again, all of these children will benefit from a CAC and/or a child abuse specialist team to guide your care.

Evidence-Based Management

Prevention Is Key

Child maltreatment is extremely detrimental to children. As healthcare providers, it is important to focus on prevention and to recognize the risk factors early on for our patients. Advocating for children and families is the key to prevention!

Remember: All Healthcare Providers Are Mandated Reporters

You do not have to decide whether or not a child is being maltreated – that is the responsibility of CPS. You are mandated to report if you have a reasonable suspicion of abuse or neglect. There are certain physical or behavioral indicators that should raise a red flag about the possibility. The history must always be integrated together with behavioral and physical indicators. Clearly, some of these indicators may be the result of other stressors in a child's life. Any one indicator is not.

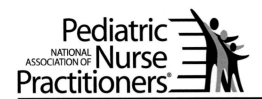

Information for Parents on Child Maltreatment

Important Facts

Child abuse and neglect is defined as causing non-accidental injury or not providing for a child's basic needs. About 3 million reports are filed every year on children that someone suspects may have been abused or neglected. It is unusual for a child that is not walking yet to sustain a lot of bruises, burns or other physical injuries. You should have a high level of concern if you see these in a child and call the child's healthcare provider.

Child sexual abuse is any use of a child for the sexual gratification of an adult. This includes touching a child's genitals, making a child touch someone else's genitals, pornography, and exposing a person's genitals to a child.

Domestic violence is closely related to child abuse. Millions of children witness domestic violence every day. The risk of these children being abused doubles if the mother is being battered. Girls raised in violent homes are at risk for becoming victims of violence as they grow older, while boys are at risk for growing up to be aggressive and violent. Many times the abuser does not intend to hurt the child. Often, they are a loving parent or caregiver who loses control and has unrealistic expectations of the child. Child abuse and violence happens on every level of society. However, it tends to be more frequent in homes that have a lot of stressors.

It also is important to know that the majority of children who are sexually or physically abused are violated by someone they know, often being one of their caretakers.

How You Can Protect Your Children and Adolescents

- There are some behavioral signs in children that may indicate a child is being abused. However, some of these can be the result of other stressors in a child's life. Any one sign doesn't mean the child is being abused, but the presence of several of these signs should raise concern.
- Appetite changes
- Nightmares/change in sleeping habits
- Mood swings including aggression (especially if child is hurting other people or animals), depression, anxiety, or self-mutilation
- Suicidal ideation
- Provocative behavior
- Extreme fears
- Regression of behavior
- Alcohol/drug abuse
- School problems
- Frequent complaints of headaches, stomachaches, or other illnesses that seem to be excessive and lacks a medical foundation

In addition to behavior signs, here are some physical signs to alert you:

- Frequent bruising, especially in a young infant or on the face, chest, back, or genitals
- Pain, extreme redness, discharge, or lesions in the genital region

- Injuries/fractures that are inconsistent with the description of the injury
- Poor weight gain, excessive weight gain, inappropriate clothing, no medical care for a child

If you are concerned about any behavioral or physical signs of abuse, please call your primary care provider. He or she can guide you through the process of how to figure everything out.

- It is important to teach children about safety and protecting themselves as they get older. Here are some things that you and your family can do to prevent abuse:
- Adults must watch for signs of abuse as young children cannot protect themselves.
- Be alert to changes in their behavior and discuss it with them.
- Teach your children how and when to say "no." They need to know that they can say no if someone makes them uncomfortable or scared.
- Set privacy boundaries within your family.
- Teach children that special secrets about touching or physical harm are not okay.
- Teach children the correct names of body parts.
- Make sure to keep the lines of communication open. LISTEN AND TALK to your children and adolescents all the time. Make sure they know they can talk to you.
- Do not confuse children with the "stranger danger" concept. This message is not effective, as danger to children is greater from someone they know.
- Screen all caregivers carefully, such as babysitters, day care providers, and coaches.
- Teach your children and adolescents how to get out of a threatening situation. Make a family safety plan!
- Supervise Internet use -- many sexual predators use this to connect with children.
- Make arrangements ahead of time to be available for your children when they go out with friends. They need to know they can call you for a ride if they find themselves in an uncomfortable position or if they have used substances and feel unsafe to drive home.
- Always report anything suspicious.

Be a parent that is involved in your children's lives. Take the time to listen to your children, which will help them to develop their sense of security. Communication is key. Also, find ways to help yourself if you are feeling stressed. Remember, your stress affects your children.

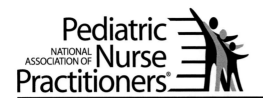

Information for
Adolescents on Child Maltreatment

Important Facts

There are many different forms of child abuse and neglect. It can happen to any child, at any age, including adolescents. Here are some things that could be child abuse:

- An adult is hurting you physically, such as hitting you, especially if it is with an object.
- An adult is touching you in private places such as the breast or genitals, or having any form of genital or oral sex with you.
- One of your friends tries to have sex with you after you have said "NO."
- A boyfriend/girlfriend is physically or emotionally abusive to you.
- You don't have a warm place to stay.
- You don't receive medical care.
- There isn't enough food in the house.
- Your parents keep you out of school.
- Emotional abuse can happen if your caregivers are always mean to you and make you feel bad about yourself.

Adolescents are the group of people most often victimized in the United States. This is especially true for girls. Here are some things that you should be aware of:

- Adolescent girls are the most frequent victims of sexual assault.
- More than 50% of all rape victims are under 18 years old.
- One in 4 college women have been raped or have experienced attempted rape.
- 93% of juvenile sexual assault victims knew their attacker.
- Many sexual assaults are in the victim's home or a friend's home
- The impact of rape includes physical trauma, genital trauma, pregnancy, sexually transmitted infections, psychological symptoms, or economic implications.
- Many teenagers experience a lot of problems after being sexually abused or assaulted.

These include:

- Substance abuse
- Depression and anxiety
- Difficulty with close relationships
- Suicidal thoughts
- Violent behavior
- Nightmares and difficulty sleeping
- Frequent headaches, stomachaches, and other medical problems

How can you prevent this from happening to you?

- Tell a trusted adult or friend if someone is hurting you emotionally, physically or sexually at home.

- Tell a trusted adult or friend if another person in your peer group is forcing you to have sex or hurting you physically.

- Never go out alone! There is always safety in numbers. Don't hitchhike!

- Make sure that an adult knows where you are going and with whom.

- Be careful of the Internet. It is NEVER a good idea to meet a stranger with whom you have been communicating online.

- Be very careful about information that you put on Face book or other social media.

- Never send pictures of yourself partially or fully undressed on your cell phone, even if it is to a friend or boyfriend. This is illegal and you could end up with a federal offense and in lots of legal trouble.

- Don't go to parties or gatherings where there is no adult present. Although it may sound fun and very grown up, there can be lots of activities going on that you aren't ready for, such as alcohol, drug use, and sexual activity.

- Make arrangements with a trusted adult before you go out with friends to be able to call for a ride if you find yourself in an uncomfortable position. This would also work if you have been using drugs or alcohol and feel unsafe to drive home. Remember, **NEVER** get in a car with anyone who has been using drugs or drinking.

- Don't let food or beverages out of your sight! Someone may tamper with it by adding drugs.

- Remember that if someone abuses or assaults you, **IT IS NOT YOUR FAULT!!**

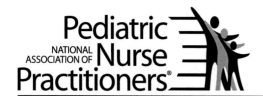

Information on Child Abuse and Neglect for School-Age Children

There are many different ways that a child your age may be abused. Child abuse means that an older child, teenager, or adult is hurting you. It may be one of your parents or someone else that you care about in your family, or even a family friend. It may even be a friend or someone that you know around your age.

Here are some things that could be child abuse or neglect:

- An adult/teenager/ or another child is hitting you, biting you, or giving you burns.

- Someone is touching you in your private areas, such as your penis (where boys pee from), rectum (where you poop from), breasts, or urethra/vagina (where girls pee from).

- If they touch you over your clothes or under your clothes, it is not okay.

- It is not okay to touch you in any of your private places with their fingers, any parts of their body, or any kind of object.

- Someone shows you their private parts or asks you to touch them or shows you movies with people that have their clothes off.

- Your parent/guardians do not send you to school.

- There is no heat in your house.

- There is not enough food in your house.

- You do not have enough clothes to keep you warm.

- Your parents/guardians do not bring you to the doctor when you are sick or hurt.

Here are some things that you can do if someone is hurting you or touching you in a way that doesn't seem right:

- You can say "**NO**" very loudly when that person tries to touch you, and then tell an adult whom you trust.

- Tell someone whom you trust what is happening. Some ideas are teachers, school nurses, police, your doctor or nurse practitioner, other family members, or the other parent that isn't hurting you.

- If someone tells you to keep a secret about hurting or touching, that would be important to tell an adult whom you trust.

- Never get into anyone's car that you don't know very well. If someone tries to force you, yell very loudly and try to run away.

- If you get lost when you are out in public, go to a salesperson or checkout counter or security person and tell them you are lost – don't tell just anyone that you see.

- Never go out alone, and make sure a trusted adult knows where you are at all times.

- Learn your address and phone number.

Remember that if someone is doing something to hurt you or make you feel bad in any way, you need to TELL!!!

IT IS NEVER YOUR FAULT.

Your body is your private area; NOBODY has the right to touch it.

Internet Resources

National Clearinghouse on Child Abuse and Neglect
www.nccanch.acf.hhs.gov

The National Clearinghouse on Child Abuse and Neglect Information is a service of the Children's Bureau, Administration for Children and Families, U.S. Department of Health and Human Services. The mission of the Clearinghouse is to connect professionals and concerned citizens to practical, timely, and essential information on programs, research, legislation, and statistics to promote the safety, permanency, and well-being of children and families. It collects, organizes, and disseminates information on all aspects of child maltreatment.

Prevent Child Abuse America
www.preventchildabuse.org

Prevent Child Abuse America has led the way in building awareness, providing education, and inspiring hope for everyone involved in the effort to prevent the abuse and neglect of children. Working with chapters in 39 states and the District of Columbia, this organization provides leadership to promote and implement prevention efforts at both the national and local levels. The organization provides many local programs, prevention initiatives, and events to help to create awareness of this problem and communicate that prevention is possible. It comprises friends, professionals, volunteers, donors, and parents who are preventing child abuse and neglect before it ever starts.

Rape, Abuse, & Incest National Network (RAINN)
www.rainn.org

RAINN is the nation's largest anti-sexual assault organization. RAINN operates the National Sexual Assault Hotline at 1.800.656.HOPE and carries out programs to prevent sexual assault, help victims and ensure that rapists are brought to justice.

National Children's Alliance
www.nationalchildrensalliance.org/

National Children's Alliance is a professional membership organization dedicated to helping local communities respond to allegations of child abuse in ways that are effective and efficient. It provides training, support, technical assistance and leadership on a national level to local children's and child advocacy centers and communities responding to reports of child abuse and neglect.

The Shaken Baby Alliance
www.shakenbaby.com

The mission of the Shaken Baby Alliance is to provide support for families of shaken baby syndrome (SBS) victims (including adoptive and foster parents), advocate for justice for SBS victims, and increase SBS awareness.

REFERENCES

Adams, J., Kaplan, R., Starling, S., et al. (2007). Guidelines for medical care of children who may have been sexually abused. *Journal of Pediatric & Adolescent Gynecology,* 20(3), 163-172.

Bergman, D., Plsek P., Saunders, M. (2006). A high-performing system for well-child care: a vision for the future. *The Commonwealth Fund.*

Dubowitz, H., Feigelman, S., Lane, W., et al. (2007). Screening for depression in an urban pediatric primary care clinic. *Pediatrics,* 119(3), 437-443.

Dubowitz, H., Lane, W., Semiatin, J., Magder, L. (2012). The SEEK Model of Pediatric Primary Care: Can child maltreatment be prevented in a low risk population? *Academic Pediatrics.* 12(4), 259-267.

Emans, S.J. & Laufer, M. (2012). *Pediatric & Adolescent Gynecology.* 6th Ed. Lippincott, Philadelphia, PA: Williams & Wilkins.

Flaherty, E., Sege, R., Price, L., Christoffel, K., Norton, D., O'Connor. (2006). Pediatrician characteristics associated with child abuse identification and reporting: Results from a national survey of pediatricians. *Child Maltreatment,* 11(4), 361-369.

Flaherty, E., Sege, R., Mattson, C., Binns, H. (2002). Assessment of suspicion of abuse in the primary care setting. *Ambulatory Pediatrics.* 2(2), 120-126.

Flaherty, E., Sege, R., Binns, H., Mattson, C., Christoffel, K., (2000). Health care Providers' experience reporting child abuse in the primary care setting. *Archives of Pediatric and Adolescent Medicine.* 154(5), 489-493.

Hagen, J., Shaw, J., Duncan, P. (Eds.). (2008). *Bright Futures.* Third Edition. Elk Grove Village, American Academy of Pediatrics.

Harris, T. (2010). Bruises in children: normal or child abuse? *Journal of Pediatric Health Care,* 24(4), 216-221.

Hornor, G. (2012). Medical evaluation for child physical abuse: what the PNP needs to know. *Journal of Pediatric Health Care,* 26(3), 163-174.

Kellogg, N. & The Committee on Child Abuse & Neglect. (2007). Evaluation of suspected child physical abuse. *Pediatrics.* 119(6), 1232-1241.

Kellogg, N. & The Committee on Child Abuse & Neglect (2005). Evaluation of sexual abuse in children. *Pediatrics,* 116(2), 506-512.

SECTION 13
Victoria von Sadovszky

Sexuality

Fast Facts

- **Sexual Risk Behaviors:**
    - 47% have had sexual intercourse
    - 6% have had sexual intercourse prior to the age of 13 years
    - 15% have had sex with four or more people
    - 40% did not use a condom at their last sexual intercourse
    - 77% did not use contraception before their last sexual intercourse
    - If sex is initiated during the early teen years, these teens are likely to have several sex partners during their teenage years and are less likely to use condoms.
    - Oral and anal sex in teens is on the rise and there is a misperception that these are a safe form of sex.

- **Teen Pregnancy**
    - Although teen pregnancy rates have been decreasing, teen births still represent 10% of all births in this country.
    - Rates of teen births in the United States are still higher than in other countries.
    - The majority of teenage girls have intercourse for 18 months before seeking contraception.

- **Sexually Transmitted Infections (STIs) and HIV**
    - Similarly, rates of STIs in teens are higher in the United States than in other countries.
    - Each year, 4 million US teens contract an STI.
    - Approximately 25% of new cases of HIV infection occur in teens younger than 20 years of age.
    - Although individuals aged 18-25 years make up less than 25% of all sexually experienced Americans, they comprise more than 50% of all STI cases.

- **Lesbian, Gay, Bisexual and Transgender (LGBT) Adolescents**

    o Up to 4.5% of adolescents identify as lesbian or gay; up to 4% more are not sure of their sexual identity

    o LGBT adolescents are more likely to experience verbal and physical violence at school and more likely to experience as a result of isolation, peer ridicule, abuse, assault, rejection by others, and lack of self-acceptance.

    o LGBT youth suicides account for 30% of all youth suicides.

    o LGBT youth experiencing rejection from parents or adults:

        ▪ Are nearly 6 times more likely to experience depression compared to heterosexual adolescents

        ▪ Are more than 8 times as likely to have attempted suicide

        ▪ Are more than 3 times as likely to use illegal drugs

        ▪ Are more than 3 times as likely to participate in sexual risk behaviors

- **Dating Violence**

    o By the time adolescents reach adulthood, nearly 23% of women and 15% of men have experienced some form of partner violence between the ages of 11 and 17 years.

    o Adolescents who are victims of dating violence are more likely to be depressed, do poorly in school, use drugs and alcohol, have eating disorders, think about or attempt suicide, and are at a higher risk for victimization in college.

    o Many adolescents will not report dating violence because of fear.

Brief Review of Timing of Pubertal Development

Girls

- More girls are showing signs of breast development at age 8 years; although this age is earlier than 30 years ago, it is not statically significant. Puberty is considered early if it is before 8 years of age.

- Growth of pubic hair, as well as armpit and leg hair, begins at age 9 or 10 years and reaches adult patterns usually by 13-14 years.

- The average age of menarche is 12½ years. Menarche typically occurs 2 years following the development of breast and pubic hair.

- African American girls tend to develop 1½ years earlier than white girls; however, Caucasian girls are closing this gap today. Reasons why the onset of puberty has shifted to earlier ages are unknown at this time.

Boys

- Testicular enlargement is usually the first sign of puberty in boys and occurs on average at age 9 years. Soon after, the penis will lengthen. By the age of 16-17 years, the genitals typically have reached adult size and shape.

- Growth of pubic hair, as well as armpit, leg, chest, and facial hair, begins around 12 years of age and reaches adult patterns by about 15-16 years.

- Spermarche (onset of sperm emission) occurs on average at age 14½ years, but can typically start anywhere from 13-17 years.

- African American boys appear to enter puberty sooner than their white counterparts.

Parent and Adolescent Sexual Development and Sexuality

- Sexuality is a normal part of childhood and adolescence, though it changes throughout childhood into adulthood.

- Parents often view sexuality as the big issue for adolescents, and one that is an uncomfortable issue.

- Parents can and should be the key in helping youngsters develop a healthy sense of their own sexuality.

Role of Healthcare Providers

- Primary care providers (PCPs) must talk to their adolescent patients about sexuality at every health maintenance visit and at other appropriate times.

- Many teens perceive that their providers are uncomfortable or lack communication skills to discuss sexuality adequately.

- In one study, fewer than half of PCPs asked adolescents about sexual activity and even fewer asked questions about STIs, condom use, sexual orientation, number of partners, or sexual abuse (Killebrew & Garofalo, 2002)

- **TALKING TO TEENS ABOUT SEXUALITY DOES NOT PROMOTE SEXUAL ACTIVITY.**

- **Healthcare providers need to realize that only 21 states and the District of Columbia mandate sexuality education in schools; only 18 states require that this education be "medically accurate."**

- Healthcare providers should begin discussions with children and parents about the changes of puberty before the onset, approximately age 7 for girls and 9 or 10 for boys – depending on race or family history of pubertal timing. By opening up the discussion in your office, parents will be more likely to continue the discussion with their children.

- Make sure that parents know that even though their older children and teens may seem uninterested in what they think, parents actually have more influence over their children than anyone else does. Research shows that young people want to get information about sexuality from their parents and that young people whose parents speak to them about sexuality early before they become sexually active are more likely to delay their sexual debut and be responsible when they become sexually active.

What should the healthcare provider do when a problem is disclosed?

The teen discloses that he/she is gay, bisexual, or transgender:

- Ask whether the teen has disclosed this to his/her family. If yes, what was their reaction?

- Question carefully about depression and suicidality, as these teens are at higher risk. Refer for mental health services as needed.

- Provide anticipatory guidance around risks that homosexual youth may face and discuss concerns about disclosure with teens who have not disclosed to their families. Refer for mental health services as needed.

- Be familiar with resources in the community for teens and parents, such as Parents, Families, and Friends of Lesbians and Gays (**www.pflag.org**), Healthy Initiatives for Youth (**www.hify.org**), and The Human Rights Campaign (**www.hrc.org**), among others.

What should the healthcare provider do when the teen discloses current or former sexual abuse or date rape?

- If the abuse is current, the provider must take the steps required legally for reporting abuse and the teen should be examined by someone certified as a sexual assault nurse/forensic examiner.

- If the abuse or rape was in the past, in addition to providing appropriate physical examination and testing, the provider must ascertain whether the teen has disclosed this before and whether or not he/she received counseling.

- The provider should reassure the teen that what happened was not his/her fault. This reassurance is a key step in providing care to the teen.

- Discuss the option of counseling.

Legal Issues

- Most states entitle minors (younger than 18) to receive reproductive healthcare without parental consent or notification. Check the laws in your state.

Evidence-Based Interventions

- PREVENTION is the key; Interventions must begin BEFORE sexual activity is initiated.

- Behavioral interventions are effective in promoting condom use and reducing STIs.

- Abstinence education must be paired with information about consistent and correct condom use. Abstinence education alone is ineffective in reducing sexual behaviors and STIs.

- Most effective preventive interventions for teens contain the following components:
  - Are delivered by trained instructors
  - Use a behavioral change theory as a guide for education
  - Are age-appropriate
  - Include components on:
    - Skills-building (information, motivation, behavior-change strategies)
    - Support of health behaviors in school and other environments
    - Involvement of parents, youth-serving organizations, and health organizations

- Adolescents need easy access to confidential, healthcare services, as this increases screening and treatment rates.

Interventions in Primary Care Settings

- Discuss sexual health and sexual development (prior to adolescence).

- Discuss healthy behaviors.

- Facilitate communication between parents and children/teens.

- Conduct an annual Pap smear and Chlamydia screening on all sexually active teens.

- Start the human papillomavirus (HPV) vaccine series in girls and boys ages 11-12 years.

- Use a developmental approach to the first pelvic exam. Remember, how the first pelvic exam is conducted will have an influence on further compliance with future pelvic exams.

- Guidelines and up-to-date specific treatments of sexually transmitted diseases (STDs) are available at www.cdc.gov/std/treatment/2010/.

Screening Tools/Questions for Adolescent Sexuality

Screening Questionnaires

Before taking a history, it is important to inform the adolescent that you will be asking personal questions and that you are asking these questions so you can provide the best possible care. It also is important to let the teen know that you ask these questions of all adolescents.

The number 1 reason that adolescents do not confide in their healthcare providers about their sexuality and sexual risk-taking behaviors is that they have not been assured about confidentiality.

Before beginning the interview, it is important to tell the teen that what he or she tells you is confidential between the two of you unless you are told that someone has hurt him or her or that he or she wants to hurt him/herself. Under those circumstances, you need to tell the teen that if this type of information is disclosed, you will have to make a report to another professional.

It is of great importance that the discussion is open and nonjudgmental. The provider's role is to provide information on healthy behaviors, not to judge the behaviors of the teen. Teens are very sensitive and will not likely come back if they feel they are being judged.

The HEADSS (Home, Education, Activities, Drugs, Sexuality, Suicide/Depression) assessment is a good instrument for taking a psychological history from adolescents. Refer to Section 1 for additional information about the HEADSS Assessment.

Questions about sexual behaviors include:

- Have you ever been in a romantic relationship? Tell me about the people you have dated.

- Have any of your relationships been sexual relationships? (Define oral, anal, and vaginal sex so that they are clear on what constitutes a sexual relationship.)

- Are your sexual activities enjoyable?

- What does the term "safer sex" mean to you?

- Do you use anything, or have you used anything in the past, to prevent infections or pregnancy? Are/were you satisfied with your method?

- Do you use condoms? Always? Sometimes? Once in a while? Some people are attracted to guys, some to girls, and some to both. What about you?

- Have you ever been forced to have sex?

- Have you ever been pregnant (or gotten a girl pregnant)?

- Have you ever been told you have a sexually transmitted disease?

These questions were adapted from: Goldenring, J.M. & Rosen, D.S. (2004). Getting into adolescent heads: an essential update. *Contemporary Pediatrics*, 21, 64-90.

- The Guidelines for Adolescent Preventive Services (GAPS) Questionnaire also contains questions about sexuality. These are similar to the HEADSS questions. The GAPS Questionnaire can be completed by the teen while waiting to see the provider, which can save time in a hurried clinical setting. (The GAPS forms are contained in this guide under the Screening and Assessment Section). A URL for the questionnaire is listed under Resources for Providers, on the next pages.

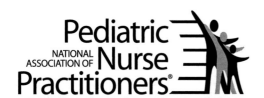

Centers for Disease Control and Prevention. (2012). Parents and guardian resource: Helping your teen make health choices about sex. http://www.cdc.gov/teenpregnancy/Parents.htm.

The Mayo Clinic. (2011). Sex education: Talking to your teen about sex. http://www.mayoclinic.com/health/sex-education/CC00032.

Richardson, J. & Schuster, M. (2004). Everything You Never Wanted Your Kids to Know About Sex (But Were Afraid They'd Ask) The Secrets to Surviving Your Child's Sexual Development from Birth to the Teens. Pittsburgh, PA: Three Rivers Press.

Roffman, D. (2001). Sex and Sensibility: The Thinking Parent's Guide to Talking Sense about Sex. Jackson, TN: Perseus Press.

Roffman, D. (2002). But How'd I Get in There in the First Place? Talking to Your Young Child about Sex. Jackson, TN: Perseus Press.

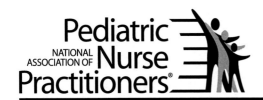

The Family Project
www.familiesaretalking.org

The Family Project, which includes the Families Are Talking Website and newsletter, is a project of the Sexuality Information and Education Council of the United States (SIECUS). This project began in 2000 to empower parents and caregivers to communicate with their children about sexuality-related issues, to provide tools to help families communicate about these issues, and to encourage parents, caregivers, and young people to become advocates on the local, state, and national levels for sexuality-related issues including comprehensive sexuality education programs in the schools.

Go Ask Alice!
www.goaskalice.columbia.edu

This is a health question-and-answer Internet service produced by **Alice! Columbia University's Health Education Program** — a division of **Health Services at Columbia**.

The Teen Health Initiative (THI)
http://www.nyclu.org/thi/frames/thi_frameset.html

The THI was created in 1997 under the auspices of the New York Civil Liberty Union's Reproductive Rights Project (RRP) to work to remove the barriers that prevent young people from accessing critical reproductive health services and information. The THI staff increases awareness of minors' rights to receive confidential reproductive and other healthcare.

Internet Resources for Healthcare Providers

The Alan Guttmacher Institute (AGI)
www.agi-usa.org/

This institute is a non-profit organization focused on sexual and reproductive health research, policy analysis, and public education.

The Centers for Disease Control and Prevention (CDC) Sexual Health
http://www.cdc.gov/sexualhealth/

The CDC provides a wealth of information, including outstanding educational handouts on multiple topics related to sexual health. It also has the current guidelines for STDs.

Guidelines for Adolescent Preventive Services (GAPS) Implementation Materials
www.ama-assn.org/ama/pub/category/1981.html

This site contains multiple resources for how to implement the GAPS tools into clinical practice.

The National Campaign to Prevent Teen Pregnancy
www.teenpregnancy.org/

Founded in February 1996, this is a non-profit, non-partisan initiative supported almost entirely by private donations. Its mission is to improve the well-being of children, youth, and families by reducing teen pregnancy.

SIECUS – the Sexuality Information and Education Council of the United States
http://www.siecus.org/

This council has served as the national voice for sexuality education, sexual health, and sexual rights for almost 40 years.

Talking with Kids about Tough Issues
www.talkwithkids.org

This is a national campaign by Children Now and the Kaiser Family Foundation. This Website offers practical, concrete tips and techniques for talking easily and openly with young children ages 8 to 12 about some very tough issues, such as sex, HIV/AIDS, violence, drugs, and alcohol. Outstanding educational handouts for dissemination are available.

REFERENCES

Biro, F. M., Galvez, M. P., Greenspan, L. C., et al. (2010). Pubertal assessment method and baseline characteristics in a mixed longitudinal study of girls. *Pediatrics*, 126(3), e583-90.

Centers for Diesease Control and Prevention. (2012). *Sexual Health.* http://www.cdc.gov/sexualhealth/.

Jellinek, M., Patel, B.P., & Froehle, M. (2002). *Bright Futures in Practice: Mental Health- Vol I. Practice Guide.* Arlington, VA: National Center for Education in Maternal and Child Health.

Jellinek, M., Patel, B.P., & Froehle, M. (2002). Bright Futures in Practice: Mental Health- Vol II. Tool Kit. Arlington,VA: National Center for Education in Maternal and Child Health.

McEvoy, M. & Coupey, S.M. (2002). Sexually transmitted infection. A challenge for nurses working with adolescents. *Nursing Clinics of North America*, 37(3), 461-474.

Melnyk, B.M., Brown, H., Jones, D.C., Kreipe, R., & Novak, J. (2003). Improving the mental/psychosocial health of U.S. children and adolescents. Outcomes and implementation strategies from the national KySS summit. *Journal of Pediatric Healthcare*, 17(6 Suppl 1), S1- S24.

Russell, S.T. & Joyner, K. (2001). Adolescent sexual orientation and suicide risk: evidence from a national study. *American Journal of Public Health*, 91(8), 1276-1281.

SECTION 14
Barbara Jones Warren

Substance Abuse and Addiction Spectrum

Fast Facts

- Children and adolescents make up approximately 27% of all persons in the United States (SAMSHA, 2011). The majority of them have normal and healthy developmental processes. However, 21% of them incur a mental illness or addiction that impairs their ability to develop normally, function every day and contribute to society as adults (SAMHSA, 2011).

- Screening and early identification are critical to the appropriate treatment of children and adolescents who use and/or abuse addictive substances. It is also imperative that culturally inclusive, evidence-based screening, identification and treatment strategies be utilized in order to support caregivers, schools and communities (Poland et al., 2008; Warren, 2012, 2010; Warren & Broome, 2011).

- Most people use drugs for the first time when they are teens. There are 8,100 new users of illicit drugs on a daily basis with 57% of them being under the age of 18 years.

- Drinking by persons between the ages of 12-20 years has declined from 28.8% to 26.3% between 2002 and 2010. This includes binge drinking (from 19.3% to 17.0%) and heavy drinking (from 6.2% to 5.1%).

- The use of inhalants and crack-cocaine has decreased for the years 2010 – 2011.

- Ecstasy and steroid use is on the rise among 12th graders, with teens viewing these drugs as safe or less dangerous.

- Marijuana use is on the increase with 7.2% of 8th graders, 17.6% of 10th graders, and 22.6% of 12th graders using marijuana within the past month. This is an increase of 5.7%, 14.2% and 18.8%, respectively, since 2007. Fewer teens smoke cigarettes than marijuana.

- In 2011, 18.5% of 12th graders have used hookah water pipes and another 19.5% report smoking small cigars.

- 6.6% of 12th graders report using marijuana daily.

- The use of synthetic marijuana, known as spice or K2, is a combination of herbal mixtures laced with cannabinoids. K2 is a serious concern in that adolescents perceive it as a safe drug. 11.4% of 12th graders reported using K2 within the past year.

- The non-medical use of prescription drugs is a serious problem for teenagers. In 2011, 15.2% of 12th graders used a prescription drug non-medically in the past year. The most commonly abused drugs include Vicodin and Adderall.

- Early marijuana use by children and teens creates a higher risk for the development of depression, anxiety, and attention deficit disorders (Robertson et al., 2003; SAMHSA, 2011).

- Experimentation may occur for children and teens when they use a substance on a few occasions because they are curious as to "how it feels." This often occurs at parties in response to peer pressure.

- Failure to identify and intervene with child and adolescent use can evolve into abuse and dependence (Boyd, 2012; Gance-Cleveland & Mays, 2008).

- The level of use, abuse, and dependence is contingent upon the child's and adolescent's developmental stage, chronological age, and level of protective and risk factors (Boyd, 2012; Lusk & Melnyk, 2011).

Differences Between Use and Abuse

- Use means that a child or teen is regularly using a substance every few weeks or more that affects their functioning.

- Abuse means that a child or teen is using a substance extensively, daily functioning is affected, and negative consequences are occurring within a child's or teen's life.

- Dependence means that the child or teen psychologically and physically needs the substance and that getting the substance becomes the center of their existence (APA, 2000).

The child and adolescent brain (into the middle 20s) is in a developmental stage that creates an increase in behavior aimed at increasing learning, expanding social life, and the need for exploration and limit testing (Arnett, 2006; Compass, 2009). It is critical that adults create an environment that fosters these growth patterns but at the same time helps children and teens to avoid destructive behaviors that may lead to substance use and subsequent abuse with co-occurring mental health problems (SAMHSA, 2011). Resilience is an important protective factor within the lives of children and adolescents. Resilience is the child's or adolescent's ability to bounce back from difficulties or hardships by maintaining their sense of health and well-being (Brown & Waite, 2005; Brown & Wells, 2006). The level of protective and risk factors is an important determinant of where screening and assessment strategies need to be targeted (Hamric & Deering, 2012).

Protective Factors

- Strong bond between children, teens, and their families

- Parental or guardian involvement in a child's or teen's life

- Supportive parenting or guardian presence that meets financial, emotional, cognitive, and social needs of children and teens

- Clear and consistent approaches for discipline

- Success in academics, involvement in extra-curricular activities and/or religious-based activities

Risk Factors

- Association with peers who have problem behaviors such as aggression toward others, use of alcohol and other drugs

- Drug availability

- Poor socioeconomic status with lack of community attachment and support

- Presence of a caregiver who abuses substances, has an untreated mental illness, or engages in criminal behavior

- Chaotic family environment

- Lack of a significant relationship with a supportive adult if parents are unavailable

- Physical and sexual abuse and trauma

- Bullying occurrences

- Homelessness

- Poverty

- Lack of parenting support and supervision

- Poor or inadequate coping and stress management skills

- Poor self-esteem

- Major transitions in life such as puberty, loss of a parent, moving
- Co-occurring mental health disorders (Goebert et al., 2011; Hamric & Deering, 2012; McGuinness & Schneider, 2007; Mylant et al., 2002; Warren, 2011; Williams & Godfrey, 2011)

Findings from studies indicate that approximately one in four children or adolescents are exposed to abuse by parents before she or he is 18 years of age (Gance-Cleveland & Mays, 2008). The presence of poverty and homelessness coupled with a parent who is a substance abuser increases a child's or adolescent's risk to engage in risky behaviors including substance use and promiscuous sexual exploration (McGuinness & Schneider, 2007).

Common Presenting Signs of Abuse

- Changes in peer group

- Decrease in school performance

- Drop in school attendance

- Disciplinary actions at school

- Changes in sleep patterns

- Avoidance of family activities

- Frequent respiratory and stomach complaints

- Change in overall physical appearance (loss of weight, sloppy appearance, looking fatigued)

- Stealing money or valuables from others (Calvert et al., 2010; SAMSHA, 2011)

The prevention of drug-related problems for children and adolescents is critical to address as it minimizes the damage that can occur once children and adolescents become addicted to substances and develop physiological and psychological problems. Screening within schools, community and primary care environments can help to identify at-risk children and adolescents or those within the early stages of addictive behaviors.

Screening and Assessment

The choice of screening, identification, and assessment tools has to be based on the needs of the children, adolescents, caregivers, and the community being served. Public health strategies need to address all three levels of prevention care: primary, secondary, and tertiary. Primary care involves screening of all available children and adolescents within school and/or community settings. Secondary care entails screening for children and adolescents who have risk factors (e.g., as noted above under risk factors) for development of substance and addiction use spectrum disorders (Poland et al., 2008; SAMSHA, 2011).

Culturally and linguistically appropriate tools are important to use when screening children and adolescents for possible substance use. Healthcare beliefs, values, and level of literacy are essential components that healthcare providers need to be aware of when developing health and wellness strategies and protocols for children and adolescents who are culturally and ethnically diverse (Warren, 2012, 2010). Failure to incorporate culturally based strategies and protocols often results in poor healthcare outcomes because the recipients of this incompetent approach think that healthcare providers are dismissive regarding the recipients' cultural needs (Brown & Wells, 2006; Warren, 2012, 2010).

Resources on Cultural and Linguistic Competency

(Substance Abuse and Mental Health Services Administration [SAMHSA], 2011)

- **Care for Diverse Populations**
  http://www.molinamedicare.com/providers/ (see bottom of Web page)

- **Center for Health and Health Care in Schools: Caring Across Communities: Addressing the Mental Health Needs of Refugees and Immigrants (Web page)**
  http://www.healthinschools.org/Immigrant-and-Refugee-Children/Caring-AcrossCommunities.aspx

- **Culturally and Linguistically Appropriate Services: Review Guidelines (Web page)**
  http://clas.uiuc.edu/review/index.html

- **Indian Health Service (Web site)**
  http://www.ihs.gov

- **National Center for Cultural Competence: Child and Adolescent Mental Health Project (Web page)**
  http://www11.georgetown.edu/research/gucchd/nccc/projects/camh.html

- **National Network to Eliminate Disparities: Resources (Web page)**
  http://nned.net/index-nned.php/resources/

- **Screening and Assessing Immigrant and Refugee Youth in School-Based Mental Health Programs (Publication)**
  http://www.rwjf.org/files/research/3320.32211.0508issuebriefno.1.pdf

- **Technical Assistance Partnership for Child and Family Mental Health: Cultural and Linguistic Competence Community of Practice (Web page)**
  http://www.tapartnership.org/COP/CLC/default.php

What Is a Screening Tool?

A screening tool is a brief list of questions relating to a youth's behavior, thoughts, and feelings. It usually takes only 5-15 minutes to answer. A specific method is used to score the answers to the questions, and the score indicates whether the youth is at high likelihood of having a problem or is unlikely to have a problem. As with medical tests, the language used to refer to the results of screening may be confusing. When a score indicates a likely problem, it is called a *positive finding*; when the score indicates that a problem is not likely, it is called a *negative finding*. Like other medical tests, sometimes screening tools might miss problems or are positive when there is not a problem. For examples of a screening tool, see the Pediatric Symptom Checklist forms at http://www2.massgeneral.org/allpsych/psc/psc_forms.htm (SAMHSA, 2011).

Materials That Provide Information on the Signs of a Mental Health or Substance Use Problem (SAMHSA, 2011)

For Infants

What Is Infant Mental Health and Why Is It Important? *(Publication)*
http://www.projectabc-la.org/dl/ABC_InfantMentalHlth_English.pdf

For Children

Mental Illness and the Family: Recognizing Warning Signs and How to Cope *(Website)*
http://www.nmha.org/go/information/get-info/mi-and-the-family/recognizingwarning-signs-and-how-to-cope

For Teens—Mental Health

Mental, Emotional, and Behavioral Disorders in Teens *(Website)*
http://www.cumminsbhs.com/teens.htm

For Teens—Substance Use

Warning Signs of Teenage Drug Abuse *(Website)*
http://parentingteens.about.com/cs/drugsofabuse/a/driug_abuse20.htm

General Signs of Alcohol or Drug Use *(Website)*
http://www.adolescent-substance-abuse.com/signs-drug-use.html

For Suicide Prevention

Risk Factors for Child and Teen Suicide *(Website)*
http://www.healthyplace.com/depression/articles/risk-factors-for-child-and-teen-suicide/

Suicide Warning Signs *(Website)*
http://store.samhsa.gov/shin/content//SVP11-0126/SVP11-0126.pdf (English)
http://store.samhsa.gov/shin/content//SVP11-0126SP/SVP11-0126SP.pdf (Spanish)

Diagnosis of Substance Use and Abuse

Information regarding changes from the previous Diagnostic and Statistical Manual of Mental Disorder-IV-Text Revision (DSM-IV-TR) version and the Diagnostic and Statistical Manual of Mental Disorder-5 (DSM-5™) is important to understand in order to properly assess children and adolescents and determine which evidence-based treatment is needed for them. The 4th version defined separate diagnostic categories in a discrete way. The 5th version defines the substance use and abuse as a spectrum (e.g., Substance-Related and Addiction Disorders). This indicates the range and variety of diagnostic areas that exist within substance use, abuse, addiction, and dependence for children and adolescents. DSM-5™ addresses substance-related disorders for: Alcohol, Caffeine, Cannabis, Hallucinogen, Inhalant, Opioid, Sedative, Hypnotic, Anxiolytic, Stimulant, Tobacco, and Other-related disorders. Additional information is available at: http://www.dsm5.org/Pages/Default.aspx.

Evidence-Based Management of Substance Use and Addiction in Children and Adolescents

Treatment of substance use and addiction spectrum disorders in children and adolescents addresses the biopsychosocial components. This treatment may involve the use of skills enhancement training in the areas of communication, conflict management, and stress management. Healthcare providers need to help children and adolescents develop health and wellness behaviors that enhance good nutritional, exercise, sleep, and relaxation habits (Boyd, 2012; Lusk & Melnyk, 2011). Medication may be used to target anxiety and attention deficit issues for children and adolescents. However, with the exception of the psychostimulants, other psychiatric medications are off-label usage within this population (Boyd, 2012). Moreover, there are three primary principles that guide clinicians' use and choice of any medication within the population of children and adolescents:

- Identification of clear rationale for use of medication based on screening, assessment, and level of symptoms.

- Remember that children and adolescents are physically different from adults and hence dosage of medications needs to be aimed at their chronological age and size. Prescribing providers need to carefully document why any medication is used and what outcomes occur as a result of the medication.

- Adherence to medications is the responsibility of the parents/caregivers, so they must have education regarding the target and side effect profile for medications their children and/or adolescents are taking.

There also are community guidelines and principles that guide the evidence-based treatment for children and adolescents diagnosed with substance use and addiction spectrum disorders. These include development of the following:

- Age-related assessment of children, adolescents, parent/caregivers and peers

- Enhancement of parenting skills and training in drug education recognition

- Preschool, elementary, middle and high school programs for children and adolescents' academic and social skills enhancement

- Child and adolescent peer discussion groups and parent role playing to enhance education about drug use and abuse

- Use of research-based prevention and intervention programs within communities and across school settings (Boyd, 2012; Lusk & Melnyk, 2011; Robertson et al., 2003).

Summary

Children and adolescents comprise approximately a quarter of the US population (SAMHSA, 2011). These individuals may be at risk for development of mental health and addiction disorders. This can impair their ability to function, develop normally, and become productive members within society (Poland et al., 2008). The spectrum of substance use is an area in which healthcare providers may be instrumental in the assessment and development of interventions and strategies for prevention and treatment for children, adolescents, and their caregivers. Community programs need to be developed within school systems and healthcare settings. Children, adolescents, their caregivers, and teachers all have layers of culture that help to define their belief systems and guide their healthcare behaviors. It is important that healthcare providers develop treatment strategies and protocols that are culturally inclusive in order to maximize quality and appropriate health and wellness outcomes at primary, secondary, and tertiary levels of care (SAMSHA, 2011).

CRAFFT SCREENING TEST
(J.R. Knight)

The **CRAFFT** is a tool that can be used by healthcare providers to assess adolescent risk taking behaviors and their feelings related to alcohol and drug use (Knight et al., 2002). The CRAFFT is recommended for use with children and adolescents under the age of 21. It consists of a series of six questions:

C – Have you ever ridden in a CAR driven by someone (including yourself) who was "high" or had been using alcohol or drugs?

R – Do you ever use alcohol or drugs to RELAX, feel better about yourself, or fit in?

A – Do you ever use alcohol/drugs while you are by yourself, ALONE?

F – Do you ever FORGET things you did while using alcohol or drugs?

F – Does your family or FRIENDS ever tell you that you should cut down on your drinking or drug use?

T – Have you gotten into TROUBLE while you were using alcohol or drugs? (Knight et al., 2002).

Please see the Web page for more information: http://archpedi.jamanetwork.com/searchResults.aspx?q=drug%20abuse%20screening%20test&gclid=CNmA8J_MrLQCFSpnOgodgRcAQA in order to get more information about the tool.

The CAGE Questionnaire for Alcohol Use
(J.A. Ewing)

The CAGE Questionnaire was developed by Ewing (1984) for clinicians' assessment of an adult's or adolescent's (e.g., over the age of 16 years) use of alcohol. The CAGE may be self- or clinician-administered. An additional use of "or drug use" has been added to the CAGE to assess drug usage. Each question is worth one point for a yes response and zero for a no response. Answering yes indicates a possible problem. Answering yes to two or more questions indicates a possible alcohol or drug abuse problem.

The **CAGE** involves the following questions:

C – Have you ever felt you should cut down on your drinking or drug use? . . . (Yes or No)

A – Have people annoyed you by criticizing your drinking or drug use?. . . . . (Yes or No)

G – Do you ever feel bad or guilty about your drinking or drug use? . . . . . . (Yes or No)

E – Have you ever had a drink or used drugs first thing in the morning to steady your nerves or get rid of a hang over?. . . . . (Yes or No)

Indications for Use: Self-report screening instrument that is well suited for use in busy medical settings where there is limited time for patient interviews. It uses four straightforward yes/no questions that clinicians can easily remember. CAGE can be self-administered or conducted by a clinician and has proven utility for use in routine health screening of adults and adolescents over the age of 16. The screen may identify individuals with alcohol problems that may have been otherwise missed. The CAGE screen may fail to detect low but risky levels of drinking.

Time to Administer: *1 minute*
Scoring:

Score 1	Score 2 or greater:	Score 3 or greater:
Evidence of AT RISK. Indicates need for further clinical investigation, including questions on amount and frequency, etc.	Evidence of CURRENT PROBLEM. Indicates need for further clinical investigation and/or referral as indicated by clinician's expertise. (Score of 2 or greater associated with SENSITIVITY of 74% and SPECIFICITY of 91%.)	Evidence of dependence until ruled out. Evaluate, treat, and/or refer as indicated by clinician's expertise.
Additional information regarding the CAGE may be accessed at: http://pubs.niaaa.nih.gov/publications/inscage.htm		

Source Reference

Ewing, J.A. (1984). Detecting alcoholism: The CAGE questionnaire. JAMA: Journal of the American Medical Association, 252(14), 1905-1907.

Supporting References

Reynaud, M., Schwan, R., Loiseaux-Meunier, M.N., Albuisson, E. & Deteix, P. (2001).

Patients admitted to emergency services for drunkenness: Moderate alcohol users or harmful drinkers? American Journal of Psychiatry, 158(1), 96-99.

Aertgeerts, B., Buntinx, F., Fevery, J., & Ansoms, S. (2000). Is there a difference between CAGE interviews and written CAGE interviews. Alcoholism: Clinical and Experimental Research, 24(5), 733-736.

Fiellin, D.A., Reid, M.C., & O'Connor, P.G. (2000). Screening for alcohol problems in primary care: systematic review. Journal of General Internal Medicine, 15(Suppl 1), 65-66.

Mayfield, D., McLeod, G., & Hall, P. (1974). The CAGE questionnaire: Validation of a new alcoholism instrument. American Journal of Psychiatry, 131(10), 1121-1123.

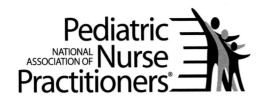

Important Information For Parents on Substance Use Disorders in Children and Teens and How to Prevent Them

- Fifty-two Percent of high school students admit to using alcohol in the past month, and 33% reported binge driving (5 or more drinks at a time). One quarter used marijuana in the past month, and 20% said they had sniffed or inhaled intoxicating substances. More than one third of high school students reported smoking cigarettes within the past month.

- Rates of substance use increase with age are slightly higher for males and for white adolescents. Other mental health problems (e.g., anxiety and depression) frequently coexist with substance use and abuse. Adolescents might use substances in an attempt to treat these and help themselves feel better.

- Common signs of substance use include changes in peer group, decrease in school performance, changes in sleep patterns frequent respiratory and gastrointestinal complaints, and an increase in behavior problems, including stealing money or other valuables.

- Risk Factors

  Peer group use of alcohol and other drugs
  Family conflict, substance abuse, parenting problems
  Physical or sexual abuse
  Lack of other activites
  Poor coping skills
  Poor self-esteem

Children/teens with substance use disorders need evaluation and treatment:

Substance abuse is defined in the *Diagnostic and Statistical Manual of Mental Disorders, Fourth Edition*, as; "A maladaptive pattern of substance use leading to clinically significant impairment or distress, and manifested by 1 or more of the following, occurring within a 12-month period:

1) Recurrent substance use resulting in failure to fulfill major role obligations at work, school, or home,

2) Recurrent substance use in situations in which it is physically hazardous,

3) Recurrent substance-related legal problems

4) Continued substance use despite having persistent or recurrent social interpersonal problems caused or exacerbated by the effects of the substance."

Differences between Use and Abuse:

- Children/teens that use substance on a few occasion are typically curious about "how it feels."

- Experimentation can be described as using a substance more than a few times; usually this occurs at parties or in response to peer pressure

- Regular use is when a child/teen uses substances every few weeks or more and it begins to affect functioning.

- Abuse is extensive use that impacts daily functioning with negative consequences.

- Dependency is when a child's/teen's life revolves around getting and using substances (the child/teen can be psychologically or physiologically dependent).

If you believe that your child is using or abusing alcohol or drugs, talk to his/her health care provider about it right away.

How to Help Prevent Substance Use in Your Child:

- Help your child learn to problem-solve and find resources to address their challenges.

- Define position on at-risk behaviors (e.g., zero tolerance for drug or alcohol use).

- Frequently communicate expectations to children regarding behaviors and school performance.

- Get to know your child's friends and parents of their friends.

- Requre at least 48 hour advance notice for sleep over events as most drug parties fall together at the last minute.

- Be available for your child; take time to listen.

For more information, access www.familysamsha.gov and www.moniteringthefuture.org

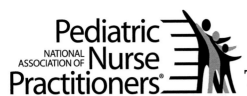

Important Information For
Teens about Alcohol and Other Drugs

- As you get older, you may find that more of your peers are trying alcohol and other drugs. Even though the dangers of alcohol and other drug use are well known, about half of high school students admit to using alcohol in the past month, and one third report binge drinking (more than 5 drinks in one sitting).

- More than one third of high school students reported smoking cigarettes within the past month. A smaller number of young people admit to using illegal drugs, such as marijuana ("pot", "grass") and cocaine. Today, we are seeing more problems in young people related to use of "designer" drugs such as Ecstasy.

- Serious problems also happen when young people use substances (like airplane glue) that are meant for other uses, or if they take someone else's medication.

- Young people who use alcohol and other drugs often have other mental health problems (such as depression, anxiety, ADHD). Young people sometimes use substances to try to help them with symptoms of the other mental health problem. This is very risky.

- You know that you or a friends may be having a problem if you or they start "hanging out" with peers who use alcohol or other drugs, have a drop in grades, or start getting into trouble due to drug or alcohol use (arrests, suspensions, etc). Any young person who beings to lose control over her or his drinking or drug use is headed for problems. Young people who begin to go out of their way to get and use drugs or alcohol, or continute to use even after there have been problems, has a substance abuse issue.

- Young people who are most at risk for alcohol and other drug use may also have problems with:

  Family conflict
  Physical or sexual abuse
  Lack of other activities
  Poor coping skills
  Poor self-esteem
  Depression

- Some young people are also worried about the alcohol or other drug use of a family member, possibly a parent.

Help is Available.

If you are stressed about something or worried that you may have a problem with alcohol or drugs, talk to someone you trust (e.g., your parent, doctor or nurse practitioner, or someone at school).

Don't turn to alcohol or drugs as an answer to your problems; they will just make things worse

The following Web sites might also be helpful: www.family.samhsa.gov and www.monitoringthefuture.org.

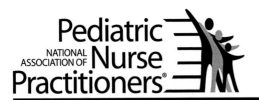
NO DRINKING AND DRIVING CONTRACT

I _____ , promise to keep myself safe. If I or a friend uses any alcohol or drugs and we are driving a motor vehicle, I will call _____ to pick

Name of Parent/Legal Guardian

me up and drive me home.

_____
Signature of Adolescent

_____
Signature of Provider or
Parent/Guardian

_____
Date

REFERENCES

American Psychiatric Association. (2000). *Diagnostic and Statistical Manual of Mental Disorders-Fourth Edition-Text Revision* (DSM-IV-TR). Washington, DC: APA.

Arnett, J. (2006). *Emerging adults in America: Coming of age in the 21st century.* Washington, DC: The American Psychological Association.

Boyd, M. A. (2012). Psychiatric disorders of childhood and adolescence. In M.A. Boyd (Ed.), *Psychiatric Nursing: Contemporary Practice (5th ed.)* (Ch. 35, pp.679-707). Philadelphia, PA: Wolters Kluwer, Lippincott Williams & Wilkins.

Brown, E. J. & Waite, C. D. (2005). Perceptions of risk and resiliency factors associated with rural African American Adolescents' substance abuse and HIV behaviors. Journal of the American Psychiatric Nurses Association, 11(2), 88-100.

Brown, E. J. & Wells, S. (2006). A faith-based integrated substance abuse and HIV prevention program for rural African American adolescents. *Journal of the American Psychiatric Nurses Association*, 11(6), 344-350.

Calvert, W. J., Bucholz, K. K., & Steger-May, K. (2010). Early drinking and its association with adolescents' participation in risky behaviors. *Journal of the American Psychiatric Nurses Association*, 16(4), 239-251.

Compass, B. E. (2009). Coping, regulation and development during childhood and adolescence. *New Directions for Child and Adolescent Development*, 124, 87-99.

Ewing, J. A. (1984). Detecting alcoholism: The CAGE questionnaire. *Journal of the American Medical Association* (JAMA), 252(14), 1905-1907.

Gance-Cleveland, B. & Mays, M. Z. (2008). School-based support groups for adolescents with a substance-abusing parent. *Journal of the American Psychiatric Nurses Association*, 14(4), 297-309.

Goebert, D., Matsu, C., Chung-Do, J., & Chang, J.Y. (2011). The impact of cyber bullying on substance use and mental health in a multiethnic sample. *Maternal Child Health Journal*, 15(8), 1282-1286.

Hamric, V. & Deering, C. G. (2012). Mental health assessment of children and adolescents. In M.A. Boyd (Ed.), *Psychiatric Nursing: Contemporary Practice (5th ed.)* (Ch.34, pp.661-678). Philadelphia, PA: Wolters Kluwer, Lippincott Williams & Wilkins.

Knight, J. R., Sherritt, L., Shrier, L. A., Harris, S. K., & Chang, G. (2002). Validity of the CRAFFT substance abuse screening test among adolescent clinic patients. *Archives of Pediatric and Adolescent Medicine*, 156(6), 607-614.

Lusk, P. & Melnyk, B.M. (2011). COPE for the treatment of depressed adolescents. Lessons learned from implementing an evidence-based practice change. *Journal of the American Psychiatric Nurses Association*, 17(4), 297-309.

McGuinness, T. M. & Schneider, K. (2007). Poverty, child maltreatment, and foster care. *Journal of the American Psychiatric Nurses Association*, 13(5), 296-303.

Mylant, M. Ide, B., Cuevas, E., & Meehan, M. (2002). Adolescent children of alcoholics" Vulnerable or resilient? *Journal of the American Psychiatric Nurses Association*, 8(4), 57-64.

Poland, M. R., Whitlock, E. P., Nygren, P., & Bougatsos, C. (January 2008) *Screening in primary care settings for illicit drug use: Staged systematic review for the U. S. Preventive Services Task Force. Evidence Synthesis No. 58, Part I.* AHRQ Publication No. 08-05108-EF-s. Rockville, MD: Agency for Healthcare Research and Quality.

Robertson, E. B., David, S. L., & Rao, S. L. (2003). *Preventing drug use among children and adolescents: A research-based guide for parents, educators and community leaders (2nd ed.).* Bethesda, MD: U.S. Department of Health and Human Services National Institutes of Health.

Substance Abuse and Mental Health Services Administration (SAMHSA). (2011). *Identifying mental health and substance abuse use problems of children and adolescents: A guide for child-serving organizations* (HHS Publication No. SMA 12-4670). Rockville, MD: SAMSHA.

Warren, B. J. (2012). Depression: Management of depressive disorders and suicidal behavior. In Boyd, M. A. (Ed.), *Psychiatric Nursing: Contemporary Practice (5th ed.)* (Ch.24, pp.401-425). Philadelphia, PA: Wolters Kluwer, Lippincott Williams & Wilkins.

Warren, B. J. (2011).Two sides of the coin: the bully and the bullied. *Journal of Psychosocial Nursing & Mental Health Services*, 49(10), 22-29.

Warren, B. J. (2010). Cultural competence in psychiatric nursing. In Keltner, N. L., Schwecke, L. H., & Bostrom, C. E. (Eds.) (Ch. 14, pp. 164-172), *Psychiatric Nursing (6th ed.).* St. Louis, MO: Mosby.

Warren, B. J. (2008). Ethnopharmacology: the effect on patients, healthcare professionals and systems. *Urologic Nursing*, 28(4), 292-295.

Warren, B. J. & Broome, B. (2011). CNE Series: The culture of adolescents with urologic dysfunction: Mental health, wellness, and illness awareness. *Urologic Nursing*, 31(2), 95-104.

Williams, S. G. & Godfrey, A. J. (2011). What is cyberbullying & how can psychiatric-mental health nurses recognize it? *Journal of Psychosocial Nursing & Mental Health Services*, 49(10), 36-41.

SECTION 15
Mary Muscari

Bullying and Violence

Fast Facts

- Police arrest a child/teen for a violent crime every 5 minutes.

- Homicide remains the second leading cause of death in teens. In 2007, 5764 young people ages 10 to 24 were murdered, which is an average of 16 each day.

- In 2008, juveniles accounted for 16% of all violent crime arrests and 26% of all property crime arrests.

- Arrests of girls increased more/decreased less than arrests of boys for most types of offenses so that by 2004, girls accounted for 30%of all juvenile arrests.

- 15% of all spinal cord injuries are a result of intentional trauma.

- Gun violence takes a child/teen's life almost every 3 hours.

- According to the 2011 Youth Risk Behavior Surveillance System by the Centers for Disease Control and Prevention (CDC), 20% of students in grades 9–12 experienced bullying.

- School shooters, including Kip Kinkel and Luke Woodham, engaged in animal cruelty prior to their shooting rampages.

- Bullying and animal cruelty are two possible characteristics of conduct disorder.

- Youth violence prevention is one of the oldest fields in violence, and there are many evidence-based violence prevention programs that have shown positive effects.

Risk Factors for Violence

The CDC compiled several factors that place youth at risk for violence and categorized these factors into 4 clusters: individual, family, peer/school, and community. These risk factors are listed below.

Individual Risk Factors

- History of violent victimization

- Attention deficits, hyperactivity or learning disorders

- History of early aggressive behavior

- Involvement with drugs, alcohol or tobacco

- Low IQ

- Poor behavioral control

- Deficits in social cognitive or information-processing abilities

- High emotional distress

- History of treatment for emotional problems

- Antisocial beliefs and attitudes

- Exposure to violence and conflict in the family

Family Risk Factors

- Authoritarian child-rearing attitudes
- Harsh, lax or inconsistent disciplinary practices
- Low parental involvement
- Low emotional attachment to parents or caregivers
- Low parental education and income
- Parental substance abuse or criminality
- Poor family functioning
- Poor monitoring and supervision of children

Peer/Social Risk Factors

- Association with delinquent peers
- Involvement in gangs
- Social rejection by peers
- Lack of involvement in conventional activities
- Poor academic performance
- Low commitment to school and school failure

Community Risk Factors

- Diminished economic opportunities
- High concentrations of poor residents
- High level of transiency
- High level of family disruption
- Low levels of community participation
- Socially disorganized neighborhoods

Conduct disorder, which is a formal diagnostic category, has been associated with child abuse, parental drug addiction or alcoholism, family conflict, genetic defects, and poverty. It is more common in males, often associated with attention deficit hyperactivity disorder (ADHD), and may be an early sign of depression or bipolar disorder.

Common Presenting Complaints

While most children do not present with violence-related complaints, there are warning signs that may become apparent in during the history. These signs may be associated with conduct disorder.

Warning Signs of Potential Violence

Recognizing the following warning signs betters the chance of detecting the potential for violence in children as young as toddlers. For some children, combinations of behaviors and events may lead to violence.

- Fire setting
- Animal cruelty
- Excessive tantrums
- Gradual withdrawal from social contacts, and eventually complete withdrawal

- Expresses feelings of isolation and being alone
- Expresses feelings of being rejected
- Irrational beliefs and ideas
- Fascination with weaponry or explosives
- Unreciprocated romantic obsession
- Drastic change in belief system
- Family or fellow students feel fear because of your child
- Violence toward inanimate objects
- Sabotages projects or equipment
- History of being a victim of violence, including physical and sexual abuse, at home, in school, or in the community
- Low interest in school
- Expresses violence in drawings or writings; listens to music with violent themes
- When doing school projects, displays "dark side" that shows anger or frustration
- Demonstrates patterns of impulsive and chronic hitting, intimidating, and other bullying behaviors
- History of being bullied
- History of disciplinary problems
- Past history of violent or overt behavior, including fire setting, vandalism, lying, and cheating
- Intolerance to differences when doing school projects; prejudicial attitudes toward others based on race, ethnicity, religion, language, gender, sexual orientation, ability, or physical appearance
- Inappropriate access to firearms
- Brings weapon to school
- Increased risk-taking behaviors

Warning Signs of Imminent Violence

These signs, listed by the Center for the Study and Prevention of Violence, indicate that a child is dangerously close to behaving violently and require immediate action. The safest action would be to contact police immediately.

- Serious physical fighting with peers or a family member
- Severe property destruction
- Severe rage for apparently minor reason
- Possession or use of firearms or other weapons
- Detailed plan to commit a violent act or serious threats
- Self-injurious behaviors or suicidal threats

Two of the warning signs, **fire setting and animal cruelty**, consistently correlate with violence toward humans. In a horrifying and recent example, Kip Kinkel, the 15-year-old from Springfield, Oregon, who was accused of killing his parents and two fellow students, bragged about stuffing firecrackers into cats' mouths.

Watch for a drastic change in a child's belief system, irrational beliefs, feelings of isolation or rejection, unreciprocated romantic obsession, fire setting, vandalism, a fascination with weaponry or explosives, and intolerance to differences or prejudicial attitudes.

Potentially violent children may also gradually withdraw from social contacts. Other signs include: family or peers feeling fear because of the child, violence toward inanimate objects, sabotaging of projects or equipment, violence in drawings or writings, and an obsession with music with violent themes.

Screening for the Condition

The *Structured Assessment of Violence Risk in Youth (SAVRY)* is composed of 24 items in three risk domains (Historical Risk Factors, Social/Contextual Risk Factors, and Individual/Clinical Factors), drawn from existing research and the professional literature on adolescent development, and violence and aggression in youth. Each risk item has a three-level rating structure with specific rating guidelines (*Low, Moderate, or High*). The tool also contains six Protective Factor items that are rated as either Present or Absent. The SAVRY is useful in the assessment of adolescents between the ages of 12 and 18 years, and may be used by professionals in a variety of disciplines who conduct assessments and/or make intervention or supervision plans concerning violence risk in youth. The SAVRY is not a formal test or scale; there are no assigned numerical values nor are there any specified cutoff scores. Instead, it helps assist in structuring an assessment so that the important factors will not be missed and, thus, will be emphasized when formulating a final professional judgment about a youth's level of risk.

Assessment

Assessments for Bullying
Bully:

- *Overt bullies* behave in an active, outgoing, aggressive manner, using brute force or open harassment, rejecting rules, and rebelling to feel superior and secure.

- *Covert bullies* behave in a more reserved and deceptive manner, not wanting to be recognized as bullies.

- Both types have the same underlying characteristics -- interest in their own pleasure, desire for power over others, willingness to manipulate others to get what they want, and the inability to see things from another's perspective.

- Detecting bullies can be difficult because they are adept at hiding their mistreatment of others.

- They may act cocky, arrogant, and self-assured, and they may have difficulty accepting authority. When asked about bullying, they are apt to be condescending about responding to questions.

- Because most bullies lack empathy, they also tend to appear pleased or amused when providers ask them how they feel about other children getting hurt.

- Bullies may also exhibit depression, anxiety, psychosomatic symptoms, and substance abuse problems.

- Repeated bullying may be a sign of conduct disorder.

Victim:

- *Passive victims* tend to be insecure, reacting passively and anxiously to situations. They may be physically smaller than their peers, cautious, sensitive, socially isolated and quiet. They have a negative view of themselves, seeing themselves as failures and feeling lonely, stupid, ashamed, and unattractive. Other vulnerable populations are children with learning disorders, children with physical disabilities, and children who are experiencing a family crisis or who are actually neglected. In general, it appears that the children who already have much to cope with in terms of physical, emotional, or social disadvantage become victims of bullies.

- *Provocative victims* are usually be quick-tempered and try to fight back if they feel insulted or attacked. They may be hyperactive and have difficulty concentrating. Children who tend to be restless and irritable and who tease and provoke others can become victims. Provocative victims frequently display the social-emotional problems of victimized children, as well as the behavioral problems of bullies, which may create challenges for treatment.

- Victims may be fearful of walking to and from school or riding the bus. Subtle sign may be present; however, these signs can indicate other disorders, such as depression and substance abuse, which should be ruled out. Possible signs of victimization include the following:

    o Depression

    o Suicidal ideation

    o Anxiety

    o Moodiness

    o Withdrawal from family interaction

    o Loss of interest in school

    o Aggression

    o Unexplained bruises or injuries

    o Disappearance of personal belongings or pocket money

    o Waiting to use the bathroom at home or enuresis

    o Nightmares

    o Mysterious illnesses invented to avoid going to school

    o Outright refusal to go to school

    o Changes in sleep or eating patterns

    o Desire to carry a weapon for protection

Electronic Aggression (Cyberbullying)

- Electronic aggression, which encompasses cyberbullying, refers to any kind of aggression perpetrated through technology.

- Acts include harassment or bullying (teasing, telling lies, making fun of someone, making rude or mean comments, spreading rumors, or making threatening or aggressive comments) that occur through email, a chat room, instant messaging, a website (including blogs), or text messaging.

- Victims of cyberbullying may exhibit the same symptoms as those who are victimized by traditional bullying. They may not tell their parents about the problem due to their fear of losing their technical devices; they may simply suffer in silence.

Stop Cyberbullying (**www.stopcyberbullying.org**) describes five types of cyberbullies:

- Vengeful Angels believe they are righting wrongs, or protecting themselves or others from the "villain" they are victimizing. They may have been the victims of bullying or may be acting out to protect a friend who has been bullied.

- Power-Hungry Cyberbullies want to control others and get them to obey their commands. They brag and crave attention to the point that they may escalate their actions to get it.

- Revenge of the Nerds Cyberbullies usually target single victims and keep their actions secretive. They rarely appreciate the impact of their actions, and, because of their level of technical skills, can be the most dangerous of cyberbullies.

- Mean Girls are typically egotistical, immature, and bored. They use cyberbullying as entertainment and tend to act as a group because they require an audience. This form of cyberbullying is typically fed by admiration, cliques, and the silence of others who let it happen. Mean Girls quit when the entertainment value dissipates.

- Inadvertent Cyberbullies may be pretending to be tough or role playing. They don't lash out intentionally and instead behave without thinking.

Assessment for Juvenile Animal Cruelty

- Children as young as age 4 may harm animals, but cruelty is most common during adolescence.

- Animal cruelty may be a sign of conduct disorder.

- Cruelty is often associated with poor academic performance, low self-esteem, few friendships, bullying, truancy, vandalism and other antisocial behaviors.

- Ascione provide a typology of juvenile animal abusers:

  - Exploratory/curious animal abusers are usually young children who are poorly supervised and lack training on the physical care and humane treatment of animals. They abuse animals out of innocent exploration and do not intend to cause harm. Children with cognitive developmental disabilities may also fit into this category.

  - Pathological animal abusers are usually older (but not necessarily). They may be symptomatic of psychological disturbances of varying severity, and/or may have a history of physical abuse, sexual abuse or exposure to domestic violence. These children intend to cause harm to the animals.

  - Delinquent animal abusers are typically adolescents with other antisocial behaviors, including substance abuse. These children intend to cause harm and may derive pleasure from the animal's suffering.

DSM-5™ Diagnostic Criteria for Conduct Disorder

A. A repetitive and persistent pattern of behavior in which the basic rights of others or major age-appropriate societal norms or rules are violated, as manifested by the presence of at least three of the following 15 criteria in the past 12 months from any of the categories below, with at least one criterion present in the past 6 months:

Aggression to People and Animals

1. Often bullies, threatens, or intimidates others.

2. Often initiates physical fights.

3. Has used a weapon that can cause serious physical harm to others (e.g., a bat, brick, broken bottle, knife, gun).

4. Has been physically cruel to people.

5. Has been physically cruel to animals.

6. Has stolen while confronting a victim (e.g., mugging, purse snatching, extortion, armed robbery).

7. Has forced someone into sexual activity.

Destruction of Property

8. Has deliberately engaged in fire setting with the intention of causing serious damage.

9. Has deliberately destroyed others' property (other than by fire setting).

Deceitfulness or Theft

10. Has broken into someone else's house, building, or car.

11. Often lies to obtain goods or favors or to avoid obligations (i.e., "cons" others).

12. Has stolen items on nontrivial value without confronting a victim (e.g., shoplifting, but without breaking and entering; forgery).

Serious Violations of Rules

13. Often stays out at night despite parental prohibitions, beginning before age 13 years.

14. Has run away from home overnight at least twice while living in the parental or parental surrogate home, or once without returning for a lengthy period.

15. Is often truant from school, beginning before age 13 years.

B. The disturbance in behavior causes clinically significant impairment in social, academic, or occupational functioning.

C. If the individual is age 18 years or older, criteria are not met for antisocial personality disorder.

Specify whether:

312.81 (F91.1) Childhood-onset type: Individuals show at least one symptom characteristic of conduct disorder prior to age 10 years.

312.82 (F91.2) Adolescent-onset type: Individuals show no symptom characteristic of conduct disorder prior to age 10 years.

312.89 (F91.9) Unspecified onset: Criteria for diagnosis of conduct disorder are met, but there is not enough information available to determine whether the onset of the first symptom was before or after age 10 years.

Specify if:

With limited prosocial emotions: To qualify for this specifier, an individual must have displayed at least two of the following characteristics persistently over at least 12 months and in multiple relationships and settings. These characteristics reflect the individual's typical pattern of interpersonal and emotional functioning over this period and not just occasional occurrences in some situations. Thus, to assess the criteria for the specifier, multiple information sources are necessary. In addition to the individual's self-report, it is necessary to consider reports by others who have known the individual for extended periods of time (e.g., parents, teachers, co-workers, extended family members, peers).

Lack of remorse or guilt: Does not feel bad or guilty when he or she does something wrong (exclude remorse when expressed only when caught and/or facing punishment). The individual shows a general lack of concern about the negative consequences of his or her actions. For example, the individual is not remorseful after hurting someone or does not care about the consequences of breaking rules.

Callous - lack of empathy: Disregards and is unconcerned about the feelings of others. The individual is described as cold and uncaring. The person appears more concerned about the effects of his or her actions on himself or herself, rather than their effects on others, even when they result in substantial harm to others.

Unconcerned about performance: Does not show concern about poor/problematic performance at school, at work, or in other important activities. The individual does not put forth the effort necessary to perform well, even when expectations are clear, and typically blames others for his or her poor performance.

Shallow or deficient affect: Does not express feelings or show emotions to others, except in ways that seem shallow, insincere, or superficial (e.g., actions contradict the emotion displayed; can turn emotions "on" or "off" quickly) or when emotional expressional are used for gain (e.g., emotions displayed to manipulate or intimidate others).

Specify severity:

Mild: Few if any conduct problems in excess of those required to make the diagnosis are present, and conduct problems cause relatively minor harm to others (e.g., lying, truancy, staying out after dark without permission, other rule breaking).

Moderate: The number of conduct problems and the effect on others are intermediate between those specified in "mild" and those in "severe" (e.g., stealing without confronting a victim, vandalism).

Severe: Many conduct problems in excess of those required to make the diagnosis are present,or conduct problems cause considerable harm to others (e.g., forced sex, physical cruelty, use of a weapon, stealing while confronting a victim, breaking and entering).

Evidence-Based Management

Information on pharmacological management of aggression is found in the behavior disorders section of this manual.

Violence

- The American Academy of Pediatrics (AAP) Connected Kids **(http://www2.aap.org/connectedkids)** program addresses violence prevention and is a systematic method for enhancing the violence prevention anticipatory guidance that is made up of four elements:

  1. The Clinical Guide provides an overview to the entire program.

  2. The color-coded Counseling Schedule is designed for 3 separate age groups: GREEN for infancy to early childhood; BLUE for middle childhood; and RED for adolescence. The schedule recommends topics to be introduced, topics to be reinforced, and brochures to be distributed for each health supervision visit.

  3. Educational Brochures have been designed for parents and children to reinforce each of the topics covered in Connected Kids.

  4. The PowerPoint presentation offers an alternative presentation of the material in the Clinical Guide. This presentation may be helpful for personnel in-service training before implementing Connected Kids.

- Healthcare providers can participate in prevention strategies such as the CDC's *Best Practices for Violence Prevention.* This plan identifies four strategies for combatting the problem of youth violence and offers specific suggestions for implementation:

  1. Family-based strategies that combine training in parenting skills, education about child development, and exercises to help parents develop skills for communicating with their children and resolving conflict non-violently.

  2. A home visiting strategy that brings community resources to at-risk families in their homes, especially for pregnant and first-time parents.

  3. A social-cognitive strategy that helps children develop the skills they need to deal effectively with difficult situations by teaching nonviolent methods for resolving conflict and establishing (and strengthening) nonviolent beliefs in young people.

  4. A mentoring strategy that emphasizes the importance of a positive adult role model in reducing risk for violence and delinquent behavior.

- The Office of Juvenile Justice and Delinquency Prevention (OJJDP) developed *The National Juvenile Justice Action Plan* that emphasizes five key areas of best practice for communities developing a response to violence:

  1. Mobilizing communities

  2. Strengthening the juvenile justice system

  3. Decreasing gangs, guns, and drugs

  4. Creating opportunities for youth

  5. Breaking the cycle of violence through family strengthening and parent education

Bullying

Management of bullying should be multidisciplinary, involving the parents, primary healthcare provider, teachers, school administrators, school counselors, and other mental health professionals as needed.

Bullies: Intervening with bullies can be a difficult undertaking because both the parent and child may be reluctant to admit to bullying. Like victims, bullies benefit from learning appropriate social skills. Thus, they too should be encouraged to participate in small group activities, preferably with older children, so that they can engage in cooperative tasks. Adult supervision is warranted during these groups, and bullies should receive positive reinforcement each time they engage in prosocial or caring behaviors, which enables them to learn more positive ways of gaining attention and affection.

Victims: Encourage children and their parents to verbalize their feelings about the bullying. Victims and their parents need reassurance that the healthcare provider can help them find effective ways to respond to bullying and to change the children's behavior to prevent them from being bullied in the future.

Juvenile Animal Cruelty

Animal cruelty is not part of normal development. All episodes of abuse, even those done out of curiosity, warrant intervention. Interventions can be based on typology:

* Exploratory/curious animal abusers: Humane education is likely to be sufficient intervention; however, age should not be the only determining factor as animal cruelty is one of the earliest signs of conduct disorder.

* Pathological animal abusers: Professional counseling is warranted.

* Delinquent animal abusers: Both psychiatric and judicial interventions may be required.

RESOURCES

Violence

* American Medical Association's Connecting the Dots to Prevent Youth Violence: A Training and Outreach Guide for Physicians and Other Health Professionals www.ama-assn.org/ama/pub/physician-resources/public-health/promoting-healthy-lifestyles/violence-prevention/youth-violence-prevention-training-outreach-guide.shtml

* Best Practices of Youth Violence Prevention: A Sourcebook for Community Action www.cdc.gov/ncipc/dvp/bestpractices.htm

* Centers for Disease Control and Prevention Youth Violence: www.cdc.gov/violenceprevention/youthviolence/schoolviolence/index.html

* Early Warning, Timely Response A Guide to Safe Schools: www.ncjrs.gov/pdffiles1/172854.pdf.

* School Health Guidelines to Prevent Unintentional Injuries and Violence (CDC): www.cdc.gov/mmwr/PDF/rr/rr5022.pdf.

Bullying

* Bullying: American Academy of Child & Adolescent Psychiatrists
* www.aacap.org/cs/root/facts_for_families/bullying
* Bullying: Medline Plus: www.nlm.nih.gov/medlineplus/bullying.htmlCenter for Safe and Responsible Internet Use: www.cyberbully.org
* Connected Kids Clinical Guide: www.aap.org/connectedkids/ClinicalGuide.pdf
* Connected Kids Program: www.aap.org/ConnectedKids/default.htm

- Electronic Media and Youth Violence: A CDC Issue Brief for Educators and Caregivers www.cdc.gov/ViolencePrevention/pdf/EA-brief-a.pdf
- Helping Kids Deal with Bullies: http://kidshealth.org/parent/emotions/behavior/bullies.html
- National Crime Prevention Council Cyberbullying: www.ncpc.org/cyberbullying
- Stop Bullying Now: http://stopbullyingnow.hrsa.gov
- Stop Cyberbullying Now: www.stopcyberbullying.org

Animal Cruelty

- American Humane Society: www.americanhumane.org
- American Society for the Prevention of Cruelty to Animals: www.aspca.org
- Humane Society of the United States First Strike Program: www.hsus.org/firststrike
- Latham Foundation: www.latham.org
- National Association for Human and Environmental Education: http://nahee.org/
- People for the Ethical Treatment of Animals: www.peta.org
- Society and Animal Forum: http://www.societyandanimalsforum.org/

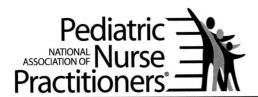

How to Raise a Nonviolent Child: Information for Parents

Know the Difference Between Normal and Abnormal Behaviors & Emotions

All children behave in a negative manner at some time or another, and parents need to be able to tell the difference between behaviors that are appropriate for a child's age (imaginary warfare during the school-age years) from those that are not (biting after age 2). Although it is not unusual for children to show some aggressive behaviors, it is socially unacceptable. If your child shows these types of behaviors, it is important to set limits on them.

Provide Your Child with Plenty of Love and Attention

Lack of attention causes increased aggression in children and places children at risk for becoming hostile, difficult, and hard to manage. Children need attention, even if only 15 to 20 minutes of special time with you every day. Tell your children you love them often, and provide them with a safe and secure home.

Foster Positive Self-Esteem

Children with positive self-esteem typically have an easier time handling conflicts and resisting negative pressures. Praise your children often. Catch your children being good.

Talk With Your Child, Not at Him or Her

Families with poor communication skills are at higher risk for raising violent children. Teach your children good, basic communication skills.

Supervise Your Child Closely

A critical factor in teen violence is lack of parental supervision, especially not knowing the whereabouts of children. Children with minimal parental monitoring have higher levels of problem behaviors than children with proper monitoring. Always know where your child is, with whom, and what they are doing.

Set Limits with Your Child

Children misbehave to get attention, assert power, or act out their frustration, anger, depression, or pain. They misbehave when rules are not clear or consistent. Therefore, parents need to set limits and make sure that their children understand them. Discipline is not the same as punishment; it is teaching children what behaviors are acceptable and not acceptable. Time out as a method of discipline works well for younger children. Appropriate consequences for negative behaviors in older children and teens might include not allowing them to watch TV, play computer games, or spend time with a friend. Be consistent in setting limits with your child.

Teach Responsibility

When children have a number of responsibilities, they learn how to establish priorities and organize their time. Have your child help with household chores and participate in community service activities.

Teach Your Child How to Problem-Solve and Make Decisions

Encourage your child to problem-solve through play if he or she is younger. Older children should be encouraged to make age-appropriate decisions, such as planning what to wear for the week.

Help Your Child to Decrease Stress

Stress overload can cause children to be anxious, withdrawn or depressed.

Help your child to recognize signs of stress and develop ways to deal with stress (e.g., hobbies, humor, relaxation techniques, and pet therapy). Exercise also is a wonderful outlet for stress in children. Remember, your level of stress affects your child.

Help Your Child to Deal with their Anger in Positive Ways

Teach your child how to recognize their own angry feelings, express anger in positive ways, and learn positive ways for dealing with their anger (e.g., counting to 10; blowing the anger away, writing in a journal, exercising).

Teach Tolerance

Help your child to understand and appreciate differences among people.

Enforce Family Values

Share your values with your child regularly (e.g., honesty, compassion, self-discipline).

Minimize the Effects of Peer Pressure

Know your child's friends and tell your child that being part of a group does not require them to give in to their every desire. Choose battles wisely by compromising on minor issues, such as hairstyles and pierced ears, and by holding firm on the major issues, such as shoplifting, alcohol or drug use.

Monitor What Your Child Watches and the Games He/She Plays

Do not allow your children to watch violent shows or play violent video games. Studies have shown that watching violence can lead to an increase in violent behavior.

Keep Your Child Away from Alcohol and Drugs

Teens under the influence of drugs, especially alcohol, are more likely to commit acts of violence than teens who do not use drugs. Start talking to your child about alcohol and drugs at an early age. Set a zero tolerance for their use.

Keep Guns Away from Your Child

Do not keep guns in your home. If guns are in the home, they must be kept locked away in safe storage. Teach your child what to do if they come across a gun.

Be a Responsible Role Model for Your Child

Children learn best by what they see, not what they hear, and parents serve as their most important role models. Therefore, it is important for you to show your child a healthy self-esteem and healthy ways to handle life's challenges.

Get Involved in Your Child's School and Activities

Involved parents send a strong, positive message to their children, and decrease the change that their children will engage in risk-taking behaviors.

Decrease Bullying Behaviors

If your child gets bullied, help him or her to stand up to those who are bullying him or her and report the problem to the proper authorities.

Know the Warning Signs of Violence

Be aware of the warning signs of violence and teach your children the signs as well.

Get Help When Needed

Talk to your child's physician or nurse practitioner and get counseling for your child if he or she is showing problem behaviors.

Adapted with permission from: Muscari, M. (2002). Not My Kid: 21 Steps to Raising a Nonviolent Child. Scranton, PA: University of Scranton Press.

REFERENCES

American Academy of Pediatrics Committee on Injury, Violence, and Poison Prevention. (2009). Role of the Pediatrician in Youth Violence Prevention. *Pediatrics*; 124 (1), 393-402.

American Psychiatric Association (2000). *Diagnostic and Statistical Manual of Mental Disorders, Fourth Edition* (DSM-IV). Washington, DC: APA.

Arseneault, L., Walsh, E., Trzesniewski, K., Newcombe, R., Caspi, A., Moffitt, T. E. (2006). Bullying victimization uniquely contributes to adjustment problems in young children: a nationally representative cohort study. *Pediatrics*, 118(1),130-138.

Ascione, F. (2001). Animal abuse and youth violence. OJJDP Juvenile Justice Bulletin, NCJ 188677. **www.ncjrs.org/html/ojjdp/ jjbul2001_9_2/contents.html**.

Centers for Disease Control and Prevention. (2010). Understanding School Violence Fact Sheet. **www.cdc.gov/violenceprevention/pdf/SchoolViolence_FactSheet-a.pdf**

Centers for Disease Control and Prevention. (2008). Youth Violence Prevention Scientific Information: Risk and Protective Factors. www.cdc.gov/NCIPC/dvp/YVP/YVP-risk-p-factors.htm

David-Ferdon C, Hertz MF. (2007). Electronic media, violence, and adolescents: an emerging public health problem. *Journal of Adolescent Health*, 41(suppl 1):S1-S5.

Lamb, J., Pepler, D., & Craig, W. (2009). Approach to bullying and victimization. *Canadian Family Physician*, 55(4), 356-360.

Lemstra, M., Nielsen, G., Rogers, M., Thompson, A., & Moraros, J. (2012). Risk indicators and outcomes associated with bullying in youth aged 9-15 years. *Canadian Journal of Public Health*, 103(1), 9-13.

Melnyk, B.M., Brown, H., Jones, D.C., Kreipe, R., & Novak, J. (2003). Improving the mental/psychosocial health of U.S. children and adolescents. Outcomes and implementation strategies from the national KySS summit. *Journal of Pediatric Healthcare*, 17(6: Suppl 1), S1-S24.

Peeters, M., Cillessen, A., & Scholte, R. (2010). Clueless or powerful? Identifying subtypes of bullies in adolescence. *Journal of Youth Adolescence*, 39(9), 1041–1052.

Resnick, M. D., Ireland, M., & Borowsky, I. (2004). Youth violence perpetration: what protects? What predicts? Findings from the National Longitudinal Study of Adolescent Health. *Journal of Adolescent Health*, 35(5), 424.e1–e10.

Sekol, I. & Farrington, D. (2010). The overlap between bullying and victimization in adolescent residential care: Are bully/victims a special category? *Children and Youth Services Review*, 32(12), 1758-1769.

Wasserman, G., et al. (2003). Risk of protective factors of child delinquency. *Child Delinquency Bulletin Series, April*, 1-14. Office of Juvenile Justice and Delinquency Prevention.

SECTION 16
Diana Jacobson, Leigh Small, and Bernadette Mazurek Melnyk

Overweight and Obesity

Fast Facts

- Although obesity is considered a medical condition, not a psychological disorder, many researchers and clinicians argue that the psychological and social impact of living with obesity is a risk factor in the development and persistence of mental health problems.

- There is much research evidence that supports the predictive relationship of child emotional and behavioral problems (i.e., high levels of internalizing and externalizing behaviors) and the later life development of obesity or overweight.

- Psychological and social comorbidities associated with excess body weight in childhood and adolescence includes depression, poor body image and self-esteem, and decreased social competence and academic achievement.

- Routine calculation of body mass index (BMI) of all children 2 years of age and older is essential to identify all children who may be overweight or obese. Although not a perfect indicator of body fatness, BMI is a useful tool as an initial screen to classify health risks. Children less than 2 years of age should be routinely assessed for excess body weight through use of weight for height calculations that are age and gender adjusted.

- National estimates indicate that 32% of children and adolescents ages 2 to 19 years are overweight or obese as defined by a BMI greater than the 85th percentile for age and gender. Child obesity is defined as having a BMI >95th percentile.
  - 27% of preschool children, 2-5 years, are overweight or obese.
  - 33% of school aged children, 6-11 years, are overweight or obese.
  - 34% of teens, 12-19 years, are overweight or obese.

- Waist circumference and waist-by-height ratio is yet another measure of obesity that is an independent predictor of associated severe and chronic comorbid health problems.

- The cardiovascular and metabolic consequences of obesity during childhood are well known and include insulin resistance, type 2 diabetes, hypertension, dyslipidemia, and atherosclerosis.

- Other known health comorbidities of excess body weight include polycystic ovary disease, musculoskeletal pain and injury, gastroesophageal reflux, non-alcoholic steatohepatitis, sleep apnea, and increased asthma symptoms.

Risk Factors

- Ethnic and minority status (e.g., Hispanic/Latino, African American, Native American)
- Parental educational level
- Family socioeconomic status
- Children exhibiting maladaptive internalizing (e.g., withdrawal, depression, and somatization) or externalizing (e., hyperactivity and aggression) behaviors
- Parental or first generation relative who is overweight or obese
- Family history of first generation or second generation diabetes (gestational or type 2 diabetes), insu-

lin resistance or metabolic syndrome, hypertension, hyperlipidemia, or cardiovascular disease

- History of low birth weight, large birth weight and formula feeding in infancy
- Rapid weight gain in the first 4-12 months of life
- Adiposity rebound, normally occurring in children who are 5-7 years, is a critical time during which risk factors can be easily identified and they include:
  - Children with a high BMI during adiposity rebound
  - Children who experience early adiposity rebound
  - Children with rapidly accelerating BMI during adiposity rebound
- History of psychotropic medications used to treat mental health disorders
- History of sleep disturbances

Common Presenting Complaints
- Sleep disturbances
- Increased asthma symptoms
- Shortness of breath with activity
- Depression and/or anxiety; low self-esteem
- Acanthosis nigricans, striae or fungal infections of the skin
- Dysmenorrhea, irregular periods and hirsuitism
- Gastrointestinal reflux symptoms
- Hip, knee and/or foot pain or injury
- Elevated blood pressure

Screening for the Condition
- Children <2 years of age: Determination of age- and gender-adjusted Height for Recumbent Weight percentile
- Children 4-8 years: Waist circumference >90 percentile and/or Waist-by-Height ratio greater than 0.5
- Children >2 years of age: Determination of child/adolescent height and weight with calculation of age and gender absolute BMI and adjusted BMI percentile
- The United States Preventive Services Task Force (USPSTF) recommends that clinicians screen children aged 6 years and older for obesity and offer them or refer them to comprehensive, intensive behavioral interventions to promote improvement in weight status (see http://www.uspreventiveservicestaskforce.org/uspstf/uspschobes.htm). The USPSTF found adequate evidence that BMI was an acceptable measure for identifying children and adolescents with excess weight.

Assessment
- Historical information to determine modifiable lifestyle factors
  - Overall dietary quality and quantity (e.g., portion sizes, balance of macronutrients [carbohydrates, fats, saturated fats, protein], meal frequency, and snacking)
  - High intake patterns of energy dense foods and sweetened beverages including fruit juice and sodas
  - High frequency of fast food and fast/frozen meal consumption
  - Limited home cooked family meals
  - Low dietary intake of fruits and vegetables, calcium and fiber

- o Limited frequency of breakfast consumption
- o High frequency of meals and/or snacks consumed while involved in screen time activities
- o Presence of binge eating, boredom eating, emotional eating, and night eating
- o Assessment of average screen time (i.e., television, computer, gaming and cell phone texting) use per day
- o Assessment of the average quality and quantity of physical activity per day
- o Distractions from adequate sleep (i.e., TV in bedroom, access to cell phones or technology at night, irregular bedtime routines)
- Historical information to identify risk for physical comorbid health problems

  - o Snoring, daily fatigue, sleep difficulties, or daytime sleepiness
  - o Respiratory complaints of shortness of breath, exercise intolerance, frequent coughing or wheezing
  - o Abdominal pain (recurrent or non-specific), heartburn or chest pain, constipation and/or encopresis and/or right upper quadrant abdominal pain
  - o Polyuria, polyphagia, and polydipsia
  - o Nocturia, enuresis, and incontinence
  - o Menstrual irregularities and dysmenorrhea
  - o Unexplained headache
  - o Lower limb pain or frequent injuries
  - o Acne, striae, hirsutism, skin rash and/or skin problems
- Historical information to identify risk for comorbid psychosocial/mental health problems

  - o Recipient of weight-related victimization (i.e., bullying or teasing) at home, school or childcare
  - o Avoidance of social situations appropriate for age, social exclusion, peer rejection or difficulties with social interactions
  - o Reluctance or avoidance to participate in physical activities (i.e., home, family- associated, or group)
  - o Decreased confidence in ability to be physically active
  - o Poor academic achievement or underachievement
  - o School avoidance and school absences for illness or truancy
  - o Sleep problems (i.e., delayed sleep onset, frequent awakenings, early rising, nightmares, insomnia, or hypersomnia)
  - o History or potential for sexual, physical or emotional abuse
  - o Binge eating with or without self-induced vomiting
  - o Fatigue, listlessness, withdrawn, flat affect, depressive symptoms or apathy
  - o Increased worries relative to other children and/or anxiety
  - o Body dissatisfaction
  - o Low self-esteem or self-neglect
  - o Anger, aggression, irritability, or hyperactivity

- Assessment of child and/or parent/caregiver's readiness to change and increase healthy lifestyle behaviors

- Consistent with the principles of Motivational Interviewing, assess the felt importance of the problem, desire to change behaviors and confidence in ability to change behaviors

- Identify personal, familial, social, contextual and environmental barriers to making behavioral change (i.e., potential and actual)

- Identify personal and familial attributes, as well as social, contextual and environmental facilitators of behavior change

- Determine the degree of supportiveness in the relationship between the parent and child (parent-child "fit") and potential need for alternative support systems

- Identify the child's temperament and/or personality style which may influence the type and methods of environmental and behavioral change strategies

- Physical examination findings to assess for health comorbidities

  - Blood pressure using the correct cuff size to evaluate for hypertension

    - Diagnostic parameters: $\geq$95th percentile for age, gender and height on $\geq$3 separate occasions

  - Acanthosis nigricans

  - Tonsillar hypertrophy

  - Goiter

  - Genu varum, genu valgum, pes planus

  - Abnormal gait: limited hip range of motion or pain elicited during exam

  - Fundoscopic examination to rule out papilledema

  - Liver span assessment

  - Tanner stage to examine for precocious or delayed puberty onset; micropenis; undescended testes

  - Acne, striae and/or hirsutism

  - Assessment of waist circumference at the umbilicus and superior spine of the iliac crests.

  Determine waist circumference percentile. Intervention initiation indicated if calculated waist-by-height ratio is greater than 0.5 regardless of BMI.

  - Serum blood analyses are evaluated depending upon family history, age and risk.

    - Children $\geq$10 years of age with a BMI of 85th to 94th percentile should have a lipid panel ordered and if other risk factors are present (i.e., family history of hyperlipidemia) should, additionally, have a fasting glucose, ALT and AST levels ordered. These test(s) are repeated every 2 years.

    - Children $\geq$10 years of age with a BMI of 95th or greater percentile should have a fasting lipid panel, fasting glucose, ALT and AST levels ordered and repeated every 2 years. If the AST and/or AST levels are above 60 U/L on two occasions, then referral to a gastroenterologist is recommended.

Diagnosis

- Age- and gender-adjusted weight for recumbent length ≥95th percentile = overweight for children ≤2 years of age

- BMI percentile ≥85th – 94th BMI percentile = overweight for children and adolescents 2-19 years of age

- BMI percentile ≥95th percentile or absolute BMI ≥30 = obese for children and adolescents 2-19 years of age

Management of Weight Goals by Age

- 2-5 years of age for those with 85-94th BMI percentile: weight maintenance until BMI is <85th percentile or demonstration of slowing of weight gain (e.g., decreasing BMI trajectory)

- 2-5 years of age for those with ≥95th BMI percentile: weight maintenance until BMI is <85th BMI percentile or gradual weight loss of no more than 1 lb. per month if the BMI is >21

- 6-11 years of age for those with 85-94th BMI percentile: weight maintenance until BMI <85th BMI percentile, slowing of weight gain, or decrease in absolute BMI

- 6-11 years of age for those with 95th - 98th BMI percentile: weight maintenance until BMI < 85th BMI percentile, slowing of weight gain, or decrease in absolute BMI (e.g., goal of approximately 1 lb. gradual weight loss per month)

- 6-11 years of age for those with ≥99th BMI percentile: weight loss (e.g., goal of weight loss is no more than 2 lbs. per week)

- 12-19 years of age for those with 85th - 94th BMI percentile: weight maintenance until BMI <85th BMI percentile, slowing of weight gain, or decrease in absolute BMI (e.g., goal of no more than 2 lbs. gradual weight loss per week)

- 12-19 years of age for those with 95th - 98th BMI percentile: weight loss of no more than 2 lbs. per week)

- 12-19 years of age for those with >99th BMI percentile: weight loss not to exceed 2 lbs. per week

- Parent, family, or other support has been empirically found to be an important element

- Behavioral strategies are a component of effective healthy weight interventions

Assessment

Formal assessment tools for bullying behavior (aggressor/perpetrator), victims of bullying and child social assessment tools are available at no cost from:

1) http://www.cdc.gov/violenceprevention/pdf/bullyCompendiumbk-a.pdf

2) Revised ProVictim Scale (Ken Rigby): available with scoring instruction at http://www.kenrigby.net/01a-Questionnaires

3) Sizing Me Up—Weight Related Quality of Life (Modi & Zeller): this instrument is available free of charge after permission is granted from the authors. Information can be found at http://www.cincinnatichildrens.org/research/divisions/b/psychology/labs/zeller/hrqol-pediatric-obesity/sizing/default/

Perpetrator and Victim Assessment tools, which are available at a cost:

1) Peer Relations Assessment Questionnaires-Revised (PRAQ-R) (Ken Rigby): available for schools to assess the presence of bullying behavior at: https://shop.acer.edu.au/acer-shop/group/PRAQR

2) Pediatric Quality of Life Inventory Child-Self Report and Parent-Proxy Report (ages 8-12) (PedsQL™)—(James W. Varni) are instruments measuring health-related quality of life and are available for clinical practice. These instruments can be found at http://www.pedsql.org/about_pedsql.html

---

Evidence-Based Overweight and Obesity Treatment/Management by Stage of Overweight/Obesity

Stage 1: Prevention Plus (Barlow & the Expert Committee, 2007)—Youth between the ages of 2 and 19 years with BMI >85th percentile

- Focus on educating families concerning basic healthy lifestyle eating and activity behaviors utilizing Motivational Interviewing techniques:
  - Consume ≥5 servings of fruits and vegetables every day
  - Eliminate sugar sweetened beverages (i.e., juice, soda, sports drinks)
  - Decrease screen time to ≤2 hours per day. No television for children under 2 years of age
  - Increase physical activity to at least 60 minutes each day
  - Prepare family meals at least 5-6 times a week to decrease fast and restaurant food consumption
  - Eat a healthy breakfast every day
  - Involve the family in all lifestyle changes respecting cultural differences and developmental age of the child/adolescent
- Motivational Interviewing principles include:
  - Express empathy
  - Avoid argumentation
  - Support self-efficacy
  - Roll with resistance
  - Develop discrepancy
- Use patient/family-centered problem-solving.
  - Identify the barriers
  - Have a patient/family generate potential strategies to work through unhealthy behaviors contributing to the child/adolescent's energy imbalance
  - Patient/family chooses initial goals to target
  - Evaluate the strategy
- Follow up for 3-6 months, meeting with the child/adolescent and the family in the office setting at mutually agreed upon times.
- If there is no improvement in lifestyle behaviors and in the child's health/weight, the provider offers the next level of weight management.

Stage 2: Structured Weight Management—Children 2-19 years of age with BMI >85th - 99th percentile.

- Lifestyle habits as in Stage 1
- Motivational interviewing techniques continue to be utilized for the family to set healthy lifestyle behavior goals for nutrition and physical activity
- Include the following as family/patient goals:
  - Three structured, balanced daily eating plan and 1-2 planned snacks of foods that are low in energy density and high in fiber; no sugar sweetened beverages.
  - Decreased screen time to ≤1 hour each day
  - Planned and supervised physical activity of at least 60 minutes each day

- o Diet and physical activity logs (e.g., diaries)
- More formal nutritional plan may require the expertise of a dietician
- Monthly follow up office visits or group sessions

Stage 3: Comprehensive Multidisciplinary Intervention—Children 2-19 years of age with BMI >95th percentile

- Maximize primary care office and specialist support given to the child/adolescent and family to increase behavior change.

- Eating and activity goals are similar to Stage 1 and 2.

- Goal setting and, food and physical activity monitoring are structured with behavior modification techniques

- Parent involvement and training in improving the home environment is imperative especially with children <12 years of age

- Child or adolescent must be assessed for mental health issues along with assistance of others in a multidisciplinary team (e.g., registered dietician, exercise specialist, counseling, social worker)

- Primary care provider continues to manage all medical problems and provide a supportive alliance with families

- Weekly multidisciplinary counseling for a minimum of 8 to 12 weeks.

Stage 4: Tertiary Care Intervention—Children >11 years of age with BMI >95th – 99th percentile

- Severely obese youth who have attempted the Stages 1 to 3 recommendations from a multidisciplinary team without success

- Medications such as sibutramine or orlistat may be initiated for children, 16 years or older, in conjunction with a structured diet and exercise program (safety and efficacy in younger children is untested)

- Very low-calorie restrictive diets and weight control surgery may be offered by the tertiary team to adolescents who have not responded to intensive Stage 3 treatment modalities

USPSTF Recommendations for Treatment

The USPSTF found that effective comprehensive weight-management programs incorporated counseling and other interventions that targeted diet and physical activity. Interventions also included behavioral management techniques to assist in behavior change. Interventions that focused on younger children incorporated parental involvement as a component.

Moderate- to high-intensity programs involved >25 hours of contact with the child and/or the family over a 6-month period and showed results including improved weight status, defined as an absolute and/or relative decrease in the BMI 12 months after the beginning of the intervention. Evidence was limited on the long-term sustainability of BMI changes achieved through behavioral interventions and on the trajectory of weight gain in children and adolescents. Interventions generally took place in referral settings, and the results can only be generalized to children who follow through on treatment (see **http://www.uspreventiveservicestaskforce.org/uspstf10/childobes/chobesrs.htm**).

Primary Care and School-Based Intervention Programs for Overweight and Obesity

- Preliminary testing of healthy weight intervention strategies have been conducted with children of various ages and their parents in primary care settings and each has demonstrated positive findings (i.e., anthropometric, emotional and behavioral). For more information, please contact: Dr. Leigh Small at **Leigh.Small@asu.edu** for a parent-directed program for healthy weight in 4-8-year old children. Dr. Diana Jacobson at **Diana.Jacobson@asu.edu** for a primary care healthy lifestyle program to improve healthy lifestyle choices and psychosocial health for school aged children and parents.

- The evidence-based COPE (Creating Opportunities for Personal Empowerment) Healthy Lifestyles TEEN (Thinking, Emotions, Exercise, and Nutrition) Program is a manualized, 15-session, cognitive-behavioral skills building intervention program for adolescents that can be integrated into high school health courses or taught in group format in primary care or specialty settings. Findings from pilot studies and a full-scale randomized controlled trial with 779 adolescents indicate that the COPE intervention: prevents overweight and obesity; improves self-esteem, social skills and academic performance; decreases alcohol use and reduces depressive symptoms (Melnyk et al., 2009; Melnyk et al., in press).

  For more information about the COPE program, contact Dr. Bernadette Melnyk at cope.melnyk@gmail.com.

Psychotropic Medication Use and Overweight/Obesity

Weight gain is associated with the use of many psychotropic medications, including antidepressants, mood stabilizers, and antipsychotic drugs (See Tables 16.1 and 16.2). Understanding the increased risk of metabolic consequences (e.g., weight gain, diabetes, dyslipidemia) of psychotropic medications is essential for healthcare providers. Several management options are available if a child or adolescent is gaining weight at an accelerated pace after the initiation of one of these therapeutic agents. When it is assessed that the child or adolescent taking psychotropic medications is gaining weight abnormally, the practitioner may choose change to another drug (e.g., collaboratively consult with mental health provider if not the prescribing provider), provide nutritional counseling and encourage increased physical activity and/or initiate or refer for behavioral treatment and management. Prevention of weight gain for children and adolescents requiring psychotropic medications is the best approach and begins by routinely choosing medications which have been shown to cause less weight gain and by educating and counseling parents and children/adolescents about the weight gain risks. Upon initiation of any psychotropic medication, routine treatment should include monitoring of weight, BMI, blood pressure, fasting glucose, fasting cholesterol and triglyceride levels and glycosylated hemoglobin (hemoglobin A1C).

Table 16.1. Psychotropic Medications Associated With Increased Risk of Weight Gain

Antidepressants	Mood Stabilizers	Atypical Antipsychotics
Paxil (paroxetine)	Lithium (i.e., *Eskalith*; *Lithobid*; *Lithostat*)	*Risperdal* (risperidone)
Tricyclic antidepressants (i.e., *Elavil* [amitriptyline]; Norpramin [desipramine] ; *Tofranil* [imipramine]; *Vivactil* [protriptyline]; *Sumontil* [trimipramine]; *Anafranil* [clomipramine])	Valproate (i.e., *Depakote*; *Depakote* ER)	*Zyprexa* (olanzapine)
Remeron (mirtazapine)		*Clozaril* (clozapine)

Table 16.2. Psychotropic Medications That Are Weight Neutral for Most Children and Adolescents

Antidepressants	Mood Stabilizers	Atypical Antipsychotics
Prozac (fluoxetine)	*Neurontin* (gabapentin)	*Abilify* (aripiprazole)
Luvox (fluvoxamine)	*Topamax* (topiramate)	*Geodon* (ziprasidone)
Lexapro (escitalopram)		
Zoloft (sertraline)		
Celexa (citalopram)		
Wellbutrin (buproprion)		
Cymbalta (duloxetine)		
Effexor (venlafaxine)		

Resources for Parents and Providers

American Academy of Pediatrics, Prevention and Treatment of Childhood Overweight and Obesity: http://www2.aap.org/obesity/

- Creates awareness for parents of simple techniques that will improve both the nutritional intake and physical activity level of children and teens

Centers for Disease Control and Prevention, Child Obesity Facts: http://www.cdc.cov/healthyyouth/obesity/facts.htm
Provides parent and providers information concerning obesity and the importance of measuring and plotting BMI

Center for Disease Control and Prevention, Injury Prevention & Control: Violence Prevention http://www.cdc.gov/violenceprevention/pub/measuring_bullying.html

- Provides a compendium of bullying assessment tools to assess the behavior of perpetrators, victims and bystanders

Institute of Medicine, Accelerating Progress in Obesity Prevention: http://www.iom.edu/Reports/2012/Accelerating-Progress-in-Obesity-Prevention.aspx

- Reports on the state of the science in the most efficacious prevention of overweight and obesity interventions

Let's Move: http://www.letsmove.gov/

- Provides parents, providers and communities recommendations for food and nutrition and physical activity for children and families

Mental Health Medications, National Institutes of Mental Health: http://www.nimh.nih.gov/health/publications/mental-health-medications/complete-index.shtml

- Provides information for parents and providers concerning the medications that are commonly prescribed for mental health disorders

Robert Wood Johnson Foundation, Childhood Obesity: http://www.rwjf.org/en/about-rwjf/program-areas/childhood-obesity.html

- Discusses the state of improvement in nutrition policies for schools meals in the United States

United States Department of Agriculture, Choose My Plate: http://www.choosemyplate.gov/

- Nutritional information and handouts for parents and providers focused on improving meal planning and dietary intake of children and teens.

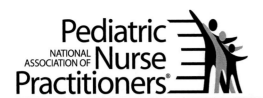

What Is Considered Overweight or at Risk for Overweight in Children and Teens?

Overweight in children is determined by their BMI percentile, not their BMI as in adults. Children found to be greater than the 85th percentile are considered to be overweight; however, children found to be greater than the 95th BMI percentile are considered to be obese. These guidelines were established by many professional organizations, including the American Academy of Pediatrics. If you are unsure whether your child or teen is overweight, have your child's healthcare provider calculate their BMI percentile for you or consult one of the many Websites that will help you to calculate this. Heavily muscled athletes may be overweight, but not overfat, and excess body fat is the primary cause of the medical complications associated with a high BMI.

How Can Overweight Affect Someone's Health?

Excessive weight can cause a wide variety of health problems, including:

- Type 2 diabetes
- High blood pressure
- Worsening of asthma
- Heart disease
- Sleep apnea
- Gastro-esophageal reflux
- Poor coping/mental health outcomes (e.g., depression, anxiety, low self-esteem)

What Causes Overweight?

The point at which a person's nutritional intake exceeds his or her activity level causes an energy imbalance. If this energy imbalance is maintained over a long period of time, a person will store the extra energy as fat and put on extra weight.

Which Children/Teens Are at Risk to Become Overweight?

Scientists who study overweight in children and teens have identified factors that place certain children and teens at high risk for overweight.

Those risk factors include:

- Overweight in the toddler and preschool years
- Sedentary lifestyle (e.g., a lot of computer or television viewing time)
- Natural parents or caretakers who are overweight or have a complication of overweight/obesity
- Dietary intake of high-calorie, often fatty, foods and/or decreased intake of fruits and vegetables

What Are the Treatments for Overweight in Children and Teens?

It is important that overweight in children and teens be treated using the following three approaches, which focus on healthy lifestyle patterns:

- Healthy dietary intake
- Regular exercise or activity
- Positive emphasis on supportive and healthy lifestyles

What Can You Do to Help Your Child with His or Her Weight?

There are a few simple guidelines that you can initiate with your child or teen to help him or her to make positive, healthy lifestyle changes:

- Decrease the amount of sugared beverages that your child drinks (e.g., soda, fruit punch, and sports drinks). Skim milk provides essential nutrients and may satisfy hunger.
- Decrease the amount of television viewing time and/or computer time to 1-2 hours per day.
- Provide a moderately low fat diet.
- Provide healthy snacks for your family.
- Engage in healthy family activities on a regular basis.
- Do not restrict your child's/teens dietary intake only, rather than changing the whole family's diet to a healthy one.
- Be a positive and supportive influence on your child/teen and model regular healthy eating and activity habits.
- Build your child's self-esteem by focuses on his special characteristics and strengths.
- Help your child build his beliefs/confidence that he or she can engage in healthy behavior

REFERENCES

Ahn, S. & Fedewa, A. L. (2011). A meta-analysis of the relationship between children's physical activity and mental health. *Journal of Pediatric Psychology* 36(4), 385-397. doi: 10.1093/jpepsy/jsq107

Anzman-Frasca, S., Stifter, C. A., & Birch, L. L. (2012). Temperament and childhood obesity risk: A review of the literature. *Journal of Developmental and Behavioral Pediatrics*, 33(9), 732-745. doi: 10.1097/DBP.0b013e31826a119f; 10.1097/DBP.0b013e31826a119f

Barlow, S. E., & Expert Committee. (2007). Expert committee recommendations regarding the prevention, assessment, and treatment of child and adolescent overweight and obesity: Summary report. *Pediatrics*, 120(Suppl 4), S164-S192. doi: 10.1542/peds.2007-2329C

Duarte, C. S., Sourander, A., Nikolakaros, G., et al. (2010). Child mental health problems and obesity in early adulthood. The *Journal of Pediatrics*, 156(1), 93-97. doi: 10.1016/j.jpeds.2009.06.066

French, S. A., Story, M., & Perry, C. L. (1995). Self-esteem and obesity in children and adolescents: a literature review. *Obesity Research*, 3(5), 479-490.

Greco, L. A., & Morris, T. A. (2005). Factors influencing the link between social anxiety and peer acceptance: contributions of social skills and close friendships during middle childhood. *Behavior Therapy*, 36(2), 197-205.

Griffiths, L. J., Dezateux, C., & Hill, A. (2011). Is obesity associated with emotional and behavioural problems in children? Findings from the millennium cohort study. *International Journal of Pediatric Obesity*, 6(2-2), e423-e432. doi: 10.3109/17477166.2010.526221; 10.3109/17477166.2010.526221

Gunnarsdottir, T., Njardvik, U., Olafsdottir, A. S., Craighead, L. W., & Bjarnason, R. (2012). Teasing and social rejection among obese children enrolling in family-based behavioural treatment: Effects on psychological adjustment and academic competencies. *International Journal of Obesity*, 36(1), 35-44. doi: 10.1038/ijo.2011.181; 10.1038/ijo.2011.181

Hamburger, M. E., Basile, K. C., & Vivolo, A. M. (2011). Measuring bullying victimization, perpetration, and bystander experiences: A compendium of assessment tools. Centers for Disease Control and Prevention, National Center for Injury Prevention and Control; Atlanta, GA.

Hebebrand, J. & Herpertz-Dahlmann, B. (2009). Psychological and psychiatric aspects of pediatric obesity. *Child and Adolescent Psychiatric Clinics of North America*, 18(1), 49-65. doi: 10.1016/j.chc.2008.08.002

Hills, A. P., King, N. A., & Armstrong, T. P. (2007). The contribution of physical activity and sedentary behaviours to the growth and development of children and adolescents: Implications for overweight and obesity. *Sports Medicine*, 37(6), 533-545.

Jacobson, D. & Melnyk, B. M. (2012). A primary care Healthy Choices Intervention program for overweight and obese school-age children and their parents. Journal of Pediatric Health Care, 26(2), 126-138. *Impact Factor =1.163*. DOI: 10.1016/j.pedhc.2010.07.004

Janicke, D. M., Harman, J. S., Kelleher, K. J., & Zhang, J. (2008). Psychiatric diagnosis in children and adolescents with obesity-related health conditions. *Journal of Developmental and Behavioral Pediatrics*, 29(4), 276-284. doi: 10.1097/DBP.0b013e31817102f8

Janicke, D. M., Marciel, K. K., Ingerski, L. M., et al. (2007). Impact of psychosocial factors on quality of life in overweight youth. *Obesity*, 15(7), 1799-1807. doi: 10.1038/oby.2007.214

Jelalian, E. & Saelens, B. E. (1999). Empirically supported treatments in pediatric psychology: *Pediatric obesity. Journal of Pediatric Psychology*, 24(3), 223-248.

Keeley, T. J. H. & Fox, K. R. (2009). The impact of physical activity and fitness on academic achievement and cognitive performance in children. *International Review of Sport and Exercise Psychology*, 2(2), 198-214.

Krebs, N. F., Himes, J. H., Jacobson, D., Nicklas, T. A., Guilday, P., & Styne, D. (2007). Assessment of child and adolescent overweight and obesity. *Pediatrics*, 120(Suppl 4), S193-228. doi: 10.1542/peds.2007-2329D

Maloney, A. E. (2010). Pediatric obesity: A review for the child psychiatrist. *Child and Adolescent Psychiatric Clinics of North America*, 19(2), 353-370. doi: 10.1016/j.chc.2010.01.005

Mamun, A. A., O'Callaghan, M. J., Cramb, S. M., Najman, J. M., Williams, G. M., & Bor, W. (2009). Childhood behavioral problems predict young adults' BMI and obesity: evidence from a birth cohort study. *Obesity*, 17(4), 761-766. doi: 10.1038/oby.2008.594

Melnyk, B.M., Jacobson, D., Kelly, S., et al. (in press). Promoting healthy lifestyles in high school adolescents. *American Journal of Preventive Medicine*.

Melnyk, B.M., Jacobson, D., Kelly, S., O'Haver, J., Small, L., & Mays, M.Z. (2009). Improving the mental health, healthy lifestyle choices and physical health of Hispanic adolescents: A randomized controlled pilot study. *Journal of School Health*, 79(12), 575-584.

Ogden, C. L., Carroll, M. D., Curtin, L. R., Lamb, M. M., & Flegal, K. M. (2010). Prevalence of high body mass index in US children and adolescents, 2007-2008. *The Journal of the American Medical Association*, 303(3), 242-249. doi: 10.1001/jama.2009.2012

Paluska, S. A. & Schwenk, T. L. (2000). Physical activity and mental health: Current concepts. *Sports Medicine*, 29(3), 167-180.

Parfitt, G. & Eston, R. G. (2005). The relationship between children's habitual activity level and psychological well-being. *Acta Paediatrica*, 94(12), 1791-1797. doi: 10.1080/08035250500268266

Parsons, T. J., Power, C., Logan, S., & Summerbell, C. D. (1999). Childhood predictors of adult obesity: A systematic review. *International Journal of Obesity Related Metabolic Disorders*, 23(Suppl. 8), S1-107.

Puder, J. J. & Munsch, S. (2010). Psychological correlates of childhood obesity. *International Journal of Obesity*, 34(Suppl 2), S37-S43. doi: 10.1038/ijo.2010.238

Seeyave, D. M., Coleman, S., Appugliese, D., et al. (2009). Ability to delay gratification at age 4 years and risk of overweight at age 11 years. *Archives of Pediatrics & Adolescent Medicine*, 163(4), 303-308. doi: 10.1001/archpediatrics.2009.12; 10.1001/archpediatrics.2009.12

Sjoberg, R. L., Nilsson, K. W., & Leppert, J. (2005). Obesity, shame, and depression in school-aged children: a population-based study. *Pediatrics*, 116(3), e389-392. doi: 10.1542/peds.2005-0170

Small, L., Sidora-Arcoleo, K., Vaughan, L., Capsel, J., Chung, K. Y., & Stevens, C. (2009). The addition of photographs to dietary diaries: one method to enhance dietary intake assessment of young children. Infant, *Child & Adolescent Nutrition*, 1(1), 27-36.

Spear, B. A., Barlow, S. E., Ervin, C., et al. (2007). Recommendations for treatment of child and adolescent overweight and obesity. Pediatrics, 120(Suppl. 4), S254-S288. doi: 10.1542/peds.2007-2329F

Strauss, R. S. & Pollack, H. A. (2003). Social marginalization of overweight children. *Archives of Pediatric & Adolescent Medicine*, 157(8), 746-752.

Vila, G., Zipper, E., Dabbas, M., et al. (2004). Mental disorders in obese children and adolescents. *Psychosomatic Medicine*, 66(3), 387-394.

Vollrath, M. E., Stene-Larsen, K., Tonstad, S., Rothbart, M. K., & Hampson, S. E. (2012). Associations between temperament at age 1.5 years and obesogenic diet at ages 3 and 7 years. *Journal of Developmental and Behavioral Pediatrics*, 33(9), 721-727. doi: 10.1097/DBP.0b013e31826bac0d; 10.1097/DBP.0b013e31826bac0d

White, B., Nicholls, D., Christie, D., Cole, T. J., & Viner, R. M. (2012). Childhood psychological function and obesity risk across the lifecourse: Findings from the 1970 British cohort study. *International Journal of Obesity*, 36(4), 511-516. doi: 10.1038/ijo.2011.253; 10.1038/ijo.2011.253

Williams, L. R., Degnan, K. A., Perez-Edgar, K. E., et al. (2009). Impact of behavioral inhibition and parenting style on internalizing and externalizing problems from early childhood through adolescence. *Journal of Abnormal Child Psychology*, 37(8), 1063-1075. doi: 10.1007/s10802-009-9331-3

Zeller, M. H. & Modi, A. C. (2006). Predictors of health-related quality of life in obese youth. *Obesity*, 14(1), 122-130. doi: 10.1038/oby.2006.15

Zeller, M. H., Reiter-Purtill, J., & Ramey, C. (2008). Negative peer perceptions of obese children in the classroom environment. *Obesity*, 16(4), 755-762. doi: 10.1038/oby.2008.4

SECTION 17
Neil Herendeen

Reimbursement

Fast Facts

- Getting reimbursed for the time and effort that you spend caring for children with psychosocial and mental health issues requires a working knowledge of the diagnostic coding system and local practices of your third-party payers.

- There are two parts to your billing submission, the service code and the diagnosis code. The Current Procedural Terminology (CPT) code set is maintained by the American Medical Association and describes medical, surgical, and diagnostic services. It is designed to communicate uniform information about medical services and procedures as well as help to establish reimbursement values for each type of service. The CPT code is often referred to as the level of billing.

- The International Classification of Diseases (ICD) coding book is updated yearly (the deadline for transition to ICD-10 in the United States is slated for publishing in October 2014) and has thousands of **diagnostic** codes from which to choose. Although these are nationally accepted tools, you may risk a rejected claim if your local insurers have restrictions on certain codes. In some areas, time-based codes for counseling can only be used by mental health providers, not by primary care providers. The list below is meant to save time from sorting through the entire coding book, but you may want to ask your local insurance company if they recognize a specific code before you submit your bill.

Routine Evaluation and Management Codes for Office Visits

The documentation guidelines established for each level need to be followed, including history of present illness, review of symptoms, past medical history, social history, physical exam, and medical complexity. These are the same codes used for "medical" office visits.

For "established patients," the CPT codes are:

99211 level one, minimal severity

99212 level two, low severity

99213 level three, moderate severity

99214 level four, high severity

99215 level five, very complex

Time-Based Codes for Counseling

Documentation includes diagnosis and management as well as the time spent with the patient and/or family but may not require a physical exam component. A good way to state this in your note is: "I spent 40 minutes total time and more than 50% of the visit was spent in counseling and coordination of care with the patient."

For preventive medicine counseling and/or risk factor reduction:

Individual	Group Visits
99401 approximately 15 minutes	
99402 approximately 30 minutes	99411 approximately 30 minutes
99403 approximately 45 minutes	
99404 approximately 60 minutes	99412 approximately 60 minutes

For the delivery of brief cognitive-behavioral skills building programs for depression and anxiety:

The delivery of brief cognitive-behavioral skills building intervention programs, such as the COPE (Creating Opportunities for Personal Empowerment) program for children, teens, and college youth (see Brief Interventions Section), can be billed as 99214.

99214 is the code assigned to the medical service that meets the following requirements:

1. The patient is an established one; this is not his or her first visit.

2. It must be an outpatient visit.

3. It must meet or exceed two of the following three points: A) a detailed medical history, B) a detailed medical exam, and C) a medical decision that entails moderate complexity.

4. The level of severity of the problem that brings the patient to the clinic must be from a moderate to a high one.

5. The provider and the patient should have a maximum of 25 minutes face time.

Can I code for reviewing screening tools/forms?

96110: "Developmental Testing—Limited"
At this time, this is the only CPT code available for the non-interactive screening and rating scales used in mental healthcare. Rating scales should be scored and scanned into the patient's chart. Expectation is that the screening tool will be completed by a nonphysician staff member and reviewed by the provider. Reimbursement is meant to cover the practice costs only (not provider time).

Common Diagnoses Used in Primary Care Pediatrics

These are some of the more common diagnoses that you will use when caring for the psychosocial needs of your pediatric patients:

ICD 9 code

300.0	Anxiety state: unspecified
300.02	Generalized anxiety disorder
300.9	Suicide ideation
300.4	Dysthymia
309.0	Brief depressive reaction
311	Depressive disorder, chronic
296.80	Bipolar disorder, unspecified
313.81	Oppositional disorder
309.24	Adjustment disorder with anxious mood
309.4	Adjustment disorder with mixed emotions and conduct
309.3	Adjustment disorder with conduct disturbance
309.0	Adjustment disorder with depressed mood
309.82	Adjustment disorder with physical symptoms
309.81	Post-traumatic stress disorder
780.30	Sleep disturbance, unspecified
313.83	Academic underachiever disorder
314.01	Attention deficit disorder with hyperactivity
314.0	Attention deficit disorder without hyperactivity
278.01	Obesity, morbid
278.0	Obesity, unspecified
785.1	Abnormal (excessive) weight gain
783.21	Weight loss
783.42	Delayed developmental milestones
299.0	Austism
V61.20	Counseling for parent/child problem
V65.5	Feared condition, not present
799.9	Other unknown and unspecified cause (still trying to figure it out)
995.2	Adverse effects of medication, NOS

SECTION 18
Pamela Lusk and Bernadette Mazurek Melnyk

Brief Evidence-Based Interventions for Child and Adolescent Mental Health Disorders

Fast Facts

- One in four to five children and adolescents in the United States experiences mental health problems, and 75% of children with diagnosed mental health disorders are now seen in the primary care setting (Merikangas et al, 2010; http://nihcm.org/pdf/PediatricMH-FINAL.pdf).

- Building on long-standing relationships with children and their families along with an emphasis on development, early intervention and prevention, pediatric practices are the ideal setting for the integration of mental health into primary care.

- Federal, organizational, and professional initiatives strongly support integration. The American Academy of Pediatrics and private foundations are supporting initiatives to develop the evidence base and provide tools for primary care providers (PCPs) to implement mental health services in order to improve access and evidence-based treatment.

- The primary care setting is ideal for initiating services for children with emerging developmental and behavioral problems as well as common mental health disorders.

- One model for working with families that is being used successfully in many healthcare settings is SBIRT. SBIRT information is located on the Substance Abuse and Mental Health Services Administration (SAMHSA) – HRSA Integrated Health Solutions Website. The SBIRT model grew out of an Institute of Medicine recommendation that called for community-based screening for health risk behaviors, including substance use.

- SBIRT stands for:

  Screening

  Brief Intervention

  Referral

  Treatment

- In the SBIRT model, effective strategies for intervention are started in primary care prior to more extensive or specialized treatment.

- As with other approaches that started as models for alcohol/drug prevention and intervention in primary care, the SBIRT approach is being endorsed by mental health organizations to address other mental health concerns, such as depression and anxiety.

- Use of screening tools for children and teens (e.g., the Pediatric Symptom Checklist, Vanderbilt ADHD parent form) is the first step in the SBIRT model and is easily incorporated into pediatric outpatient practices as an evidence-based way to assess patients for mental health problems.

- Referral to and consultation with mental health professionals for specialty psychiatric treatment is always a consideration in primary care, depending on the presentation of the child and family and the availability of psychiatric treatment providers in the community. In many communities, there are long waiting lists for child psychiatric evaluation and treatment, which is why equipping pediatric healthcare providers with excellent skills in preventing, screening, assessing, and providing evidence-based treatment for common mental health disorders is so important.

- Ideally, the intensity of the services will match the intensity of the child's needs.

The **brief interventions** presented in this section are evidence-based interventions that can be provided by PCPs in the context of brief office visits or several standard office visits. Brief interventions can be used as a stand-alone treatment for those at risk, as well as a vehicle for engaging those in need of more intensive specialized care.

With brief interventions, the clinician can begin to actively address the family's mental health concerns within the time constraints of busy outpatient practices even as the child is awaiting psychiatric services.

Some Important Points About Brief Interventions

- Commonly used by clinicians to talk to patients about health issues or medication adherence
- Designed for use in busy clinical settings
- Can be started right away with the resources found in outpatient practices
- Generally 5-15 minutes in duration, but no more than 30 minutes
- Can be used as stand-alone treatment as well as a vehicle for engaging those in need of more intensive specialized care
- Include behavioral approaches, supportive counseling, parent-focused interventions, motivational interviewing, and cognitive behavioral therapy (CBT) based skills building techniques.

From: The National Institute on Alcohol Abuse and Alcoholism (NIAAA) and SAMHSA at http://www.samhsa.gov/prevention/SBIRT/index.aspx and http://nihcm.org/pdf/PediatricMH-FINAL.pdf, respectively

When Delivering Brief Interventions

- Use an empathetic, non-confrontational style when delivering brief interventions.
- Engage the patient/family and offer choices.
- Emphasize patient responsibility.
- Convey confidence in the patient's or family's ability to change.

Mental Health Promotion and Early Intervention With Parents

The one evidenced-based change in practice that can provide the greatest impact for children and families is modifying the parents' perception of their child – i.e., how that child compares with other children – by emphasizing the child's individual positive strengths.

Parent-based interventions are evidence-based for many common child and adolescent mental health disorders (American Academy of Pediatrics – Evidence-Based Psychosocial Interventions).

It has long been recognized that parents' perceptions of their children (i.e., how they see their children compared to other children) may be a powerful determinant in a child's future well-being.

It is often the case that modifying the parents' perception of their child (cognitive reframing) can make a huge difference in the quality of the parent-child relationship and significantly improve that child's life (Yearwood, Pearson, & Newland, 2012).

Parents value the expertise and opinion of their PCP and generally want to be seen as "good" parents. They are accustomed to anticipatory guidance at their child's visits. Therefore, PCPs are in an ideal position to intentionally modify parents' healthy perceptions of their children.

Some individuals have struggles with parenting. There are some parents who have harsh and critical parenting styles, while others are too permissive or seem indifferent to the child. No matter what challenging behaviors the parent displays, the best way to help a child is to work hard to develop a provider/parent working relationship and "nurture" the parent into being the best parent he or she is capable of being. Sometimes, this will seem like a very slow process with only tiny glimpses of progress, but it is well worth the effort for the child.

Clinicians can leverage the parent's trust in the healthcare provider and belief in the provider's expertise in all aspects of children's health to "normalize" behaviors that concern parents but are fairly common at certain developmental stages. If there are diagnosable mental disorders, it is important to de-stigmatize those disorders as having a neurodevelopmental base.

A specific strategy for working with parents is modification of their perception of the child (cognitive reframing).

- Starting at the very first visit, the positive traits of that individual child can be identified by the provider and documented. Documentation implies importance for the parent and helps the provider keep the list of the child's strengths in the chart as important clinical data.

- This same approach is followed with the parent. The parents' particular strengths and the contributions the parents have made to the child's development of skills are recognized. Strengths in the parent/child relationship are pointed out by the clinician as they are observed. Even "super challenging" parents will have one or two positives that can be noted and reinforced.

- Not only does this approach serve to engage parents into a working alliance, but it provides an opportunity to role model the positive approach employed with the child. This intervention can be used with children of all ages at all stages, even the very young.

Cepeda (2010) writes in the *Clinical Manual for the Psychiatric Interview of Children and Adolescents*: "Engagement is boosted when the clinician expresses empathy for the child's or family's circumstances and when the practitioner identifies with the child's or family's perspectives. Engagement is facilitated when the provider gives the child positive feedback for behaving adaptively or in a developmentally appropriate manner or when the examiner praises the parent for opportune and sensitive redirection during the interview."

Clinicians can role model at every visit – focusing on the child's unique strengths (instead of only talking about problem behaviors) with the goal of guiding the parent into changing negative perceptions of the child to a more positive view.

Clinical Example of the Cognitive Reframing Technique for Parents

The parent says: "Johnny is tearing up everything in the house. He takes apart everything, his toys, his sister's things, the vacuum cleaner, everything. . . ."

The provider might say, "Johnny seems to be very curious and that can be an outstanding trait. Probably famous inventors like Edison or the new inventors of smartphones were boys like that. Johnny – what do you learn from taking toys apart; have you discovered the parts inside the toys? Are you good with tools?" Then the parent can be asked, "Who in the family shares Johnny's curiosity? Who else is good with their hands and tools?"

"Is there a way to promote Johnny's curiosity, but not have other family members' things taken apart?" "Let's set a rule today about what is off limits for Johnny's toolkit, and then when he comes in for his next appointment, he can tell me about some new discovery he has made."

Pediatric healthcare providers can serve as the parents' support and coach and, in the SBIRT model, provide referral information (along with brief intervention) to connect that family with support services and a network of other parents in a similar situation. Providing written materials for home reading also reinforces what the clinician is teaching.

Brief Interventions Provided Routinely by Pediatric Practitioners

Pediatric healthcare providers routinely provide brief psychosocial interventions in their practices. The literature increasingly supports the importance of brief psychosocial interventions in increasing families' ability to problem solve. Psychosocial interventions include:

- Active monitoring - when a symptom or concern first presents, the PCP often uses screening tools and reschedules the family for a return visit, which is sooner than would normally be scheduled, so that active monitoring of the child's symptom can occur. The PCP counsels the family about developmental parameters, when to ignore the child's symptoms, and when the presentation requires immediate attention.

- Behavioral interventions - most pediatric clinicians have an assortment of favorite behavior strategies that they use in counseling parents about behavior management: Checklist/ monitoring, Reward charts, Special times, Logical consequences, Planned ignoring, Goal setting/ target behaviors, Positive and negative reinforcements, and Time-outs and time-ins.

- Supportive counseling related to developmental changes or significant losses, such as loss by death of a family member or pet or environmental stresses (e.g., moving, or changing schools).

As more practices move toward integration of mental health/behavioral healthcare into primary care, professionals in the practice will be educated in specific brief evidence-based interventions, such as motivational interviewing and cognitive behavioral approaches.

Motivational Interviewing to Modify Health Behaviors in Primary Care

One approach that has been used successfully to change or modify health behaviors in primary care settings is motivational interviewing. Motivational interviewing has been used to address many of the basic health concerns we see with young people of all ages (e.g., alcohol use, exercise, unhealthy eating) (Gance-Cleveland, 2007).

Motivational interviewing is a counseling intervention, based on the Stages of Change Theory and Rogerian client-centered psychotherapy, which has been found to be effective in eliciting behavior change to promote health and reduce risk in adults. Evidence is accumulating to support similar effects of motivational interviewing with adolescents – especially in the area of substance abuse prevention and early intervention (Barnett et al., 2012), but also with peer violence and overweight/obesity. Although risky behaviors are a leading cause of preventable morbidity and mortality, behavioral counseling interventions to address them are not commonly used in healthcare settings.

Developmentally, young people are likely to be receptive to self-guided behavior change strategies, a cornerstone of brief interventions.

What Is Motivational Interviewing?

Motivational interviewing is a "client-centered, directive method for enhancing intrinsic motivation to change by exploring and resolving ambivalence" (Miller & Rollnick, 2002). Originally, it was designed for multiple sessions of 30 minutes or longer, but it has been adapted for brief (5-15 minute) encounters in a variety of settings.

Essential Principles of Motivational Interviewing

- Express empathy
- Develop discrepancy
- Roll with resistance
- Support self-efficacy

Spirit of Motivational Interviewing

- Readiness to change is a state (such as depression), not a trait (such as optimism)

- Change comes from the client

- Resolving ambivalence is the client's task

- Helping client explore ambivalence

  — Avoid direct persuasion

  — Quiet, eliciting, respectful style

- Provider-client partnership

How Do Clinicians Facilitate Change?

Providers need to understand why people do change, do not change, and how they change.

Why People Do Not Change

People do not change when the sum of the forces discouraging change is greater than the sum of the forces encouraging change (e.g., when what a person likes about smoking is greater than what they don't like about smoking, or their fear about quitting may be greater than the imagined benefits of quitting).

Why People Change

People change when the sum of the forces encouraging change is greater than the sum of the forces discouraging change (e.g., when the perceived negative consequences of drinking outweigh the benefits of drinking).

How People Change

Stages of Change	Intervention by Healthcare Provider
Pre-contemplation – not considering change	Increase awareness
Contemplation – considering change, but ambivalent	Facilitate resolution of ambivalence
Preparation – willing to accept direction, anxious about change	Help the client develop an action plan
Action – learning the new behavior	Solve problems related to new behavior
Maintenance – stable in the new behavior	Review successes, reinforce healthy behavior
Relapse – reappearance of old behavior (a process, not an event)	Move into action once again

Tools for Motivational Interviewing

- Agenda Setting – client determines priorities, e.g., "What would you like to talk about today?"

- Getting Permission –e.g., "I'd like to spend a few minutes talking about…Is that OK with you?"

- Open-ended questions to get started – e.g., "Tell me about……" "Help me understand….."

- Reflective Listening- e.g., "It sounds like you are feeling"; "It sounds like that is important to you."

- Summarizing – e.g., "So it sounds like you have two strong reasons why you want to quit, but on the other hand you worry that you will experience stress during the quitting process."

- Eliciting Self-Motivational Statements – change talk.

- Willing – e.g., "On a scale of 1 to 10 – with 0 being not willing to 10 being very willing, how willing (motivated, interested) are you to walk the dog every day?"

- Importance – e.g., "On a scale of 0 to 10 with 0 being not confident at all to 10 being very confident, assuming you decided to … (begin exercising, quit smoking), how confident are you that you can succeed?"

Eliciting Strengths and Barriers

Example: "You said your confidence to change is a 7. Why did you say 7 instead of 0 or 1"?

Example: "You said your level of interest was 5. Why isn't it a 9 or 10. "

Providing Information Without Interpreting for the Client

Example: "Chlamydia can increase a woman's risk of pelvic infections and infertility. What do you think about that?"

Closing the Deal

Example: "Where does that leave you?"; "Where do we go from here?"

Markers of a Productive Motivational Interviewing Encounter

- Client does most of the work
- Client accepts the possibility of change
- Client accepts the responsibility for change
- Upward slope of commitment language within or between sessions
- Dancing not wrestling

Cognitive Behavior-Based Brief Interventions

Below is the American Academy of Pediatrics' (AAP) **EVIDENCE-BASED CHILD AND ADOLESCENT PSYCHOSOCIAL INTERVENTIONS** chart. The interventions in the AAP chart generally represent treatment protocols that involve 60-minute visits over a period of time in specialty practices that have been replicated in university and community settings. The interventions that have the strongest research evidence to support them are listed, and it is clear that there is strong support for cognitive behavioral approaches for a variety of mental health conditions in children and adolescents.

- Cognitive behavioral approaches have the strongest level of evidence to support efficacy for child and adolescent anxiety, depression, substance abuse, and traumatic stress -- mental health problems that commonly present at pediatric primary care visits.

- While CBT should be conducted by mental health professionals who have appropriate education and sufficient training to conduct this type of therapy, there are key components of CBT that can be learned and incorporated into practice by other healthcare professionals (e.g., PCPs) in targeting symptoms such as stress, anxiety, and mild to moderate depression as well as assisting children and teens in coping with life stressors and learning to problem-solve and goal set.

- Cognitive behavioral concepts combined with skills-building exercises can be delivered in primary care and pediatric settings as a brief intervention.

- Depending on the age and developmental level, parents will be involved in the CBT-based intervention in different ways. It is important that the parent understand how these interventions can benefit their child and family.

EVIDENCE-BASED CHILD AND ADOLESCENT PSYCHOSOCIAL INTERVENTIONS

ADDRESSING Mental Health CONCERNS IN PRIMARY CARE A CLINICIAN'S TOOLKIT

This report is intended to guide practitioners, educators, youth, and families in developing appropriate plans using psychosocial interventions. It was created for the period November 2012–April 2013 using the PracticeWise Evidence-Based Services (PWEBS) Database, available at www.practicewise.com. If this is not the most current version, please check the American Academy of Pediatrics mental health Web site (www.aap.org/mentalhealth) for updates.

Problem Area	Level 1- BEST SUPPORT	Level 2- GOOD SUPPORT	Level 3- MODERATE SUPPORT	Level 4- MINIMAL SUPPORT	Level 5- NO SUPPORT
Anxious or Avoidant Behaviors	Cognitive Behavior Therapy (CBT), CBT and Medication, CBT with Parents, Education, Exposure, Modeling	Assertiveness Training, Attention, CBT for Child and Parent, Cultural Storytelling, Family Psychoeducation, Hypnosis, Relaxation, Stress Inoculation	Contingency Management, Group Therapy	Biofeedback, CBT with Parents Only, Play Therapy, Psychodynamic Therapy, Rational Emotive Therapy	Assessment/Monitoring, Attachment Therapy, Client Centered Therapy, Eye Movement Desensitization and Reprocessing (EMDR), Peer Pairing, Psychoeducation, Relationship Counseling, Teacher Psychoeducation
Attention and Hyperactivity Behaviors	Behavior Therapy and Medication, Biofeedback, Parent Management Training, Self-Verbalization	Contingency Management, Education, Parent Management Training (with Problem Solving, or with Teacher Psychoeducation), Physical Exercise (with or without Relaxation), Social Skills and Medication, Working Memory Training	Biofeedback and Medication	Parent Management Training and Social Skills, Relaxation, Self-Verbalization and Contingency Management, Social Skills	Attention Training, Client Centered Therapy, CBT, CBT and Anger Control, CBT and Medication, Family Therapy, Parent Coping/Stress Management, Parent Management Training and Self-Verbalization, Problem Solving, Psychoeducation, Self-Control Training, Self-Verbalization and Medication, Skill Development
Autism Spectrum Disorders	Intensive Behavior Therapy, Intensive Communication Training	Parent Management Training, Peer Pairing, Physical/Social/Occupational Therapy	None	Cognitive Behavior Therapy, Massage, Social Skills	Auditory Integration Training, Biofeedback, Eclectic Therapy, Hyperbaric Treatment, Modeling, Structured Listening
Delinquency and Disruptive Behavior	Anger Control, Assertiveness Training, CBT, Multisystemic Therapy, Parent Management Training, Parent Management Training and Problem Solving, Social Skills	Communication Skills, Contingency Management, Functional Family Therapy, Parent Management Training and CBT, Parent Management Training and Classroom Management, Problem Solving, Rational Emotive Therapy, Relaxation, Therapeutic Foster Care, Transactional Analysis	Client Centered Therapy, Family Therapy, Moral Reasoning Training, Outreach Counseling, Peer Pairing, Self-Control Training	CBT and Teacher Training; Parent Management Training, Classroom Contingency Management, and CBT; Parent Management Training and Self-Verbalization; Physical Exercise; Stress Inoculation	Behavioral Family Therapy, Catharsis, CBT and Anger Control, CBT with Parents, Collaborative Problem Solving, Education, Exposure, Family Empowerment, Family Systems Therapy, Group Therapy (!!), Imagery Training, Parent Management Training and Peer Support, Play Therapy, Psychodynamic Therapy, Self-Verbalization, Skill Development, Wraparound
Depressive or Withdrawn Behaviors	CBT, CBT and Medication, CBT with Parents, Family Therapy	Client Centered Therapy, Cognitive Behavioral Psychoeducation, Expressive Writing/Journaling/Diary, Interpersonal Therapy, Relaxation	None	Problem Solving, Self-Control Training, Self-Modeling	Life Skills, Play Therapy, Psychodynamic Therapy, Psychoeducation, Social Skills
Eating Disorders	None	CBT, Family Therapy, Family Systems Therapy	None	None	Client Centered Therapy, Education, Goal Setting
Elimination Disorders	Behavior Alert; Behavior Alert and Behavioral Training; Behavioral Training; Behavioral Training, Dietary Care, and Medical Care (with or without Biofeedback)	Behavioral Training and Dietary Care; Behavioral Training, Hypnosis, and Dietary Care; CBT	Behavior Alert and Medication	None	Assessment/Monitoring, Assessment/Monitoring and Medication, Behavioral Training and Medical Care, Biofeedback, Contingency Management, Dietary Care, Dietary Care and Medical Care, Hypnosis, Medical Care, Psychoeducation
Mania	None	Cognitive Behavioral Psychoeducation	None	None	Family-Focused Therapy, Psychoeducation
Substance Use	CBT, Community Reinforcement, Family Therapy	Assertive Continuing Care, CBT and Medication, CBT with Parents, Contingency Management, Family Systems Therapy, Functional Family Therapy, Goal Setting/Monitoring, Motivational Interviewing/Engagement (with and without CBT), Multidimensional Family Therapy, Purdue Brief Family Therapy	Drug Court, Drug Court with Multisystemic Therapy and Contingency Management	Goal Setting	Behavioral Family Therapy, CBT and Functional Family Therapy, Client Centered Therapy, Drug Court and Multisystemic Therapy, Education, Family Court, Group Therapy (!!), Motivational Interviewing/Engagement with CBT and Family Therapy, Multisystemic Therapy, Parent Psychoeducation, Problem Solving, Project CARE (!!), Psychoeducation
Suicidality	None	Attachment Therapy, Counselors Care, Counselors Care and Support Training, Multisystemic Therapy, Social Support Team	None	None	Accelerated Hospitalization, Counselors Care and Anger Management
Traumatic Stress	CBT, CBT with Parents	Exposure	None	EMDR, Play Therapy, Psychodrama	Client Centered Therapy, CBT and Medication, CBT with Parents Only, Interpersonal Therapy, Psychodynamic Therapy, Psychoeducation, Relaxation

Note: Level 5 refers to treatments whose tests were unsupportive or inconclusive. The symbol (!!) indicates that at least one study found negative effects on the main outcome measure. The risk of using treatments so designated should be weighed against potential benefits. This report updates and replaces the "Blue Menu" originally distributed by the Hawaii Department of Health, Child and Adolescent Mental Health Division, Evidence-Based Services Committee from 2002–2009.

The recommendations in this publication do not indicate an exclusive course of treatment or serve as a standard of medical care. Variations, taking into account individual circumstances, may be appropriate. Original document included as part of Addressing Mental Health Concerns in Primary Care: A Clinician's Toolkit. Copyright © 2011 American Academy of Pediatrics, revised October 2012. All Rights Reserved. The American Academy of Pediatrics does not review or endorse any modifications made to this document and in no event shall the AAP be liable for any such changes.

American Academy of Pediatrics
DEDICATED TO THE HEALTH OF ALL CHILDREN™

Used with permission of the American Academy of Pediatrics, Addressing Mental Health Concerns in Primary Care: A Clinician's Toolkit.

Copyright © 2011 American Academy of Pediatrics, revised October 2012.

Introduction to Cognitive Behavioral Skills Building

Cognitive theory (CT). The cognitive theory of depression and psychotherapy as developed by Aaron Beck (Beck et al., 2011) focuses on identifying and correcting "cognitive distortions" or automatic negative thoughts.

Beck proposed a negative cognitive triad -- a negative view of:

a. Oneself

b. One's environment

c. The future

This pattern of thinking leads to hopelessness, anxiety, and depression.

Seligman's learned helplessness theory proposes that depression results from experiencing uncontrolled negative events with the belief that one cannot influence the outcomes with behavior.

From the cognitive theoretic perspective, a person who has negative thoughts or beliefs is more likely to have negative emotions (e.g., anxiety and depression) and display negative behaviors (e.g., risk taking and poor school performance).

Cognitive Behavioral Therapy is rooted in cognitive theory of depression as developed by Beck and also adds behavioral theories, as developed by Skinner and Lewinsohn.

- Lewinsohn stressed that the lack of positive reinforcement from pleasurable activities and other people leads to negative thought patterns.

- Behavior theory suggests that individuals are depressed/anxious not only because of a lack of positive reinforcements, but also a lack of skills to elicit positive reinforcement from others or to terminate negative reactions from others.

- CBT consists of cognitive restructuring (i.e., understanding the connection between thoughts and feelings as well as behaviors), problem solving, and behavioral change.

Active Components of CBT include:

- Reducing negative thoughts (cognitive restructuring)
- Increasing pleasurable activities (behavioral activation)
- Improving assertiveness and problem-solving skills

Important Points About CBT

- Homework is an essential component of CBT so that individuals can put into practice the skills that they are learning.

- Important skills in CBT are positive reappraisal ("Okay, I'm not at my ideal weight, but with healthy eating and exercise, I can get there") and positive self-talk ("I can learn to eat healthy and exercise; I am able to deal with stress well.")

- In CBT, individuals are taught to become aware of antecedent events (e.g., a trigger event, such as being called ugly by a friend) as well as physical symptoms being experienced, so that cognitive reappraisal and behaviors to reduce negative symptoms can be instituted early in the process.

- CBT emphasizes collaboration and active participation.

- CBT is goal oriented and problem focused.

- CBT initially emphasizes the present and focuses on present concerns.
- CBT sessions are structured.
- CBT uses a variety of techniques and exercises to change thinking, mood, and behavior.

The Thinking, Feeling, and Behaving Triangle: Individuals are taught that how they think is related to how they feel and how they behave.

- By changing (reframing) the thinking about a situation, emotions and subsequent behaviors can be positively impacted.
- Everyone is prone to negative thoughts and perceptions of ourselves or others. Many of our negative thoughts are automatic, almost reflexive. We develop these automatic negative thoughts through our life experiences, and we practice thinking this way so much that we assume the thoughts are true.
- The good news is that with brief cognitive behavioral-based intervention, thoughts can be changed to be more positive.
- By reframing our thoughts from negative to positive, we can respond more positively to situations and feel better.
- **This core concept of cognitive theory is used when parents are assisted to reframe negative perceptions of their child to more positive perceptions (like the earlier example of helping the parents see their son as a "curious boy" versus a destructive child).**

The core concept of Cognitive Behavioral Theory is that thinking affects emotions and behaviors, otherwise known as **the thinking, feeling, behaving triangle.**

How a person thinks is related to how he or she feels and acts.

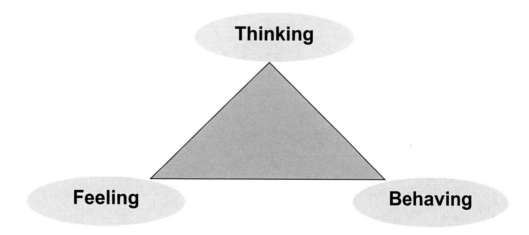

Illustration from the COPE for Teens Manual (copyright, Bernadette Melnyk)

The following is an example of a segment from a brief cognitive behavior skills building session by a healthcare provider (HP) with a depressed teen from the COPE Program for Adolescents by Bernadette Melnyk.

The Clinical Case

Anna is a 15-year-old girl who has been mildly depressed for the past few weeks, according to her mother. She does not want to go to her gymnastics class or hang out with her friends (new behaviors for her). Her appetite also has not been good lately. On interview, you find out that she received a D on a math test she took a couple of weeks ago, which seems to be a major cause of how she is feeling. It also did not help that a couple of her friends laughed at her score on the test.

During her interview, you discover that she believes that she is stupid (see below), which is causing her to feel depressed and to not want to study anymore.

HP: Anna, I understand from your mom that you have been feeling down lately.	Anna: I sure have.
HP: On a scale of 0 to 10, with 0 meaning "not at all" to 10 meaning "a lot," how down or depressed have you been feeling over the past 2 weeks?	Anna: A 9.
HP: Anna – I'm going to continue to ask you some questions that will seem very personal, but all of the questions have to do with your health. What you tell me is confidential between the two of us, unless you tell me that you want to hurt yourself or that someone else has hurt you. Then, I need to tell another professional about it. I also want you to know that I ask all teens who are feeling down this questions.	Anna: Okay.
HP: Have you ever wished that you were dead or thought about hurting yourself?	Anna: Yes, one time -- last week.
HP: Did you think about how you would hurt yourself, that is, did you make a plan?	Anna: No, I really wouldn't ever try to kill myself because my parents would never forgive me.
HP: What do you think is causing you to feel so down lately?	Anna: I just feel I can't do anything right lately. A couple of weeks ago, I got a D on my math test when I studied for it. My close friends laughed at me, saying that I was getting dumber by the year. I don't even want to try anymore because I think "what's the use?"
HP: I can understand how you feel. I have felt the same way at times in my life, but you know what I found? Thinking like that only makes you feel down and depressed, and then you give up and don't try as hard. That only makes things worse.	Anna: I guess that's true, but I don't know what to do. Everything I do lately seems to go wrong.
HP: Anna, I could teach you a few tips on how you can start to feel better – not so down. Do you want to hear about them?	Anna: Sure.
HP: There is something called the "thinking, feeling, behaving triangle." What that means is how you think affects how you feel and how you behave. For instance, if something bad happens, like getting a D on your test, you believe that you are stupid, which makes you feel bad and not want to try anymore. Can you think of another example?	Anna: Yeah. When my dad screams at me because I didn't clean my room, and I think "I flubbed up again," then I feel rotten about myself.
HP: That's right. Can you think of how you can turn that negative thought (i.e., "I flubbed up again") into a positive one?	Anna: Well, I guess I could think, "Okay, I put off cleaning my room, but that's okay; I'll get it done now."
HP: That's great, Anna. Now you are getting it. You have to start to monitor the way you are thinking when things happen and change the negative thought around as soon as it starts to happen into a positive thought, which will help you to feel a lot better. I'd like you to keep a log this week of all the things that happen that start making you have negative thoughts. I want you to write those down – the event that happened that triggered you to have a negative thought – and then, I want you to write a positive thought that could replace the negative thought you had. Would you be willing to do that?	Anna: Sure, but do you really think this will help me?

Although designed for mental health professionals, the following are useful resources that provide examples of cognitive-behavioral skills building with teens:

The Adolescent Coping with Stress Course (for teens at high risk for depression)
The Adolescent Coping with Depression Course (for teens who are depressed)

These are both available at http://www.kpchr.org/public/acwd/acwd.html.

COPE: A Cognitive Behavioral Skills-Building Intervention (CBSB)

COPE (Creating Opportunities for Personal Empowerment) is a 7-session, manualized, CBSB intervention developed by Bernadette Melnyk for children and adolescents (child version for 7- to 11-year-olds; teen version for 12- to 18-year-olds; and young adult version for 18- to 25-year-olds). The program is designed to be feasible for delivery by healthcare providers or teachers in a variety of settings, including primary care, schools as well as community mental health clinics and in-patient psychiatric settings. Findings from studies support that COPE, delivered individually, in group format, or integrated into school curricula, reduces anxiety, depressive symptoms, and anger as well as improves self-concept (Lusk & Melnyk, 2011; Melnyk et al., 2007; Melnyk et al., 2009; Melnyk et al., in press).

Information About COPE

- The COPE program is delivered exactly as written in the manual in 7 sessions.

- The sessions fit nicely into 20-minute office visits for individual children and teens; 30 to 45 minutes if delivered in group format.

- The COPE 7-session manual is developmentally appropriate and covers all of the elements of successful CBT-based interventions, and also provides skills-building activities and homework assignments.

- The COPE program has "ease of use." Once a provider is trained to use COPE, when the child or teen arrives, the manual is ready to use and has everything the provider needs to implement the program, including the homework assignments.

- COPE, as with other CBT interventions, is designed to be time limited.

- COPE is goal oriented and problem-solving focused.

- COPE emphasizes collaboration and active participation by the child or teen.

- COPE can be delivered to both children/teens and their parents.

- In the COPE program, children and adolescents are taught the **ABCs**, including:

    Antecedent Event: Friends call me "chubbo."

    Belief that is negative: I'm fat; I'll always be fat.

    Consequences – Emotional Outcome: Depression
    Behavioral Outcome: I give up;
    I won't try eating healthy anymore

    In the ABCs, the child/teen is taught to turn the initial negative belief around (e.g., I may be overweight now, but I will change that with regular exercise and healthy eating) so that they feel better and engage in healthy behaviors.

- Incorporating skills-building activities and reinforcing the practice of these skills is a critical element in the child's/teen's improvement. (Examples of a few concepts taught in the COPE program can be found in handouts at the end of this section).

- Self-regulation of behavior is a key coping strategy reinforced throughout the program.

- COPE is a CBSB program that actively promotes mastery of child/adolescent developmental tasks by each participant. The child/teen is an active participant in the intervention and the provider maintains positive belief in their abilities with statements such as:

    "You can do it. You can develop skills to COPE with whatever you are facing. By monitoring your thoughts and changing negative thinking to positive thinking, you can change/regulate your feelings and behaviors, and feel better."

The COPE handouts contained at the end of this section are designed to facilitate talking to school-age children about their thoughts, feelings, and behaviors as well as helping them to cope with stress and worry. These handouts can be reproduced for use during office visits. However, they do not replace the COPE 7-session program. A 15-session COPE Healthy Lifestyles TEEN (Thinking, Emotions, Exercise and Nutrition) program also is available that integrates nutrition and physical activity components with the 7 cognitive behavioral skills-building sessions. Findings using the 15-session program with 779 high school teens in a randomized controlled trial revealed that adolescents who received COPE, versus those who received an attention control program, had: a) less overweight/obesity; b) higher social skills, c) higher academic performance, d) less alcohol use, and 4) less depression in those teens who started the trial with severe depressive symptoms (Melnyk et al., in press).

Training to deliver the 7- and 15-session COPE programs is available through a workshop or handbook by contacting Dr. Bernadette Melnyk at cope.melnyk@gmail.com.

Tobacco Use Among Youth

- Although the number of youth who smoke has been declining since the late 1990s, the rates of smoking in high school juniors and seniors are higher than the smoking rates among adults (American Cancer Society, 2012).

- Approximately 25% of high school seniors smoke, and almost all first use of tobacco takes place before high school graduation (U.S. Department of Health and Human Services, 2012).

- Approximately 7% of middle school students report using some form of tobacco.

- Findings from studies indicate that adolescent tobacco users are more likely to: (a) use alcohol and illegal drugs, (b) get into fights, (c) carry weapons, (d) have depression and attempt suicide, (e) have low academic achievement, and (f) engage in high-risk sexual behaviors (American Cancer Society, 2012).

- **Parental tobacco use is the most significant predictor of youth smoking**. Parents should be urged to stop smoking to prevent serious health implications for their children. Children of parents who smoke are more likely to smoke themselves.

- Parents should be encouraged to talk to their children about tobacco use, starting in the early school-age years and continuing through high school, as many children start using tobacco by age 11 and are addicted by 14 (American Cancer Society, 2012). Parents can have the greatest influence on whether or not their children start smoking.

- Clinicians should provide the following advice to parents whose children do not smoke:

  1. If loved ones have tobacco-related diseases or have died from them, let your children know.

  2. Inform your children of the adverse consequences associated with tobacco use: cancer, lung damage, heart disease, bad breath, staining of teeth and fingernails, and tooth decay and loss.

  3. Do not use tobacco around your children.

  4. Talk to your children about how to say "no" to tobacco and role play with them as peer pressure influences use behavior. Know if your children's friends use tobacco.

  5. Children of parents who smoke are much more likely to smoke themselves.

  6. Talk about the false glamorization of tobacco in the media, such as ads, movies, and magazines.

- Clinicians should provide the following advice to parents who children already smoke:

  1. Encourage and support your child to quit tobacco use. Know that mood swings and crankiness are often associated with nicotine withdrawal.

  2. Offer your child the five Ds to get through the tough times (American Cancer Society, 2012):

     - **Delay**: The craving will go away with time.

     - **Deep breath**: Take a few calming deep breaths.

     - **Drink water**: It will help flush out the chemicals.

     - **Do something else**: Find a new, healthy habit.

     - **Discuss**: Talk about your thoughts and feelings.

  3. Reward your child when he or she quits.

- Tobacco dependence experts advocate screening all pediatric and adolescent patients and their parents for tobacco use.

- Advise children, adolescents, and parents to totally abstain from tobacco use.

- Multicomponent interventions, such as mass media campaigns, comprehensive community programs, comprehensive statewide tobacco control programs, and school-based interventions, can prevent the initiation of tobacco use and reduce its prevalence among youth. Messages delivered through these venues should be reinforced by healthcare practitioners.

COPE for Children

(From the Creating Opportunities for Personal Empowerment [COPE] Program,
Original Copyright, Bernadette Mazurek Melnyk, 1990)

The Thinking-Feeling-Behaving Triangle

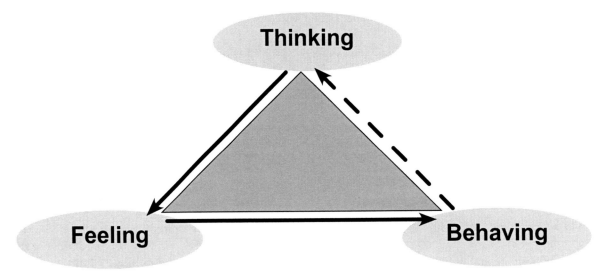

How you think affects how you feel and how you act or behave.

Here's an example:

➢ Alex is starting his first day of the school year at a new school. He is thinking that he doesn't know anybody at his new school and that maybe no one will like him. This makes him feel worried and sad. So, he acts very scared when he gets to school and doesn't talk to any other kids.

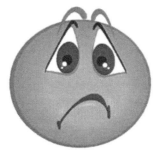

➢ How Alex thinks affects how he feels and how he acts.

Let's think of an example from your school.

We can change our thoughts from negative to positive. When we change to positive thoughts, we will feel better.

How we think affects how we feel (and how we act follows)

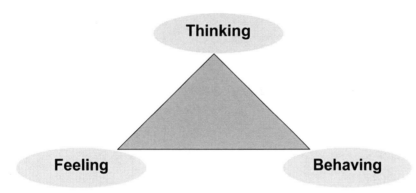

Let's change the thought (negative) to positive on the triangle. How might Alex feel with a different thought?

COPE for Children

(From the Creating Opportunities for Personal Empowerment [COPE] Program,
Original Copyright, Bernadette Mazurek Melnyk, 1990)

Healthy Coping for Stress and Worry

Healthy coping is when you deal with stressful things in positive ways that don't hurt you or other people.

Did you know that your body tells you when you are stressed?

Here are some different ways that our bodies can respond when we are feeling worried or sad:

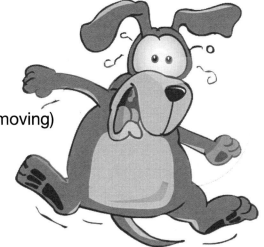

- Heart beating fast or pounding

- Breathing fast

- Sweating

- Anger

- Restlessness (feeling like you have to keep moving)

- Headaches

- Stomachaches

- Not being hungry

- Tightness in your neck or shoulders

- Problems thinking clearly

- Trouble sleeping or sleeping too much

- Feeling tired all the time

How does your body feel when you're stressed?

Here are some ideas for healthy coping:

- Talking about how you feel
- Exercise/playing outside
- Going to family or friends for help
- Writing your thoughts and feelings in a journal/diary
- Changing a negative thought into a positive one
- Using positive self-talk (positive self-statements)
- Doing relaxation exercises (we will do one today)
- Trying something new
- Doing something that you enjoy (like reading or drawing)

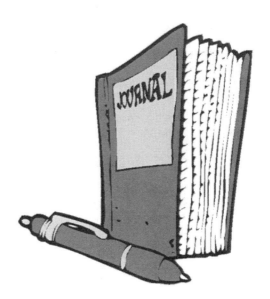

Write down 3 healthy coping skills/activities that sound fun to you.

1. _____

2. _____

3. _____

Resources for Healthcare Providers and Parents

Evidence-based treatment programs, which offer training for clinicians and resources for parents.

Collaborative Problem Solving: Clinicians find this approach helpful in addressing the very challenging disruptive behaviors of children. http://www.livesinthebalance.org/

Incredible Years (IY) is a program with several levels. There is some evidence that reading the IY manual can be helpful for parents who cannot engage in the program. Incredible Years also has CDs that cover key concepts and that may be a help. http://www.incredibleyears.com/

COPE (Creating Opportunities for Personal Empowerment) for children, teens, and young adults: Contact Bernadette Melnyk at cope.melnyk@gmail.com.

Triple P – Parenting Program: www.triplep.net/

Motivational Interviewing: www.motivationalinterview.org/

Internet Resources

American Academy of Pediatrics – Evidence-based Psychosocial Interventions http://www2.aap.org/commpeds/dochs/mentalhealth/docs/CR%20Psychosocial%20Interventions.F.0503.pdf

Guidelines for Adolescent Depression in Primary Care (GLAD-PC): http://pediatrics.aappublications.org/content/120/5/e1313.full.html

Integration of Mental Health into Pediatric Practices: http://nihcm.org/pdf/PediatricMH-FINAL.pdf

The Reach Institute: www.thereachinstitute.org/

SBIRT: http://www.samhsa.gov/prevention/SBIRT/index.aspx

Strengths and Difficulties Questionnaire: www.sdqinfo.com

Tobacco Resources

The American Cancer Society: www.cancer.org

Centers for Disease Control and Prevention (CDC): www.cdc.gov/tobacco
Office on Smoking and Health
Free quit support line, which offers information on smoking and health along with assistance to quit: 1-800-784-8669 (1-800-QUIT-NOW)

National Cancer Institute: www.smokefree.gov
Toll-free tobacco line: 1-877-448-7848 (1-877-44U-QUIT) (also available in Spanish)

Quitting information, quit-smoking guide, and phone counseling are offered, as

well as referral to state telephone-based quit programs.

QuitNet offers services to individuals trying to quit smoking: www.quitnet.com

REFERENCES

American Cancer Society (2012). *Child and Teen Tobacco Use.* **http://www.cancer.org/acs/groups/cid/documents/ webcontent/002963-pdf.pdf**, downloaded on March 17, 2013.

Barnett, E., Sussman, S., Smith, C., Rohrbach, L.A., & Spruijt-Metz, D. (2012). Motivational interviewing for adolescent substance use: a review of the literature. Addiction Behavior, 37(12), 1325-1334.

Beck, J. (2011). *Cognitive Therapy*: Basics and Beyond. New York, NY: Guilford Press.

Cepeda, C. (2010). Clinical manual for the psychiatric interview of children and adolescents.

Arlington, VA: American Psychiatric Publishing, Inc. Foy, J. (2010). Enhancing pediatric mental health care: Report from the American Academy of Pediatrics task force on mental health. *Pediatrics*, 125(Suppl 3), s69-s160.

Gance-Cleveland, B. (2007). Motivational interviewing: improving patient education. *Journal of Pediatric Health Care*, 21(2), 81- 88.

Lusk, P. & Melnyk, B.M. (2011). The brief cognitive-behavioral COPE intervention for depressed adolescents: outcomes and feasibility of delivery in 30 minute outpatient visits. *Journal of the American Psychiatric Nurses Association*, 17(3), 226-236.

Melnyk, B.M. (2003). COPE (Creating Opportunities for Personal Empowerment) for Teens: A 7-Session Cognitive Behavioral Skills Building Program. Columbus, Ohio: COPE2thrive.

Melnyk, B.M., Small, L., Morrison-Beedy, D., et al. (2007). The COPE healthy lifestyles TEEN program: Feasibility, preliminary, efficacy, & lessons learned from an after school group intervention with overweight adolescents. *Journal of Pediatric Health Care*, 21(5), 315.

Melnyk, B.M., Jacobson, D., Kelly, S., O'Haver, J., Small, L., & Mays, M.Z. (2009). Improving the mental health, healthy lifestyle choices and physical health of Hispanic adolescents: a randomized controlled pilot study. *Journal of School Health*. 79(12), 575-584.

Melnyk, B.M., Jacobson, D., Kelly, S., et al. (in press). Promoting healthy lifestyles in high school adolescents. A randomized controlled trial. *American Journal of Preventive Medicine*.

Merikangas, K. R., He, J., Burstein, M., et al. (2010). Lifetime prevalence of mental disorders in U.S. adolescents: Results from the national co morbidity survey replication – Adolescent supplement (NCS-A). *Journal of the American Academy of Child and Adolescent Psychiatry*, 49(10), 980-989.

Miller, W. R. & Rollnick, S. R. (2002). *Motivational Interviewing: Preparing People for Change (2nd)*. New York, NY: The Guilford Press.

U.S. Department of Health and Human Services. *Preventing Tobacco Use Among Youth and Young Adults: A Report of the Surgeon General*. Atlanta, GA: U.S. Department of Health and Human Services, Centers for Disease Control and Prevention, National Center for Chronic Disease Prevention and Health Promotion, Office on Smoking and Health, 2012.

Yearwood, E., Pearson, G., & Newland, J. (2012). Child and adolescent behavioral health: A resource for advanced practice psychiatric and primary care practitioners in nursing. Ames, IA: Wiley-Blackwell.

SECTION 19
Dawn Anderson-Butcher, Elizabeth Mellin, Aidyn Iachini, and Annahita Ball

Promoting Mental Health in Schools

Fast Facts

- Although healthcare professionals commonly encounter the unique mental health concerns of children and adolescents in primary care settings, estimates suggest that nearly 70% of youth who receive treatment are served in school settings.

- With increasing recognition of contextual influences (e.g., socioeconomic pressures, interpersonal relationships, discrimination) on well-being, mental health promotion has become a central theme in supporting the social and emotional development of young people across settings and especially in schools.

- Moving beyond a focus on individual mental health disorders, mental health promotion strategies involving universal prevention, early intervention, and targeted interventions focus on creating environments that support mental health and wellness. Allied healthcare professionals, educators, mental healthcare practitioners, and other professionals also are increasingly recognizing the relationship between good mental health and learning outcomes. As a result, there is a growing emphasis on mental health promotion activities in schools.

School Mental Health

The field of public health set the stage for mental health promotion-related strategies, specifically through its prevention activities focused on addressing infectious diseases. Given successes in this area, the public health prevention model now includes strategies related to addressing non-infectious diseases and chronic illnesses, including mental illness and emotional and behavioral disorders (Kutash et al., 2006; Mrazek & Haggerty, 1994). Current prevention efforts focus on health promotion/positive development strategies, universal prevention strategies aimed at entire populations of youth, selective prevention strategies focused on targeted groups, indicated prevention strategies addressing youth with significant symptoms, and treatment interventions for those with disabilities or disorders (Weisz, Sandler, Durlak, & Anton, 2005). From this, school mental health promotion has emerged, as schools are seen as ideal places for prevention.

School mental health promotion is defined as:

"Providing a full continuum of mental health promotion programs and services in schools, including enhancing environments, broadly training and promoting social and emotional learning and life skills, preventing emotional and behavioral problems, identifying and intervening in these problems early on, and providing intervention for established problems. School mental health promotion programs should be available to all students, including those in general and special education, in diverse educational settings, and should reflect a shared agenda – with families and young people, school and community partners actively involved in building, continuously improving, and expanding them" (Weist & Murray, 2007, p. 3).

School mental health promotion-related activities are often classified by the timing of the intervention (see Kutash, Duchnowski, & Lynn, 2006). For instance:

- There are school mental health programs and activities designed to prevent the onset of emotional or behavioral problems, as well as ones that target all youth in hopes of promoting general health and well-being.

- Some school mental health programs and activities target youth who are at risk and present initial signs of academic, behavioral, social and/or emotional needs. These secondary prevention programs focus on individuals and groups of young people who might benefit from early intervention to address escalating needs.

- Still others involve extensive treatments and interventions for indicated youth. These school mental health programs are implemented once a disability or disorder has been diagnosed or established.

Essentially, school mental health promotion includes all the ways in which schools allow for teachers, administrators, students, families, mental healthcare providers, community members, and others to collaborate to promote the overall well-being and academic achievement of students (see www.schoolmentalhealth.org).

The Importance of School Mental Health Promotion

Researchers have shown that well-designed school mental health promotion programs and activities impact social, emotional, and learning outcomes for youth (Durlak et al., 2011; Greenberg et al., 2003; Kutash et al., 2006; Rones & Hoagwood, 2000). Factors associated with effectiveness include the relationship between program effectiveness and consistent implementation, the use of multi-component, comprehensive strategies addressing the whole child, programming that focuses on changing specific behaviors and skills, and the integration of the programs seamlessly into the mainstream classroom (Rones & Hoagwood, 2000).

In addition to the well-recognized relationship between mental health and learning outcomes, there are several other reasons why mental health promotion activities are focused in schools:

- **Children and adolescents spend a majority of their time in schools**. From a mental health promotion framework, schools are an important environmental influence on the social and emotional well-being of young people. They also are a place where initial signs and symptoms may be identified early, allowing for intervention supports to be put in place prior to the onset of major problems and issues.

- **Schools provide unmatched access to children and adolescents for the provision of mental health services.** Estimates indicate that 20%-38% of youth are in need of some type of mental health intervention (Committee on School Health, 2004; Goodmanet al., 1997). Yet less than a third actually receive mental health services (Weist, 1997). In addition, those involved in treatment only show up for behavioral healthcare appointments 40%-50% of the time (Staudt, 2003). School mental health promotion provides increased access to care for these vulnerable youth. It also offers enhanced clinical productivity for mental healthcare providers (Flaherty & Weist, 1999).

- **Schools are also a natural environment for children and adolescents** that are not connected to stigmas associated with behavioral healthcare centers. Young people and their families are often more willing to engage in mental health services that are offered in more natural settings such as schools. School mental health may also allow for increased generalization and maintenance of treatment gains (Evans, 1999).

- **Many of the important adults** (e.g., teachers, school counselors, school support staff) **in the lives of children and adolescents are located in schools**. As a result, mental health promotion activities provided in schools create consistency among adults involved in the everyday lives of youth. A range of preventative services may also be offered to address early concerns or needs.

School mental health promotion also makes sense because school systems also organize their efforts across a learning support continuum that parallels the prevention system. Schools are focused on school-wide strategies such as high quality, effective instruction in classrooms aligned to content standards. Schools have accountability systems that allow for the ongoing assessment of achievement among students, and regularly assess student learning and provide universal, selected, and indicated strategies to promote student achievement. Schools also have learning support systems in place that address students' learning needs once they present academic and behavioral challenges, and provide more intensive instructional supports for students with significant learning problems.

Common Challenges

Despite the promise of school mental health, there are common challenges that jeopardize the success of these promotion strategies. Anecdotal accounts, practice experience, and research suggest six common challenges to school mental health promotion:

- **Differing priorities**. School and mental health systems work under different mandates that may result in competing priorities. Under the No Child Left Behind Act of 2001, schools, for example, are under enormous pressure to improve academic outcomes. School administrators may not view school mental health promotion strategies as critical to demonstrating improved academic outcomes and, as a result, they may resist efforts to address mental health in their schools.

- **Limited knowledge and planning**. Although there has been significant growth in school mental health promotion, there still is limited knowledge and understanding in the field regarding the best service delivery systems and strategies. Additionally, when school mental health services are in place, there still is limited awareness and knowledge among stakeholders with regard to the existence of these services (Weist, 1997). Additionally, sometimes services and activities are not well planned for and organized, resulting in uncoordinated strategies, service duplication, and poor sustainability.

- **Funding**. Mental health promotion necessarily encompasses a broad range of approaches, from universal prevention to indicated prevention, and these services require significant resources and funding. In a context of substantial cuts to federal, state, and local education and mental health budgets, the funding demands associated with school mental health promotion can create competition and tensions between schools and mental health systems that may jeopardize the work. Funding for school mental health promotion activities is also complicated by tensions between school and mental health systems around who pays for mental health services for youth who qualify for special education. The Individuals with Disabilities Education Act (IDEA) is largely viewed as an unfunded mandate by education professionals, while mental health professionals see IDEA as a requirement for schools to pay for services. Such different perspectives on IDEA often lead to disagreements about who is responsible for funding mental health promotion activities for students enrolled in special education services (Kutash, Duchnowski, & Lynn, 2006).

- **School infrastructure and culture**. Mental health professionals, who are often unfamiliar with school infrastructure and school culture, may have trouble identifying key contacts for starting this work. In addition, mental health professionals may struggle to "fit in" in school environments where the culture is often very different. Mental healthcare professionals, for example, often encounter more open communication about children and adolescents in schools and struggle to build relationships with teachers who do not understand the professional limits of confidentiality. Many times school mental health is seen as an "add-on" program or activity that is not central to the "real work" of schools.

- **Privacy and confidentiality**. The various systems involved in school mental health promotion each are mandated by law to maintain the privacy of their "clients." For instance, the Family Education and Privacy Act protects the privacy of student education records; whereas the Health Insurance Portability and Accountability Act of 1996 (HIPAA) protects health records. Both aim to protect privacy, but pose challenges to coordinating services and supports across different service delivery sectors.

- **Collaboration and coordination of care.** School mental health promotion activities are also challenged by interagency and interprofessional collaboration, especially when serving youth who are involved in multiple systems (e.g., healthcare, juvenile justice, child welfare). Professional turf issues, lack of trust, little support from administrators, and billing mechanisms that only reimburse for direct services represent just a few of the issues that complicate collaboration and coordination of care across systems that intersect with school mental health promotion.

Evidence-Based Management, Including Medication Management

Conceptual Models for School Mental Health Promotion

Three conceptual models of school mental health promotion (Kutash et al., 2006) provide additional context for allied healthcare providers interested in understanding how mental health services are delivered in schools. Here we briefly introduce and review The Mental Health Spectrum for Mental Disorders, Interconnected Systems, and Positive Behavior Intervention and Supports. Brief examples are offered to illustrate practical applications of each model.

- **The Mental Health Spectrum for Mental Disorders** (Mrazek & Haggerty, 1994; Weisz et al., 2005). Developed by the Institute of Medicine, the Mental Health Spectrum for Mental Disorders organizes mental health treatment on a spectrum from prevention (including universal, selective, and indicated) to treatment (including case identification, standard treatment of known disorders), and maintenance (including compliance with long-term treatment and aftercare). Organization of universal, selective, and indicated interventions at the prevention end of the spectrum is common in school mental health promotion. More recent enhancements to the model have included emphases on evidence-based practices and the interactions among schools, families, and communities within mental health service delivery. In practice, interventions such as the Promoting Alternative Thinking Strategies (universal prevention level) and Incredible Years (selective and indicated levels of prevention) are common approaches used in school mental health promotion to support positive mental health among students. (Kutash et al., 2006)

- **Interconnected Systems** (Center for School Mental Health, University of Maryland, Weist, Goldstein, Morris & Bryant, 2003; Center for Mental Health in Schools, UCLA, Adelman & Taylor, 2006). The interconnected systems framework for school mental health promotion emphasizes partnerships between school and community systems for supporting mental health among children and adolescents. Representing a person-in-environment perspective, interconnected systems seek to bridge school and community systems to support youth through the delivery of prevention, early intervention, and systems of care services. Services such as character education, graduation coaches, and trauma-focused cognitive behavior therapy (CBT) are coordinated across school and community systems, and braiding of resources is a common strategy for maximizing limited funding (Kutash et al., 2006).

- **Positive Behavior and Intervention Supports.** Positive Behavioral Supports (PBS) or Positive Behavioral Interventions and Supports (PBIS) is a system-wide prevention strategy that includes a continuum of services consisting of universal, selected, and targeted supports and interventions to ensure that all students receive effective behavior management practices (Barrett et al., 2008; Horner et al., 1999). PBIS has demonstrated effectiveness for reducing discipline referrals and suspensions as well as improving overall school climate (Taylor-Greene & Kartub, 2000). One component of PBIS is the three-tiered prevention model based on a public health approach in which programs and strategies are offered at three levels of intervention: (1) universal (school-wide) intervention; (2) targeted intervention; and (3) intensive (selected) interventions (Mrazek & Haggerty, 1994; Sugai & Horner, 2006). Summaries and examples of key practices at each level are outlined below.

Universal or School-Wide: Mental Health Promotion

Children's overall well-being may be positively impacted by the promotion of positive mental health through a variety of programs and initiatives in schools. These may include efforts to improve children's understanding of interpersonal relationships, social skills building, health awareness, and social competence development. Schools and service professionals may enhance and build upon the protective factors in children's lives that promote wellness and positive outcomes.

Children may have a variety of protective factors. Some examples include:

- Involvement in and reinforcement for prosocial activities
- Adequate adult supervision
- Strong bonds with caring adults
- Association with a prosocial peer group
- Academic achievement
- Strong bonds and connectedness to school, youth development groups, or extracurricular activities
- Feelings of support from caring adults and caregivers
- Opportunities for safe play in neighborhoods

The federal Substance Abuse and Mental Health Services Administration (SAMHSA) outlines evidence-based universal mental health promotion strategies in their National Registry of Evidence-Based Programs and Practices (http://www.nrepp.samhsa.gov/). The U.S. Department of Education also identifies exemplary programs that promote overall child well-being and safety (http://www2.ed.gov/admins/lead/safety/exemplary01). These evidence-based and exemplary programs utilize a number of strategies to address mental health on the universal level. Generally, these programs may be categorized as those that are focused on school climate, classroom-based strategies, character education, social skills training, and bullying prevention.

- **School Climate**. Positive school climate is critical for students' academic success and social-emotional well-being. School climate typically refers to the general quality of school life in four distinct areas: (1) physical and emotional safety; (2) peer and adult relationships; (3) teaching and learning; and (4) school environment (Cohen, 2009; Libby, 2004). Universal prevention and intervention strategies can promote students' mental health by addressing school climate in these four areas. For example, anti-violence initiatives promote student safety while school-wide community building activities promote connections to peers and adults.

- **Classroom-Based Strategies**. Classroom-based strategies are commonly used to provide universal intervention related to students' mental health and wellness. Typically, classroom-based strategies include curriculum-based instruction related to safe, drug-free schools, suicide awareness, social skills and problem-solving, and alcohol, tobacco, and drug use. Classroom management strategies may also prove effective as universal interventions. These strategies are typically employed by teachers to create structured, safe learning environments for all students. The use of classroom rules, reinforcement/incentive systems, and shared practices are examples of such strategies. Specifically, behavior management techniques may be included in regular classroom activities. These techniques include redirecting students who are disrupting class or providing additional outlets for student leadership and engagement.

- **Character Education**. Character education programs encompass a wide variety of techniques and curricula. Generally, these programs aim to impart positive qualities and strategies that children may use throughout their lives (e.g., leadership, trustworthiness, empathy). Several character education programs are supported in the research literature, such as Character Counts and Steps to Respect, and research continues to examine the ways in which structured character education may enhance students' mental health. Typically, a number of schools utilize aspects of character education to some extent in their regular, universal school programming.

- **Social Skills Training**. Social skills training is another universal intervention that is provided school-wide. Social skills training and character education are often provided in tandem, or social skills lessons are infused in other universal strategies (e.g., classroom instruction, physical education, health and wellness programs, etc.). A series of best practices (Dupper, 2006; LeCroy, 2006) are necessary to achieve the maximum benefits of social skills training:
    - Present the specific social skills
    - Discuss the skills
    - Provide examples to illustrate the skills
    - Allow opportunities to practice using role play
    - Create increasingly complex practice scenarios
    - Encourage practice of skills outside of group for generalization and maintenance
- **Bullying Prevention.** Bullying is of increasing concern for individual children, as well as concerning to schools in terms of overall school climate. Bullying is repeated aggressive behavior initiated by an individual or group toward another individual or group (Coloroso, 2003). Typically, bullying involves an imbalance of power that perpetuates the cycle of aggressive and passive behaviors among children. Several best practices are suggested to prevent bullying systemically:
    - Utilize assessments to understand the extent and nature of bullying: Seek input from students, teachers, student support service professionals, and families to gain information on the frequency and intensity of bullying. Identify physical areas and times of day in which bullying may be better or worse. Use these data to guide prevention and intervention strategies.
    - Focus on school-wide prevention to create a climate that discourages bullying behavior. Everyone in the school environment, including teachers, students, parents, administrators, and school staff, should promote social norms that encourage students to interact with each other in positive, prosocial ways.
    - Train school staff in bullying prevention and establish a team or committee to oversee bullying prevention and intervention efforts at the school.
    - Encourage family involvement in bullying prevention by informing parents/guardians of school norms, strategies to address bullying, or policies and procedures related to bullying in the school. Intervene consistently to stop bullying from becoming a larger problem. Adult supervision is essential, especially in areas identified as high-bullying areas. This also includes enforcing school policies consistently and appropriately.

Selected/Targeted (Early Intervention, Referral, and Linkage)

Selected and targeted strategies promote overall well-being and mental health for all students. Some children present difficulties that are identified early in their development. In addition, children may have factors in their lives that increase their risk of negative outcomes. These risk factors can be mitigated by prevention and intervention efforts.

Examples of risk factors include:

- Poor academic performance
- Antisocial behavior
- Alcohol or drug use
- Impulsivity
- Hyperactivity
- Internalizing behaviors and disorders (depression and anxiety)

- Abuse or neglect
- Inadequate adult supervision
- Family or community violence
- Association with deviant peers
- Family and community poverty

If children begin to demonstrate symptomology consistent with behavioral, mental, or developmental issues, then it is suggested that early, selected/targeted intervention is necessary. A variety of strategies and practices may be appropriate at the selected/targeted level of intervention.

- **Attendance monitoring** is often an initial strategy to engage children and families in school and support services. Students who are frequently absent or truant may suffer in their academic progress, school connectedness, peer relations, and overall satisfaction with their school experiences. Monitoring attendance on a regular basis, and using these data to identify students with frequent absences, is an effective strategy for early identification.

- **Assessments** are also integral in monitoring students' progress and identifying problems early. A number of assessments are appropriate in school settings. Those specifically related to children's mental health were identified in this section previously. Over time, school mental health professionals and other service providers may monitor students' progress to guide future interventions.

- **Individual and family counseling** is also important to address a multitude of interpersonal and social conflicts. Students may also need medication management or consultation services, often provided by a school nurse or school-based physician.

- **Case management** is another important strategy for selected/targeted intervention. Case management allows a single point of contact to monitor and facilitate services for children and families. This includes effective referral and linkage processes that connect children and families to needed services within the school and community, such as those that address basic needs (e.g., housing, food, clothing) and mental health services.

- **Student support teams** are teams of professionals that are also effective in addressing students' mental health needs at the selective/targeted tier. Student support teams financed by the districts are often effective at managing and coordinating services for children in need of targeted interventions. These teams are frequently multi-professional and may achieve maximum efficiency and greatest positive outcomes when interprofessional collaboration is a priority (see Mellin, 2009 and Mellin et al., 2009 for information on interprofessional collaboration in school mental health practice).

- **Small groups in schools.** Small therapeutic and psychoeducational groups also address children's mental health needs. Topical therapeutic groups may include groups to support students experiencing grief or trauma, family stress, peer difficulties, disruptive classroom behavior, anger, anxiety, or depression. Psychoeducation also can be an effective intervention technique for children who are first identified for support services.

Intensive Individualized Treatment/Intervention

In addition to universal and selective/targeted interventions, intensive individualized interventions are a critical component of the three-tier prevention and intervention model. These interventions target students in need of intensive services that are offered on the individual student or family level. They may include a variety of interventions and treatments that specifically address a student's mental health needs. The mode of service delivery may differ across settings and often is dependent upon available school and community resources. Examples of common service delivery strategies and interventions at the third tier include:

- **Mental health through special education** is often a necessary component of a free and appropriate educational program for students with disabilities, as required under Public Law 94-142, the Individuals with Disabilities Education Improvement Act (IDEIA). Schools are required by law to provide assessment, treatment, and education in the least restrictive education setting to students with disabilities (including emotional and behavioral disorders). As a result, education and mental health-related services are provided by special education teachers, school psychologists, and other student support personnel (i.e., school social workers) to support students' overall learning and development.

- **School-based mental health services** for intensive individualized intervention are offered by mental health providers in the school building. For example, community mental health providers may meet with students and families in the school setting. They may also consult with teachers and other school staff, as well as other healthcare providers outside of the school. One model is school-based health centers (SBHCs; of which there are more than 150 nationally; Dryfoos, 1988). SBHCs are co-located at schools and provide a range of health and mental health services for students and families. Regardless of the model, school-based mental health services operate under varying governance structures. More specifically, the school or district does not necessarily employ mental health providers that offer school-based services. These providers may be district employees, but they may also be employed by local community mental health or health agencies that are partnered with the school.

- **School-linked mental health services** that are intensive and individualized are provided outside of the school setting in partnership with the school. Schools typically contract with outside providers via formalized contracts or memoranda of understanding. In turn, treatment is provided for individual students and their families at settings outside of the school. Typically, outside providers include county mental health agencies, community mental health centers, the juvenile justice system, or child welfare agencies.

- **Systems of Care and Wraparound** sometimes exist to support students involved in multiple systems who present co-occurring problems and needs. While the education and mental health systems have been historically divided, a school-based system of care encompasses all services necessary to meet the needs of severely emotionally disturbed children. This perspective has emphasized that schools and communities must: (1) increase access to services; (2) provide individualized services in the least restrictive setting; (3) engage parents and families for service planning and delivery; and, (4) coordinate and integrate services across agencies, including schools (Leaf et al., 2003).

- **School-based mental health teams** do not provide direct service to individual students; instead, they are multidisciplinary groups that focus on coordinating services for students in need of intensive interventions. These teams are typically composed of multiple professionals, including teachers, social workers, psychologists, administrators, nurses, counselors, and other student support personnel (e.g., occupational therapists, speech pathologists). Parents and students may also serve on these teams. School-based mental health teams provide case management, triage, and referral as well.

- **Medication management services in schools** are typically led by school nurses and include the storage, administration, and tracking of medications. This service is critical to many children and adolescents who rely on medications to help manage mental health symptoms.

Overall, a number of practices and intervention strategies are supported in the existing research on school mental health. Collectively, services that are provided across the intervention continuum maximize schools' and allied health professionals' ability to address student mental health needs.

Comprehensive Approaches

The complex needs of children, families, and schools often require more comprehensive approaches to promoting children's mental health and well-being. These approaches are multi-faceted and dynamic, often including multiple disciplinary perspectives and practitioners.

- **Coordinated School Health Programs** (CSHP) involve the interaction of multiple components all centered on promoting student well-being (Centers for Disease Control and Prevention [CDC], 2007). The key CSHP components span health education and physical education, health services and nutrition services, counseling and psychological services, healthy school environment, and family/community involvement (CDC, 2007). CSHP promotes the coordination of policies, activities, and services that address these components and, ultimately, provides for the health of school students and staff while strengthening schools to be "critical facilities" for service provision and coordination (CDC, 2007, n.p.). School-based health centers (described later in this section) are one way that the CSHP has been implemented in practice.

- An **interconnected system** for meeting the needs of all students is another comprehensive approach to address student needs. In this framework, Adelman and Taylor (1999; 2006) advocate for the maximization and alignment of community and school resources and services across the learning support continuum. This work requires collaboration among jurisdictions, school districts, community agencies, and the public and private sector across the system of prevention, the system of early intervention, and the system of care. Common core standards for comprehensive systems of learning supports addressing whole child development are currently in development (Adelman & Taylor, 2012).

- **Full-service and community schools** (Dryfoos, 1998; Lubell, 2011) models have emerged in the last 20 years. These models view the school as the "hub" of community support, co-locating education, health, positive youth development, mental health, workforce development, and social services together at schools. These models exist across the country, but vary widely as some schools have a vast array of services whereas others may have only one or two service sectors represented (Dryfoos, 1994).

- The **Community Collaboration Model for School Improvement** (CCMSI) also provides an example of new models of school improvement focused on students' non-academic barriers to learning, including mental health issues (Anderson-Butcher et al., 2008; Anderson-Butcher et al., 2010). This model addresses the need for schools and educators to gain influence over students' out-of-school time and on the need for schools to further utilize existing family and community resources to optimize student learning and healthy development through the use of systematic organization of numerous improvement components. Focused on building system capacity for improvement, the CCMSI involves continuous planning and improvement processes that are evaluation-driven and anchored in "milestones" that mark developmental progress for school leaders. Five content areas guide the CCMSI expanded school improvement initiative – academic learning, youth development, parent/family engagement and support, health and social services, and community partnerships.

Often, these comprehensive approaches are rooted in more traditional school improvement processes, such as standards-based accountability and curriculum realignment. As such, local, state, and federal policy are integral in the development, implementation, and sustainability of these approaches. More specifically, several federal policy initiatives guide the promotion of mental health in schools.

Federal Policies

Current federal policy initiatives emphasize including mental health services within existing school improvement frameworks, while others promote the development and strengthening of existing mental health services in partnership with schools.

- **The Elementary and Secondary Education Act** (also known as the No Child Left Behind Act) is the federal law that funds public education, providing equal access to high-quality education for all youth. The law focuses on raising student achievement and addressing disproportionality and disparities through standards-based reforms and accountabilities. Title I is a key component of this policy, and provides additional learning supports and resources for students from disadvantaged circumstances.

- **IDEIA** is the long-standing federal policy to protect and provide intervention services for children with disabilities. Students with disabilities (physical, emotional, and learning) have the right to formalized school support services that are data-based and -driven. States are provided with partial funding to implement service strategies and systems that address students' learning needs within special education. In addition, states that receive federal funds under IDEIA are required to provide a free and public education in the least restrictive setting for all students. This is implemented via ongoing assessment, individualized education plans (IEP), appropriate accommodations and related services, and impartial hearings.

- **Section 504 of the Rehabilitation Act of 1973** prohibits discrimination based upon disability. Similar to the provisions of IDEIA, Section 504 requires that students with disabilities receive a free and appropriate education and are entitled to appropriate accommodations and related services. Written plans, termed 504 plans, are developed and enacted to specify these accommodations. 504 plans are different from IEPs, however, because any child with a disability may have a 504 plan. Only students eligible for special education services may have an IEP.

- **Race to the Top (RttT)** is a competitive grant program developed under the Obama administration to support reform and innovation in education. RttT includes funding to enhance teacher evaluation and incentive programs, school turnaround strategies, comprehensive data collection and management systems for schools, and early learning programs (U.S. Department of Education, 2012). One area of emphasis in school turnaround includes addressing the non-academic barriers that students often experience in their learning, such as mental health concerns.

- **Early Learning Challenge Fund** is a competitive grant program focused on enhancing learning opportunities during early childhood years. One key component involves the creation of early learning standards that ensure high-quality care, promote child development, and enhance kindergarten readiness. One key component of this national program focuses on assessment and screening among children from birth to age 5.

- **School-Based Health Centers** are an emerging policy priority as recent federal initiatives provide states considerable funds to establish school-based health centers. Based on the CDC's Coordinated School Health model, school-based health centers provide a myriad of health services within schools. These may include primary health care, mental health and behavioral health care, health and mental health education and promotion, case management, and crisis intervention.

Screening and Assessment Tools for School Mental Health Promotion

As part of school mental health promotion efforts, many schools utilize a wide variety of screening and assessment tools. Some screening and assessment tools are designed to assess the health and well-being of individual students, and some are designed to assess the overall school system. Examples of key constructs assessed at the individual-level include depression and suicide, bullying, alcohol and other drug use, as well as other specific social-emotional barriers to learning. School-wide assessment tools examine the overall system, specifically in relationship to improvement processes that support student learning and development.

Prior to providing examples of these individual-level and system-wide screening and assessment tools, it is important to note that schools already collect academic and behavioral data as part of normal educational practices. For example, schools not only track grades, but also track attendance and behavioral data such as suspensions and expulsions. Many schools also collect rapid assessment academic data on individual students in order to track students' trajectories over time, known as "value-added" data.

Individual-Level Screening and Assessment Tools

Individual-level screening and assessment tools allow practitioners to identify and understand the nature of problems children and adolescents might be experiencing. They also help identify related assets and strengths. Using these tools is important in practice, particularly as it ensures students are identified, referred, and provided with the best services and supports to meet their needs.

The United States Preventive Services Task Force (USPSTF) makes recommendations regarding preventative screening and other prevention services for the primary care setting (http://www.uspreventiveservicestaskforce.org/). While the focus of this section is on screening and assessment in the school setting, these recommendations are still important for nurses to consider in their practice and are presented next. Relevant Task Force recommendations for screening are overviewed here.

- Some key areas for screening and assessment in the school setting include depression, suicide, and alcohol, tobacco, and other drug (ATOD) use. With regard to depression, the USPSTF (2009) recommends screening adolescents between 12-18 years of age for Major Depressive Disorder if services and supports are available for identified students. For children (ages 7-11 years old), the USPSTF (2009) suggests there is inconclusive evidence to make a recommendation. The USPSTF (2004) also suggests there is inconclusive evidence regarding screening for suicidal risk and ATOD use in children and adolescents. The American Academy of Pediatrics (AAP, 2011), however, suggests that adolescents should be screened for alcohol, tobacco, and other drug use with psychometrically validated measures.

In addition, a variety of tools exist to screen and assess these three key areas (depression, suicide, and ATOD use):

- Some commonly used assessment tools for depression include the **Children's Depression Inventory** (CDI; Kovacs, 1992), the **Reynold's Children or Adolescent Depression Scale** (Reynolds, 1994), and the **Beck's Depression Inventory - II** (BDI - II: Beck & Steer, 1993). Both of these have demonstrated psychometric properties. They are not available in the public domain. Below are the Websites where these tools can be purchased.
  - CDI: https://ecom.mhs.com/(S(t2zxelna323yjhrr0ck2r2fj))/product.aspx?gr=cli&prod=cdi&id= overview
  - Reynold's Child Depression Scale - 2nd edition: http://www4.parinc.com/Products/Product. aspx?ProductID=RCDS-2
  - Reynold's Adolescent Depression Scale - 2nd edition:
  - http://www4.parinc.com/Products/Product.aspx?ProductID=RADS-2
  - BDI - II: http://www.pearsonassessments.com/HAIWEB/Cultures/en-us/Productdetail. htm?Pid=015-8018-370
- One widely adopted screening tool for suicide is the **Suicidal Ideation Questionnaire – Junior** (SIQ-JR: Reynolds & Mazza, 1999)
  - SIQ-Jr: http://www4.parinc.com/Products/Product.aspx?ProductID=SIQ
- AAP (2011) recommends using the **CRAFFT** as a screening measure for ATOD use. CRAFFT is a 6-item measure that can be used to screen children and adolescents, and is available free of charge from the following Website: http://www.ceasar-boston.org/CRAFFT/pdf/CRAFFT_English.pdf. This tool can also be found in Section 14 of this guide.

Another key area for assessment in the school setting is bullying. In 2011, the CDC developed a compendium of assessment tools to assess bullying. Some of these tools are available in the public domain, but others are not.

- One commonly used tool presented in this compendium with good psychometric properties is the **Olweus Bullying Questionnaire** (OBQ; Solberg & Olweus, 2003). This tool must be purchased for use.
  - OBQ: http://www.hazelden.org/OA_HTML/ibeCCtpItmDspRte.jsp?item=14432&sitex=10020:2 2372:US

In addition to measures of specific mental and behavioral health concerns, there also are other more global tools that exist. These tools assess a wide range of constructs that are of interest to school mental health promotion. Examples of these tools are presented next. All of these need to be purchased for use in the school settings. The Websites that can be accessed to purchase these tools are listed below each description of the tool.

- For example, the **Behavior Assessment System for Children (BASC-2; Reynolds & Kamphaus, 2004)** is a commonly used tool that can be completed by teachers, parents, or students. Depending on version, the BASC-2 assesses constructs such as anxiety, depression, social skills, self-esteem and attention problems.

- - BASC-2: http://www.pearsonassessments.com/HAIWEB/Cultures/en-us/Productdetail.htm?Pid=PAa30000
- Another commonly used tool is the **Child Behavior Checklist** (CBCL; Achenbach & Rescorla, 2001). The CBCL also can be completed by teachers, parents, or students. The tool assesses constructs such as social relationship competence, school competence, and youths' emotional and behavioral problems.
  - CBCL: http://shop1.mailordercentral.com/aseba/departments.asp?dept=11
- The **Developmental Assets Profile** (DAP; Search Institute, 2004) is another available tool that assesses the extent to which youth experience a range of assets across a variety of contexts, including at home, in school, and in the community.
  - DAP: http://www.search-institute.org/survey-services/surveys/DAP

Other global tools have been developed that are available for free in the public domain.

- For example, the **Community and Youth Collaborative Institute (CAYCI) School Community Surveys** (Anderson-Butcher & Amorose, 2012) assess internalizing behaviors, such as feeling anxious and worried, and externalizing behaviors such as fighting and bullying. The CAYCI surveys also assess a range of other constructs including academic motivation, school connectedness, academic press, parent involvement/support, teacher/student relationships, and community and learning supports. All of these surveys are in English and Spanish, and there are elementary and secondary youth, parent, and teacher versions of these tools. Surveys are in the public domain and may be used with permission of the author (see http://csw.osu.edu/cayci/data-services/). Please note that schools and other entities may also receive technical support related to data collection, analyses, and report generation (with normed data) for a nominal charge (http://data.mvesc.k12.oh.us/Cayci/surveysamples.aspx).

System-Level Assessment Tools

Several school-wide assessment tools also have been developed for school mental health promotion efforts. These tools are meant to identify priority areas for school-wide planning efforts, and therefore do not have validated psychometric properties.

- One relevant tool for school mental health promotion is the **School Mental Health Quality Assessment Questionnaire** (SMH-QAQ; Weist, 2006). The SMH-QAQ assesses the extent to which a school has in place a variety of SMH best practice principles, including 1) access to care, 2) funding, 3) needs assessment, 4) addressing needs and strengths, 5) evidence-based practice, 6) stakeholder involvement and feedback, 7) quality assessment and improvement, 8) continuum of care, 9) referral process, 10) clinician training, support, and service delivery, 11) competently addressing developmental, cultural, and personal differences, 12) interdisciplinary collaboration and communication, and 13) community coordination. (http://www.schoolmentalhealth.org/Resources/Clin/QAIRsrc/QAI)
- Another relevant planning tool is the CDC's **School Health Index** (SHI). The SHI assesses the eight key dimensions of the coordinated school health model. These dimensions include 1) school health and safety policies/environment, 2) health education, 3) physical education and other physical activity programs, 4) nutrition services, 5) health services, 6) counseling, psychological, and social services, 7) health promotion for staff, and 8) family and community involvement (http://www.cdc.gov/healthyyouth/shi/).
- The guidelines for school mental health, developed by the **Center for Mental Health in Schools at UCLA** (2001), also are important to consider for school-wide assessments (http://smhp.psych.ucla.edu/dbsimple.aspx?primary=2104&number=9975). Specifically, six overarching guidelines are shared related to 1) domains of intervention, 2) barriers to student learning, 3) types of services/support provided, 4) timing of interventions, 5) quality of interventions, and 6) accountability mechanisms. Examining this list and identifying the extent to which a school mental health program meets these guidelines may be a helpful step in planning efforts.

- The **CAYCI School Community Surveys** (Anderson-Butcher & Amorose, 2012) mentioned above also are useful for school-wide assessment of top priority needs and barriers to learning. Schools can explore the data collected from students, teachers, and parents together for common themes and priorities, and identify targets for system-wide improvements. This tool is listed as part of The Safe and Supportive Schools Technical Assistance Center compendium of school climate assessment tools. This Center also provides a host of other school climate assessment tools at the following website: http://safesupportiveschools.ed.gov/index.php?id=133. Again note the CAYCI surveys are in the public domain and available for use with author permission. School and district-wide data collection, analysis, and report generation is available for a small fee (see http://data.mvesc.k12.oh.us/Cayci/surveysamples.aspx).

Summary

In summary, this section highlights the value of school mental health promotion in supporting child well-being and other youth outcomes. School mental health promotion strategies focused on universal prevention, early intervention, and targeted interventions during the school day provide critical health promotion and learning opportunities, as well as valuable programs and activities to address specific mental health-related needs. Allied healthcare professionals may want to leverage the school system to assist with the treatment of child and adolescent mental health disorders. Schools' primary mission is to support healthy development, and academic learning and good mental health are key to that mission. The key points highlighted in this section will assist allied healthcare professionals in maximizing their connections with schools and creating opportunities to provide holistic treatment for children and adolescents with mental health disorders.

Resources available, including excellent Websites on the topic:

- Caring Across Communities (http://www.healthinschools.org/Immigrant-and-Refugee-children/caring-across-communities.aspx)
- Center for Health and Health Care in Schools: http://www.healthinschools.org/
- Center on School Mental Health: http://csmh.umaryland.edu/
- Family-School Partnership Lab at Vanderbilt University (http://www.vanderbilt.edu/peabody/family-school)
- Georgetown University Center for Child and Human Development http://gucchd.georgetown.edu/
- Harvard Family Research Project (www.hfrp.org)
- Mental Health-Education Integration Grant programs (www2.ed.gov/programs/mentalhealth)
- National Assembly on School-Based Health Care: www.nasbhc.org
- National Dissemination Center for Children with Disabilities: http://nichcy.org/
- National Technical Assistance Center for Children's Mental Health: http://gucchdtacenter.georgetown.edu/school.html
- National Technical Assistance Center on Positive Behavior and Intervention Supports: http://www.pbis.org/
- Research and Training Center for Children's Mental Health at USF's Louis de la Parte Florida Mental Health Institute: http://rtckids.fmhi.usf.edu/
- Safe Schools/Healthy Students (www.sshs.samhsa.gov)
- SAMHSA National Registry of Evidence-Based Programs and Practices (http://www.nrepp.samhsa.gov/)
- School-based Behavioral Health: http://www.sbbh.pitt.edu/
- School Mental Health Connection: http://www.schoolmentalhealth.org/

- Technical Assistance Center on Social Emotional Intervention for Young Children: http://www.challengingbehavior.org/
- UCLA School Mental Health Clearinghouse: http://smhp.psych.ucla.edu/clearing.htm
- USDOE Exemplary Programs (http://www2.ed.gov/admins/lead/safety/exemplary01).

Appropriate handouts with important and age-appropriate information

Presented next is a list of forms that are often helpful within school mental health promotion efforts. Each form is briefly described and a link to a template form is provided.

- **Release of Information:** This form allows parents/guardians to determine with whom professionals can share private and confidential information about their child and/or family. Until a release is signed, information should not be shared with professionals from other agencies. A template release of information can be found in the Appendix of the School Linkage Protocol (Anderson-Butcher et al., 2011) at the following Website: https://ckm.osu.edu/sitetool/sites/caycipublic/documents/USDOE/2-10-10SchoolLinkageProtocol_ForPrint.pdf.

- **Memorandum of Understanding (MOU):** An MOU, also referred to as a Memo of Agreement (MOA), is a form that ensures that all parties entering into a collaborative partnership are aware of their roles and responsibilities. In addition, an MOU outlines the time frame for the agreement. A template MOU can be found in the Appendix of the School Linkage Protocol (Anderson-Butcher et al., 2011) at the following Website: https://ckm.osu.edu/sitetool/sites/caycipublic/documents/USDOE/2-10-10SchoolLinkageProtocol_ForPrint.pdf.

- **Medication Management Checklist:** The Center for Health and Health Care in Schools has developed a brief checklist for parents to assess whether their child's school has policies in place to ensure students receive the appropriate medications at the appropriate times. This checklist can be found at http://www.healthinschools.org/Educators-and-Families/Parents/Act-Now/Helping-Children-Stay-Healthy/Medication-Management-At-School.aspx.

REFERENCES

Achenbach, T. (2009). *Child Behavior Checklist Manual for the ASEBA School-Age Forms & Profiles.* Burlington, VT: University of Vermont, Research Center for Children, Youth, & Families.

Adelman, H.S. & Taylor, L. (1999). Mental health in schools and system restructuring. *Clinical Psychology Review,* 19(2), 137-165.

Adelman, H.S. & Taylor, L. (2006). *The School Leader's Guide to Student Learning and Supports: New Directions for Addressing Barriers to Learning.* Thousand Oaks, CA: Corwin Press.

Adelman, H.S. & Taylor, L. (2012). Common core standards and learning supports.
Retrieved from http://smhp.psych.ucla.edu/pdfdocs/comcorannounce.pdf.

Anderson-Butcher, D. (2006). Building effective family support programs and interventions. In
C. Franklin, M.B. Harris, and P. Allen-Meares (Eds.), *The School Services Sourcebook: A Guide for School-Based Professionals.* New York, NY: Oxford University Press.

Anderson-Butcher, D. & Amorose, A. J. (2012). *Community and Youth Collaborative Initiative School Community Surveys technical reports.* Columbus, OH: College of Social Work, The Ohio State University.

Anderson-Butcher, D., Lawson, H.A., Bean, J., et al. (2008). Community collaboration to improve schools: Introducing a new model from Ohio. *Children & Schools,* 30(3), 161-172.

Anderson-Butcher, D., Lawson, H. A., Iachini, A., Bean, J., Flaspohler, P., & Zullig, K. (2010).
Capacity-related innovations resulting from pilot school and district implementation of a community collaboration model for school improvement. *Journal of Educational and Psychological Consultation,* 20(4), 257-287.

Barrett, S.B., Bradshaw, C.P., & Lewis-Palmer, T. (2008). Maryland statewide PBIS initiative. *Journal of Positive Behavior Intervention,* 10(2), 105-114.

Beck, A.T., Steer, R.A., & Brown, G.K. (1996). *Beck Depression Inventory – II Manual.* San Antonio, TX: Psychological Corporation.

Center for Adolescent Substance Abuse Research. (2009). *The CRAFT Screening Tool.* Children's Hospital Boston. Retrieved from http://www.ceasar-boston.org/CRAFFT/index.php

Center for Mental Health in Schools at UCLA. (2001). *Mental health in schools: Guidelines, models, resources, & policy considerations.* Los Angeles, CA: Policy Leadership Cadre for Mental Health in Schools.

Centers for Disease Control. (2007). Coordinated School Health Program. Accessed on July 16, 2008 from http://www.cdc.gov/HealthyYouth/CSHP/

Centers for Disease Control and Prevention. (2012). *School Health Index.*
Retrieved from http://www.cdc.gov/healthyyouth/shi/

Committee on School Health. (2004). School-based mental health services. *Pediatrics,* 113, 1839-1845.

Coloroso, B. (2003). *The Bully, the Bullied, and the Bystander.* New York, NY: Harper Resource.

Dryfoos, J. (1988). School based health clinics: Three years of experience. *Family Planning Perspectives,* 20, 193-200.

Dryfoos, J. (1994). *Full-Service Community schools: A revolution in Health and Social Services for Children, Youth and Families.* San Francisco, CA: Jossey-Bass.

Dupper, D. (2006). Design and utility of life schools groups in schools. In Franklin, C., Harris, M. B., and Allen-Meares, P. (Eds.), *The School Services Sourcebook: A Guide for School-Based Professionals.* New York, NY: Oxford University Press.

Durlak, J.A., Weissberg, R. P., Dymnicki, A.B., Taylor, A.D., & Schellinger, K.B. (2011). The impact of enhancing students' social and emotional learning: A meta-analysis of school-based universal interventions. *Child Development,* 82(1), 405-432.

Elias, M.J., Gager, P., & Leon. S. (1997). Spreading a warm blanket of presentation over all children: Guidelines for selecting substance abuse and related prevention curricula for use in the schools. *Journal of Primary Prevention,* 18, 41-69.

Evans, S.W. (1999). Mental health services in schools: Utilization, effectiveness, and consent. *Clinical Psychology Review,* 19, 165-178.

Flaherty, L.T., Weist, M.D., & Warner, B.S. (1996). School-based mental health services in the United States: History, current models, and needs. *Community Mental Health Journal,* 32(4), 341-52.

Goodman, S.H., Lahey, B.B., Fielding, B., Duncan, M., Narrow, W., & Rigor, D. (1997). Representatives of clinical samples of youths with mental disorders: A preliminary population-based study. *Journal of Abnormal Psychology,* 106, 3-14.

Greenberg, M.T., Weissberg, R.P., O'Briend, M.E., Zins, J.E., Fredericks, L., Resnick, H., et al. (2003). Enhancing school-based prevention and youth development through coordinated social, emotional, and academic learning. *American Psychologist*, 58(6-7), 466-474.

Hamburger, M. E., Basile, K.C., & Vivolo, A.M. (2011). *Measuring Bullying Victimization, Perpetration, and Bystander Experiences: A Compendium of Assessment Tools.* Atlanta, GA: Centers for Disease Control and Prevention, National Center for Injury Prevention and Control.

Horner, R. H., Albin, R.W., Sprague, J.R., & Todd, A.W. (1999). Positive behavior support for students with severe disabilities. In Snell, M. E. & Brown, R. (Eds). *Instruction of Students with Severe Disabilities* (5th ed. Pp. 207-243). Upper Saddle River, NJ: Merrill-Prentice-Hall.

Hoover-Dempsey, K. V., Walker, J. M. T., & Sandler, H. M., (2005). Parents' motivations for involvement in their children's education. In Patrikakou, E. N., Weisberg, R. P., Redding, S., & Walberg, H. J. (Eds.), *School-Family Partnerships for Children's Success* (pp. 40-56). New York, NY: Teachers College Press.

Kovacs, M. (1992). *Children's Depression Inventory Manual.* North Tonawanda, New York: Multi-Heath Systems, Inc.

Kutash, K., Duchnowski, A.J., & Lynn, N. (2006). *School-Based Mental Health: An Empirical Guide for Decision Makers.* Tampa, FL: The Research & Training Center for Children's Mental Health, Louis de la Parte Florida Mental Health Institute, University of South Florida.

Leaf, P.J., Schultz, D., Kiser, L.J., & Pruitt, D.B. (2003). School mental health in systems of care. In Weist, M. D., Evans, S. W., & Lever, N.A. (Eds.) *Handbook of School Mental Health: Advancing Practice and Research.* New York, NY: Springer.

LeCroy, C. W. (2006). Designing and facilitating groups with children. In Franklin, C., Harris, M. B., & Allen-Meares, P. (Eds.), *The School Services Sourcebook: A Guide for School-Based Professionals.* New York, NY: Oxford University Press.

Levy, S. J. & Kokotailo, P. K. (2011). Substance use screening, brief intervention, and referral to treatment for pediatricians. *American Academy of Pediatrics,* 128(5), doi: 10.152/peds.2011-1754

Lubell, E. (2011). *Building Community Schools: A Guide for Action.* New York, NY: Children's Aid Society.

Mellin, E. A. (2009). Unpacking interdisciplinary collaboration in expanded school mental health service utilization for children and adolescents. *Advances in School Mental Health Promotion*, 2, 5-15.

Mellin, E.A., Bronstein, L., Anderson-Butcher, D., Amorose, A.J., Ball, A., & Green, J. (2010). Measuring interprofessional team collaboration in expanded school mental health: Model refinement and scale development. *Journal of Interprofessional Care*, 24(5), 514-523.

Mrazek, P. J. & Haggerty, R. J. (1994). *Reducing Risks for Mental Disorders: Frontiers for Preventive Intervention Research.* Washington, DC: National Academy Press.

Nabors, L.A. & Reynolds, M.W. (2000). Program evaluation activities: outcomes related to treatment for adolescents receiving school-based mental health services. *Children's Services: Social Policy, Research, and Practice*, 3, 175-189.

President's New Freedom Commission on Mental Health. (2003). *Achieving the Promise: Transforming mental health care in America. Final report for the President's New Freedom Commission on Mental Health* (SMA Publication No. 03-3832). Rockville, MD: Author.

Reynolds, C. R. & Kamphaus, R. W. (2004). *BASC-2: Behavior Assessment System for Children, second edition manual.* Circle Pines, MN: American Guidance Service.

Reynolds, W. M. (1986). *Reynolds Adolescent Depression Scale.* Odessa, FL: Psychological Assessment Resources.

Reynolds, W. M. (1989). *Reynolds Child Depression Scale.* Odessa, FL: Psychological Assessment Resources.

Reynolds, W. M. (1994). Assessment of depression in children and adolescents by self-report questionnaires. In Reynolds, W. M. & Johnston, H. F. (Eds.). *Handbook of Depression in Children and Adolescents* (pp. 209-234). New York, NY: Plenum.

Rones, M. & Hoagwood, K. (2000). School-based mental health services: A research review. *Clinical Child and Family Psychology Review,* 3(4), 223-241.

Search Institute. (2004). *Developmental Assets Profile.* Minneapolis, MN: Search Institute.

Solberg, M. E. & Olweus, D. (2003). Prevalence estimation of school bullying with the Olweus Bully/Victim Questionnaire. *Aggressive Behavior*, 29(3), 239-268.

Staudt, M. M. (2003). Helping children access and use services: A review. *Journal of Child and Family Studies*, 12(1), 49-60.

Sugai, G. & Horner, R.R. (2006). A promising approach for sustaining and expanding school-wide Positive Behavior Support. *School Psychology Review*, 35(2), 245-259.

Taylor-Greene, S.J. & Kartub, D.T. (2000). Durable implementation of school-wide behavior support: The High Five Program. *Journal of Positive Behavioral Interventions*, 2(4), 233-235.

United States Department of Health and Human Services. (1999). Mental health: A report of the Surgeon General. Rockville, MD: U.S. Department of Health and Human Services, Substance Abuse and Mental Health Services Administration, Center for Mental Health Services, National Institutes of Health, National Institutes of Mental Health.

United States Preventive Services Task Force (2004). *Screening and Behavioral Counseling Interventions in Primary Care to Reduce Alcohol Misuse: Recommendation Statement.* Retrieved from http://www.uspreventiveservicestaskforce.org/3rduspstf/alcohol/alcomisrs.htm.

United States Preventive Services Task Force (2004). *Screening for Suicide Risk: Recommendation and Rationale.* Retrieved from http://www.uspreventiveservicestaskforce.org/3rduspstf/suicide/suiciderr.htm.

United States Preventive Services Task Force (2008). *Screening for Illicit Drug Use: U.S. Preventive Services Task Force Recommendation Statement.* Retrieved from http://www.uspreventiveservicestaskforce.org/uspstf08/druguse/drugrs.htm

United States Preventive Services Task Force (2009). Screening and treatment for major depressive disorder in children and adolescents: US Preventative Services Task Force Recommendation Statement. *Pediatrics*, 123, 1223-1228.

Weist, M. D. (1997). Expanded school mental health services: A national movement in progress. *Advances in Clinical Child Psychology,* 19, 319-352.

Weist, M. D., Goldstein, A., Morris, L., & Bryant, T. (2003). Integrating expanded school mental health programs and school-based health centers. *Psychology in the Schools,* 40(3), 297-308.

Weist, M.D. & Murray, M. (2007). Advancing school mental health promotion globally. *Advances in School Mental Health Promotion*, 1, 2-12.

Weist, M., Stephan, S., Lever, N., Moore, E. &, Lewis, K. (2006). *School Mental Health Quality Assessment Questionnaire (SMHQAQ).* Retrieved from http://www.schoolmentalhealth.org/Resources/Clin/QAIRsrc/QAI.

Weisz, H., Sandler, I. Durlak, J., & Anton, B. (2005). Promoting and protecting youth mental health through evidence-based prevention and treatment. *American Psychologist,* 60(6), 628-648.

Note: Page numbers followed by the letter t *refer to tables.*

A

Aberrant Behavior Checklist, 227
abuse. *See* child maltreatment
academic history, depressive disorders and, 102
active monitoring, 340
acute stress disorder, 68
ADHD. *See* attention-deficit/hyperactivity disorder (ADHD)
adjustment disorders, coding, 181–183
"Adolescent Coping with Stress and Coping with Depression," 53, 105
Adolescent Depression, Guidelines, 104
Adolescent Preventive Services, Guidelines
    about, 5, 27
    in child maltreatment screening, 268
    older adolescents, 36–40
    questionnaires, 41–44, 283
    younger adolescents, 28–35
adults. *See* parents
African-American children, health disparities, 1
Agency for Health Care Research and Quality, 54
aggression, conduct disorder, 309
alpha-adrenergic agents, 231
American Academy of Pediatrics, 54
American Medical Association (AMA), 54
anemia, ADHD and, 140
anger, 180, 196–198
animal cruelty, 305, 308, 312
anorexia nervosa, 203–204, 207, 208–209
antecedent events (trigger events), 344, 346
antipsychotics
    for autism spectrum disorder, 231
    for disruptive behaviors, 187, *188–189t*
anxiety disorders
    about, 61
    acute stress, 68
    autism spectrum disorder and, 227–228
    complicated grief vs., 239
    diagnosis, 62–63, 89
    frequency of, 1
    generalized, 67, 81–82
    KySS Worries Questionnaire, 78–80
    medical history, 63
    obsessive-compulsive, 74–75
    PTSD, 69–73
    resources. *See* resources
    SCARED screening, 83–87
    separation, 66

    signs of, 62, 88, 90–91
    State-Trait Inventory, 76–77
    treatment of, 64–65, 89
    war/terrorism, coping with, 92–93
applied behavior analysis, autism and, 228
aripiprazole (Abilify), 229, 231
Asperger syndrome, 218
assessment of mental health problems
    about, 1
    Adolescent Preventive Services, Guidelines. *See* Adolescent Preventive Services, Guidelines
    Child Behavior Checklist, 15, 26
    interviewing considerations, 5
    KySS assessments for parents, 6–12
    Pediatric Symptom Checklist, 2, 14–25, 337
    physical exams, 4
    questionnaires, 2–3
    resources. *See* resources
    risk factors, 2
    screening tools, 2–3
    special considerations, 5
    specific emotional/behavioral problems, 13
    well-child visits, 45–46
    See also *specific disorder*
atomoxetine (Strattera), 146, 231
attendance monitoring, 363
attention-deficit/hyperactivity disorder (ADHD)
    about, 139–140
    autism spectrum disorder and, 227
    diagnosis, 139, 141–143
    DSM coding changes, 144
    frequency of, 1
    information for
        children/teens, 160–161
        parents, 158–159
    medications for, 54, 145–146
    resources. *See* resources
    screening/assessment of, 147–157
    signs of, 160
Autism Diagnostic Interview, 225
autism spectrum disorder
    about, 217–219
    comorbidities, 226–228
    diagnosis, 222–223
    information for parents, 233
    managing, 228–229
    medical history, 220
    medications, 229–231
    office visit considerations, 231–232
    resources. *See* resources
    screening/assessment of, 219, 224–228

B

Beck Post-partum Depression Screening Scale, 268
Beck's Depression Inventory, 367
behavior, autism spectrum disorder and, 228
Behavior Assessment System for Children, 227, 367–368
Behavior Problem inventory, 227
behavioral indicators of abuse, 266, 271–272
behavioral interventions, 340
benzodiazepines, 65t
binge-eating/purging, 203
bipolar disorder, 103, 108, 132
bipolar I disorder, 114–117
bipolar II disorder, 118–120
body mass index (BMI), 319, 329
brief interventions, 340
Bright Futures in Practice: Mental Health, 54
Bright Futures Tool for Professionals, 123
bulimia nervosa, 203, 205–206, 207, 210–213
bullying/violence
    about, 303
    bully characteristics, 306
    conduct disorder, 309–312
    electronic aggression (cyberbullying), 307–308
    information for parents, 314–316
    interventions, 312
    presenting complaints, 304–306
    prevention, 362
    resources. *See* resources
    risk factors for, 303–304
    screening/assessment of, 306–307, 308, 323
    victim characteristics, 306–307
Buspirone (Buspar), 65t

C

caffeine, anxiety disorders and, 64, 89
CAGE Questionnaire for Alcohol Use, 296
Carbamazepine (Carbatrol, Tegretol), 189
cardiovascular consequences of obesity, 319
CARS2 (Childhood Autism Rating Scale 2), 225
case management, 363
CBCL (Child Behavior Checklist), 15, 26, 227, 368
CDC website, STDs and, 282
Center for Epidemiological Studies Depression Scale for Children, 122–123
Center for Mental Health in Schools at UCLA, guidelines, 368
change facilitation, 341–342
character education, 361

Child Behavior Checklist (CBCL), 15, 26, 227, 368
child maltreatment
    about, 265
    behavioral indicators, 266, 271–272
    diagnosis, 270
    information for
        parents, 271–272
        school-age children, 275–276
        teens, 273–274
    managing, 270
    physical indicators, 266–267
    presenting complaints, 266
    resources. *See* resources
    risk factors for, 265
    screening/assessment of, 268–269
    sexual abuse. *See* sexual abuse
Child Protective Services, disruptive behavior and, 186
Childhood Autism Rating Scale 2 (CARS2), 225
childhood disintegrative disorder, 219
children
    depression scale for, 122–123
    grief inventory, 242–243
    information for
        ADHD, 160–161
        disruptive behaviors, 194–198
    KySS Worries Questionnaire, 77–78
    maltreatment, screening for, 269
    SCARED screening, 84–85
    SSRI caution, 108
    State-Trait Anxiety Inventory, 76
    substance use, signs of, 293
    war/terrorism, coping with, 92–93
    See also school-age children
Children's Depression Inventory, 367
chromosomal abnormalities, 221
Citalopram (Celexa)
    for anxiety disorders, *65t*
    for autism spectrum disorder, 231
    for depressive disorders, *106t*
classroom-based strategies, 361
Clonazepam (Klonopin), 65t
clonidine (Catapress, Kapvay), 231
Clonidine HCl (Kapvay), 146
coding
    ADHD, 143
    adjustment disorders, 181–183
    autism spectrum disorder, 223
    bipolar disorder, 116–117, 120
    counseling, 334
    major depressive disorder, 113
    office visits, 333

pediatrics diagnoses, 335
    for screening/assessment, 334
cognition alterations, PTSD, 72
cognitive behavioral approaches, 343–348
cognitive reframing, 338–340
cohabitation, parental, 256
collateral information sources, 52
college students
    KySS Worries Questionnaire, 78–79
    State-Trait Anxiety Inventory, 77
Communication and Symbolic Behavior Scales,
    224
communication impairment, autism, 217–219,
    222–223, 232
Community and Youth Collaborative Institute
    (CAYCI) surveys, 368, 369
Community Collaboration Model for School
    Improvement, 365
competing priorities in educational systems, 359
complicated grief
    about, 239
    comorbidities with, 239
    death in the line of duty, 245
    interventions for, 244–245
    inventory for, 242–243
    misbehavior as response, 246
    risk of, 240
    screening/assessment of, 240, 241
    suicide, parental, 245
    symptoms of, 241
conceptual models of school mental health,
    360–362
conduct disorder
    about, 304
    animal cruelty as, 308
    diagnosis, 309–312
confidentiality, 5, 283, 359
Contract for Others' Safety, 135
Contract for Self Safety, 134
conversion disorder, 169
coordinated school health programs, 364–365
COPE. See Creating Opportunities for Personal
    Empowerment (COPE)
counseling in school mental health, 363
CRAFFT Screening Test, 295, 367
craniofacial abnormalities, 221
Creating Opportunities for Personal
    Empowerment (COPE)
        about, 53
        for depressive disorders, 105
        for disruptive behaviors, 186
        as evidence-based intervention, 347–348

handouts for, 350–353
    for overweight and obesity, 326
crisis plans, family, 180
cyberbullying, 307–308

D

dating violence, 280
DBC (Developmental Behavior Checklist), 227
death, loss, and grief
    about, 235
    complicated grief. See complicated grief
    grief facilitation, 236–237
    information for
        parents, 247–249
        teens, 250–251
    managing, 237–238
    resources. See resources
delayed expression, PTSD, 71, 73
Denver Early Start Model, autism and, 228
depersonalization, PTSD, 71, 73
depressive disorders
    about, 99
    autism spectrum disorder and, 228
    bipolar disorder, 103
    bipolar I disorder, 114–117
    bipolar II disorder, 118–120
    complicated grief vs., 239
    Contract for Others' Safety, 135
    Contract for Self Safety, 134
    differential diagnosis, 103
    family history, 102
    frequency of, 1
    grief vs., 248
    information
        for parents, 130–131
        for teens, 132–133
    interviewing, 102
    major, 112–113
    managing, 104–107
    medical history, 102
    medications for, 54
    persistent, 110–111
    presenting complaints, 100
    resources. See resources
    risk factors for, 100
    school history, 102
    screening/assessment of, 101, 102–103, 121–129
    signs of, 130
    social history, 102
    SSRI caution, 108–109

suicide and, 100, 103
derealization, PTSD, 71, 73
Developmental Assets Profile, 368
Developmental Behavior Checklist (DBC), 227
Dextroamphetamine (Dexedrine/Dextrostat/
    Adderall/Vyvanse), *145t*
diagnosis. See *specific disorders*
Diagnostic and Statistical Manual of Mental
    Disorders (DSM-5), 51–52, 144
        See also coding
Diazepam (Valium), *65t*
differential diagnosis. See specific disorders
disruptive behaviors
    about, 177–179
    adjustment disorders, 181–183
    diagnosis, 181
    information for
        children, 194–198
        parents, 191–193
    oppositional defiant disorder. *See* oppositional
        defiant disorder
    presenting complaints, 179
    resources. *See* resources
    risk factors for, 179
    screening/assessment of, 180
dissociative symptoms, PTSD, 72
Divalproex (Depakote), 189
divorce. *See* marital separation/divorce
domestic violence, screening for, 268
DSM-5. *See* Diagnostic and Statistical Manual of
    Mental Disorders (DSM-5)
dysthymia (persistent depressive disorder),
    110–111, 226–228

E

Early Learning Challenge Fund, 366
eating disorders
    about, 201
    anorexia nervosa, 203–204, 207, 208–209
    bulimia nervosa, 203, 205–206, 207, 210–213
    information for
        parents, 208–211
        teens, 212–213
    resources. *See* resources
    screening/assessment of, 202
    signs of, 208, 210, 212
Edinburgh Postnatal Depression Scale, 127–129,
    268
educational systems, psychopharmacological
    intervention and, 230
electronic aggression (cyberbullying), 307–308

Elementary and Secondary Education Act, 359, 365
elopement (wandering away), 228
endocrine diseases, autism association, 226
Escitalopram (Lexapro), *65t, 107t*
ethnic disparities, 1
evidence kit, sexual abuse, 269, 270
evidence-based interventions
    about, 337–338
    brief interventions, 338–339
    change facilitation, 341–342
    cognitive behavioral approaches, 343–348
    cognitive reframing, 340
    motivational interviewing in, 340–341, 342
    parent-based, 340
    psychosocial, 343
    resources. *See* resources

F

family crisis plans, 180
Family Education and Privacy Act, 359
family history, depressive disorders, 102
father-child relationships, 256
feeding challenges, 228
fetal alcohol syndrome, ADHD and, 140
fire setting, violence toward humans and, 305
Fluoxetine (Prozac)
    for anxiety disorders, *65t*
    for autism spectrum disorder, 231
    for depressive disorders, *106t*
Fluvoxamine (Luvox)
    for anxiety disorders, *65t*
    for autism spectrum disorder, 231
    for depressive disorders, 107t
4-goal model for mental health visits, 53
Fragile X syndrome, 221
full-service/community schools, 365
funding of school mental health, 359

G

GARS-2 (Guilliam Autism Rating Scale-2), 225
generalized anxiety disorders, 67, 81–82
genetic links, autism spectrum disorder, 218
genetic screening, ADHD and, 140
genitals, development of, 280
grief
    complicated grief vs., 239
    major depressive episode vs., 117
    mourning/depression vs., 248
    See also death, loss, and grief

guanfacine (Tenex, Intuniv), 146, 231
Guilliam Autism Rating Scale-2 (GARS-2), 225

H

Haloperidol (Haldol), 188
HEADSS (Home, Education, Activities, Drugs, Sexuality, Suicide/Depression), 5, 283
health disparities, 1
Health Insurance Portability and Accountability Act (HIPAA;1996), 359
healthcare providers
    overweight and obesity resources, 328
    teen sexuality and, 281, 285
HIPAA (Health Insurance Portability and Accountability Act;1996), 359
Hispanic children, health disparities, 1
HIV infection
    prophylaxis after sexual abuse, 269, 270
    risky behavior and, 279
Home, Education, Activities, Drugs, Sexuality, Suicide/Depression (HEADSS), 5, 283
home environment distress, 181
human papillomavirus (HPV) vaccine, 282
hypomanic episodes, 114–115, 118

I

IDEA (Individuals with Disabilities Education Act), 359
ideation of suicide, 104, 105
IDEIA (Individuals with Disabilities Education Improvement Act), 363–364, 365–366
illness anxiety disorder, 168–170
individual screening/assessment, 366–369
individualized treatment/intervention, 363–364
Individuals with Disabilities Education Act (IDEA), 359
Individuals with Disabilities Education Improvement Act (IDEIA), 363–364, 365–366
infants
    assessment of, 6–7
    death and grief responses, 236, 247
    depressive disorders, 100
    substance use, signs of, 293
Integrated Health Solutions website, 337
intellectual disabilities, 221
interconnected systems, 360, 365
Internet resources. See resources
interventions
    parent-based, 338
    psychosocial, 53
        See also evidence-based interventions
interviewing
    depressive disorders and, 102, 121
    importance of, 1
    motivational, 340–341
    special considerations, 5
intimate partner violence, 269

K

KySS assessment questions for parents
    of older infants and toddlers, 6–7
    of preschool children, 8–9
    of school-age children and teens, 10–12
KySS Worries Questionnaire, 78–80

L

labeling, stigma of, 52
laboratory tests
    for ADHD, 140
    for anxiety disorders, 63
    for autism spectrum disorder, 226
    for bipolar disorder, 103
    for depressive disorders, 103
    for eating disorders, 202
    genetic, 221
    for obesity, 322
    for persistent depressive disorder (dysthymia), 226
Lamotrigine (Lamictal)
    for autism spectrum disorder, 231
    for disruptive behaviors, 189
lead poisoning, ADHD and, 140
learned helplessness, 344
legal issues, reproductive healthcare, 282
Lesbian, Gay, Bisexual and Transgender (LGBT) sexuality, 280
limit-setting for parents, 56
Lithium, 189
Lorazepam (Ativan), 65t

M

major depressive disorder/episodes, 112–113, 115–116, 119
mandated reporting, child maltreatment, 270
manic episodes, 114
marital separation/divorce
    about, 255

conflict, 256
history-taking, 258
information for parents, 261
interventions, 258–259
parenting, 256
remarriage, 256
resources. *See* resources
screening/assessment of, 260
medical history, 63, 102
medications
    ADHD, *145t*, 146, 161
    anxiety disorders, 65, 89
    depressive disorders, *106–107t*
    disruptive behaviors, 187–189
    psychopharmacology, 54
    in school mental health, 364
    somatoform disorders, 171
    substance abuse/addiction, 294
    weight gain and, 326–327
    See also *specific disorders; specific medications*
mental health disorders
    diagnosis, 51–52
    management, evidence-based, 52–54
    prevention, 55–57
    psychopharmacology, 54
    resources. *See* resources
Mental Health Spectrum for Mental Disorders, 360
mental status exams, 3–4
metabolic diseases
    autism association, 226
    obesity and, 319
methylphenidate HCl (Ritalin/Methylin/
    Concerta), *145t*, 230
military deployment, impact of, 245
Modified Checklist of Autism in Toddlers
    (M-CHAT™), 224
Molindone, 188
motivational interviewing in behavior
    modification, 340–341, 342
mourning, grief vs., 248

N

National Guideline Clearinghouse, 54
negative cognitive triad, 344
negative finding, definition, 292
neurodevelopmental disorders, 217–220, 221
No Child Left Behind Act (2001), 359, 365
No Drinking and Driving Contract, 301
nonresident father-child relationships, 256
norepinephrine reuptake inhibitors, 231

O

obsessive-compulsive disorder, 54, 74–75, 225
older infants, assessment of, 6–7
Olweus Bullying Questionnaire, 367
online resources. *See* resources
oppositional defiant disorder
    about, 183
    diagnosis, 184–185
    managing, 185–187
    medications, 187–189
overweight and obesity
    about, 319
    bullying behavior. *See* bullying/violence
    comorbidities, 321–322, 329
    diagnosis, 323
    information for parents, 328, 329–330
    interventions, 326
    managing, 323, 324–325
    medical history, 321–322
    motivational interviewing in, 341
    physical exam, 322
    presenting complaints, 320
    psychotropic medication use and, 326–327
    resources. *See* resources
    risk factors for, 319–320
    screening/assessment of, 320–321

P

parents
    assessment tools for, 6–7
    consent/notification, reproductive healthcare
        and, 282
    depression impact on children, 109
    depressive disorders and, 102–103
    disruptive behaviors and, 186–187
    Edinburgh Postnatal Depression Scale, 127–129
    effectiveness training, 55
    information for
        ADHD, 158–159
        anxiety disorders, 88–93
        bullying/violence, 314–316
        child maltreatment, 271–272
        death, loss, and grief, 247–249
        depressive disorders, 130–131
        disruptive behaviors, 191–193
        eating disorders, 208–211
        overweight and obesity, 328, 329–330
        sexuality, 284
        somatoform disorders, 172–173

substance abuse/addiction, 297–298
KySS Worries Questionnaire, 80
limit-setting for, 56
perception of children, 339
resources for, 57
SCARED screening, 86–87
State-Trait Anxiety Inventory, 77
teen sexuality and, 281
tobacco use, 348–349
See also adults
Paroxetine (Paxil)
for anxiety disorders, *65t*
for depressive disorders, *107t*
Patient Health Questionnaire, 124–126
Pediatric Symptom Checklist, 2, 14–25, 337
pelvic exams, 282
perception modification, 338–340
perpetrators (bullying), 323
Perphenazine, 188
persistent complex bereavement. *See* complicated
grief
persistent depressive disorder (dysthymia),
110–111, 226–228
pervasive developmental disorder, 218
physical abuse indicators, 266–267, 269, 270,
271–272
pica (eating inedible objects), 228
Positive Behavior and Intervention Supports, 360
positive finding, definition, 292
positive reappraisal, 344
postpartum depression, 108–109
posttraumatic stress disorder (PTSD), 69–73, 239
pregnancy, 279
preschool children
assessment of, 8–9
death and grief responses, 236, 247
depressive disorders
presenting complaints, 100
screening/assessment of, 102
PRESTO plan, 185
pre-teens, death and grief responses, 236
See also school-age children; teens
preventive care
guidelines for
about, 27
older adolescents, 36–40
questionnaires, 41–44, 283
younger adolescents, 28–35
in reproductive health, 282
privacy, 5, 283, 359
property destruction, conduct disorder, 309
prophylactic medications, sexual abuse, 269, 270

psychiatric disorders. See *specific disorders*
psycho-education, 53
psychopharmacology. See medications; *specific
disorders*
psychosocial interventions, 53
PTSD (posttraumatic stress disorder), 69–73, 239
pubertal development, 280

Q

questionnaires for screening/assessment. See
specific questionnaires

R

Race to the Top (RttT), 366
REACH (REsource for Advancing Children's
Health) Institute, 54
Rehabilitation Act of 1973, 366
reimbursement, coding for, 333–335
reinforcement, positive/negative, 187
remarriage, 256
Repetitive Behavior Scale, 227
reporting mandates, child maltreatment, 270
reproductive healthcare, 282
REsource for Advancing Children's Health
(REACH) Institute, 54
resources
ADHD, 162
animal cruelty, 313
anxiety disorders, 96
assessment tools, 47–48
autism spectrum disorder, 228, 229, 233
bullying/violence, 312–313
CDC website, 282
child maltreatment, 277
depressive disorders, 109, 136–137
disruptive behaviors, 187, 190, 193, 198
eating disorders, 214
evidence-based interventions, 354
managing disorders, 53, 54, 58
marital separation/divorce, 262
overweight and obesity, 328
for parents/children, 57
school mental health promotion, 369–370
screening/assessment tools, 367–369
sexuality, 284–286
somatoform disorders, 174
substance abuse/addiction, 292, 293, 300
tobacco use, 354
restrictive eating, 203

Rett syndrome, 219, 221
Reynold's Children/Adolescent Depression Scale, 367
risk assessment (behavior), 180
risky behavior
    sexual, 279
    substance abuse. *See* substance abuse/addiction
risperidone (Risperdal), 229, 231
Rogerian client-centered psychotherapy, 340
role models, clinicians as, 339
RttT (Race to the Top), 366
rule violations, conduct disorder, 309
ruling out health conditions, 4

S

SAMHSA (Substance Abuse and Mental Health Services Administration), 337, 361
SAVRY (Structured Assessment of Violence Risk in Youth), 306
SBHCs (school-based health centers), 364, 366
SBIRT (screening, brief intervention, referral, treatment), 337–338
SCARED (Screen for Child Anxiety Related Disorders), 83–87
school climate, 361
School Health Index, 368
school mental health promotion
    about, 357–358
    challenges of, 359–360
    comprehensive approaches, 364–365
    evidence-based management, 360–362
    federal policies, 365–366
    importance of, 358–359
    individualized treatment/intervention, 363–364
    resources. *See* resources
    screening/assessment for, 363, 366–369
    selected/targeted interventions, 362–363
School Mental Health Quality Assessment Questionnaire, 368
school-age children
    assessment of, 10–12
    death and grief responses, 236, 247
    depressive disorders
        presenting complaints, 100
        screening/assessment of, 102
    information for
        child maltreatment, 275–276
        stress/anxiety, 94–95
    marital separation, responses to, 257
    parental help for, 56

resources for, 57
    See also children
school-based health centers (SBHCs), 364, 366
school-based mental health teams, 364
school-based obesity intervention, 326
school-linked mental health services, 364
Screen for Child Anxiety Related Disorders (SCARED), 83–87
screening, brief intervention, referral, treatment (SBIRT), 337–338
Screening for Autism in Two-Year Olds (STAT), 224
screening tools. *See* also *specific disorders*
    definition, 292
    parental discussions and, 1
    for primary care, 2–3
SEEK Model, child maltreatment screening, 268
seizure disorders, ADHD and, 140
selected/targeted interventions, 362–363
selective serotonin reuptake inhibitors (SSRIs)
    for anxiety disorders, 65t
    for autism spectrum disorder, 231
    for depressive disorders, 54, 105
    suicidal ideation and, 108
separation anxiety disorder, 66
Sertraline (Zoloft)
    for anxiety disorders, 65t
    for depressive disorders, 107t
sexual abuse
    evidence collection, 269, 270
    indicators of, 266
    information for
        parents, 271–272
        school-age children, 275–276
        teens, 273
    teen disclosure of, 281–282
sexuality
    dating violence, 280
    healthcare providers and, 281
    information for
        healthcare providers, 285
        parents, 284
        teens, 285
    interventions, 282
    legal issues, 282
    Lesbian, Gay, Bisexual and Transgender (LGBT), 280
    parents and, 281
    pregnancy, 279
    pubertal development, 280
    resources. See resources
    risky behavior, 279
    screening/assessment of, 283

sexually transmitted diseases (STDs)
    CDC website and, 282
    HPV vaccine, 282
    risky behavior and, 279
    sexual abuse and, 269, 270
side effects. See *specific medications*
sleep challenges, 228
Smith-Magenis syndrome, 221
Social Communication Questionnaire, 224
social history, depressive disorders and, 102
social skills training, 362
socialization impairment, autism, 217–219, 222–223
somatic symptom disorder, 166–167
somatoform disorders
    about, 165
    illness anxiety disorder, 168–170
    information for parents, 172–173
    medications, 171
    resources. See resources
    somatic symptom disorder, 166–167
Spanish language assessment tools
    Adolescent Preventive Services, Guidelines
        adolescents, 32–35, 38–40
        parent/guardian questionnaire, 43–44
    Pediatric Symptom Checklist, 18–19, 22–23, 25
special education, 363–364
SSRIs. See selective serotonin reuptake inhibitors
    (SSRIs)
Stages of Change Theory, 340, 342
STAT (Screening for Autism in Two-Year Olds), 224
State-Trait Anxiety Inventory, 76–77
STDs. See sexually transmitted diseases (STDs)
stepfather-child relationships, 256
stigma, diagnosis and, 52
stimuli avoidance, PTSD, 72
Structured Assessment of Violence Risk in Youth
    (SAVRY), 306
Substance Abuse and Mental Health Services
    Administration (SAMHSA), 337, 361
substance abuse/addiction
    about, 289
    definition, 297
    diagnosis, 293
    information for
        parents, 297–298
        teens, 299–300
    managing, 294
    motivational interviewing in, 341
    protective factors for, 290
    resources. See resources
    risk factors for, 290–291
    screening/assessment of, 291, 295–296

signs of, 291, 293
    use vs. abuse, 290, 298
suicide
    antidepressant choices, 105
    depressive disorders and, 100, 103
    parents and, 130, 245
    signs of, 293
    SSRI caution, 108
    teens' information, 132
support teams, 363
supportive counseling, 340
Swanson, Nolan and Pelham Scales, 154–157
system-level assessment tools, 368–369

T

targeted interventions, 362–363
teens
    assessment of, 10–12
    death and grief responses, 236, 247
    depressive disorders
        presenting complaints, 100
        screening/assessment of, 102
    information for
        ADHD, 160–161
        child maltreatment, 273–274
        death, loss, and grief, 250–251
        depressive disorders, 132–133
        eating disorders, 212–213
        sexuality, 285
        stress/anxiety, 94–95
        substance abuse/addiction, 299–300
    KySS Worries Questionnaire, 78–79
    maltreatment, screening for, 269
    marital separation, responses to, 257
    parental help for, 56
    Patient Health Questionnaire, 124–126
    resources for, 57
    SSRI caution, 108
    State-Trait Anxiety Inventory, 77
    substance use, signs of, 293
    war/terrorism, coping with, 92–93
    See also Adolescent Preventive Services,
        Guidelines
terrorism, coping with, 92–93
theft, conduct disorder, 309
thinking, feeling, behaving triangle, 345, 346,
    350–351
thyroid disorder, ADHD and, 140
tic disorder, 75
tobacco use, 348–349

toddlers
    assessment of, 6–7
    death and grief responses, 236, 247
    depressive disorders, 100
    marital separation, responses to, 257
toileting difficulties, 228
topical therapeutic groups, 363
toxicology screening, ADHD and, 140
training, for Pediatric Symptom Checklist, 14
traumatic brain injury, ADHD and, 140
trigger events (antecedent events), 344, 346
tuberous sclerosis complex, 221

U

universal/school-wide mental health promotion, 361–362
U.S. Department of Education programs, 361
U.S. Preventive Services Task Force
    recommendations, 3, 325, 366
use vs. abuse, substance, 290, 298

V

valproic acid (Depakote), 231
Vanderbilt ADHD parent form, 337
Vanderbilt Assessment Scale for ADHD, 147–153
victims (bullying)
    assessment of, 323
    characteristics of, 308–309
violence prevention, 311, 341
    See also bullying/violence

W

waist circumference, 319, 322
waist-by-height ratio, 319
war, coping with, 92–93
warning signs of violence, 304–306
websites. *See* resources
well-child visits, 45–46
wraparound care, 364